T0146065

Riverblindness in Africa

Riverblindness in Africa

Taming the Lion's Stare

Bruce Benton

Foreword by James D. Wolfensohn

Johns Hopkins University Press
Baltimore

© 2020 Johns Hopkins University Press
All rights reserved. Published 2020
Printed in the United States of America on acid-free paper

9 8 7 6 5 4 3 2 1

Johns Hopkins University Press
2715 North Charles Street
Baltimore, Maryland 21218-4363
www.press.jhu.edu

Library of Congress Cataloging-in-Publication Data

Names: Benton, Bruce, 1942– author.
Title: Riverblindness in Africa : taming the lion's stare / Bruce Benton ;
    foreword by James D. Wolfensohn.
Description: Baltimore : Johns Hopkins University Press, [2020] |
    Includes bibliographical references and index.
Identifiers: LCCN 2020009051 | ISBN 9781421439662 (hardcover ;
    alk. paper) | ISBN 9781421439679 (ebook)
Subjects: MESH: Onchocerciasis Control Programme in West Africa. |
    African Programme for Onchocerciasis Control. | Onchocerciasis,
    Ocular—prevention & control | Onchocerciasis, Ocular—epidemiology |
    Neglected Diseases—prevention & control | Disease Eradication—
    organization & administration | Program Evaluation | International
    Cooperation | Africa
Classification: LCC RA644.O53 | NLM WW 160 | DDC 614.5/552—dc23
LC record available at https://lccn.loc.gov/2020009051

A catalog record for this book is available from the British Library.

Special discounts are available for bulk purchases of this book. For more
information, please contact Special Sales at specialsales@press.jhu.edu.

Johns Hopkins University Press uses environmentally friendly book
materials, including recycled text paper that is composed of at least
30 percent post-consumer waste, whenever possible.

Contents

Photographs appear following page 136

Foreword

If we ever need a reminder of what is possible when people and institutions work together, we should turn to this marvelous book, which recounts the tremendous obstacles and triumphs of the work to rid Africa of riverblindness. The cornerstone of this work has been the partnership forged between donors, nongovernmental organizations, the private sector, the World Health Organization, World Bank, other UN agencies, and the African governments, along with the affected local communities within the endemic countries. This partnership worked because, despite any differences, the participants were committed to the same goal, namely, that no person throughout the continent should suffer the horrific itching, disfigurement, and loss of vision caused by riverblindness. We have not yet fully achieved that goal, but the profound reduction of transmission and prevalence of the disease from levels 50 years ago tells us we can do so, and soon.

With this excellent and important book, Bruce Benton, who managed the World Bank's Riverblindness Program for 20 years, does a great service in bringing this story to the broader audience it deserves. Benton draws upon extensive research, interviews with a large number of the surviving players, and his own personal and professional experience. His passion for the subject is evident on each page, but this doesn't prevent him from taking a hard look at the clashes and mistakes that are inevitable in an endeavor of this magnitude and duration. Benton also unpacks the pivotal actions and decisions that led to success. All of these lessons can be applied in some fashion to other partnerships and large-scale disease control efforts.

On average, a person infected with riverblindness is blind by age 30. Years are lost that otherwise would be a prime time for providing for one's livelihood, supporting a family, and contributing to the community. Instead, that person becomes heavily dependent on others, including, often, a child, who is taken out of school to serve as a guide and whose education and future earning power also suffers. The direct link between riverblindness and poverty has long been evident. Across vast endemic regions where the disease persisted, fertile lands and riverside villages were abandoned and no economic development was possible.

But besides health and economics, there was another argument—the human element. A life with this disease is a life of misery, and those of us who are in a position to implement control efforts have a moral and social obligation to do so. This obligation required a long-term commitment, both because the parasite responsible for riverblindness lives up to 14 years in the human body and continues to produce microscopic worms for more than a decade; and because the goal was so ambitious, namely, to lift this burden from tens of millions of Africans living in remote, rural areas. From the beginning of the first riverblindness program, the commitment to this goal was unstinting and durable. And today you can meet families with adults whose vision was lost to riverblindness and a child or grandchild who will never experience its devastating symptoms.

Partnership was the driving force behind this success. Within that partnership, Merck deserves a wealth of credit for donating ivermectin to the countries that need it, in perpetuity. And credit is due to the local communities, who direct the drug treatment process by electing volunteers to coordinate the schedule, keep records, and distribute tablets. The villagers themselves own the distribution network, which is exactly as it should be in a program based on inclusion and grassroots empowerment. Moreover, this system is extremely effective in scaling locally and ensuring the high treatment coverage necessary to achieve elimination of the disease.

If you walk through the atrium of the World Bank Headquarters, you will see a large statue of a boy leading a man who has lost his vision to riverblindness. The statue is dedicated to the riverblindness programs in honor of their remarkable progress, and its larger-than-life size reflects the superhuman scope of the programs' ambitions. Someday, we hope, the statue will symbolize a disease that has been eliminated. For now, its imposing presence is an inspiration and a command: keep going.

As World Bank president, I was fortunate to oversee the successful conclusion of the first program and to host the launch for the second program that widened the effort to all of Africa. These programs represented the World Bank at its best. As much as any Bank-supported operation, they exemplify the ideal and purpose of the institution and its staff, of which Bruce Benton is a shining example—achieving results where it counts, to directly and intimately improve the quality of life of the most vulnerable poor.

James D. Wolfensohn
President of the World Bank, 1995–2005

Preface

This book had its genesis in presentations I began making to the World Bank Board in the late 1990s and early 2000s on progress in eliminating riverblindness, or onchocerciasis ("oncho"), in Africa through the Onchocerciasis Control Program (OCP) and the African Program for Onchocerciasis Control (APOC). By the early 2000s, new drug donations were coming on stream for several of the major neglected tropical diseases (NTDs) in addition to onchocerciasis. My colleague Bernhard Liese and I began brainstorming on lessons learned from the OCP/APOC experience to incorporate in Board presentations. Our objective was to provide guidance to the wider development community on ways of organizing viable, sustainable control efforts for the other major NTDs for which there were new and effective drugs. Oncho was the first of the neglected tropical diseases to be addressed through a large-scale control effort. Hence, lessons learned and best practices extrapolated from the OCP/APOC experience were seen as important legacies of those two programs.

Shortly after my retirement in early 2005, I wrote up a concept note for a book that would delve into lessons learned from the then 30-year history of the oncho programs—including what worked well and pitfalls to avoid. That note was distributed to select current and retired Bank staff in hopes of generating interest and financing to enable the book to go forward. The major themes to be covered were partnership, organizational structures, regional approaches, long-term donor commitment, private–public sector collaboration (based on the Merck example), community-led drug delivery as an entry point for other health-care interventions, and socioeconomic development of the oncho-freed areas. Several World Bank vice presidents and then-retired Bank president Robert McNamara were highly receptive to the concept note. However, the unavailability of the required financing precluded proceeding with the book project at that time.

I revived the book proposal—including the themes in the concept note and the lessons learned highlighted in the Board presentations—a decade later, after several former Bank colleagues encouraged me to undertake the project. By then,

APOC had made considerable progress in eliminating oncho as a public health problem in Africa, and it appeared likely that that program would be brought to a conclusion at the end of 2015. That revived proposal became the basis for this book and for mobilizing funding to support my travel for research and interviews.

Despite the extra time and effort involved, I sought limited amounts of financing for the book from each of a variety of sources to avoid the appearance of being beholden to any one source of financing and to ensure that I retained full editorial freedom as the author. During 2014–2018, I succeeded in securing two-thirds of the required funding for the book (with the remaining financing to be covered by me) from six sources: the Mectizan Donation Program, the Kuwait Fund, philanthropist John Moores, Sightsavers International, the George & Angelina Owusu Foundation, and the Izumi Foundation. With that funding coming in, I launched the book project in late 2014 and began traveling to conduct interviews and collect documentation. Those travels eventually consisted of two trips each to West Africa (APOC headquarters in Ouagadougou; former program directors based in Lomé and Accra; Sightsavers International office in Accra), Europe (WHO headquarters in Geneva; Organization for the Prevention of Blindness headquarters in Paris), and the United Kingdom (Sightsavers International headquarters; London School of Hygiene and Tropical Medicine; Liverpool School of Tropical Medicine; GlaxoSmithKline headquarters), as well as around the United States (Merck headquarters in New Jersey; the Task Force for Global Health, Centers for Disease Control and Prevention, The Carter Center, and Emory University in Atlanta; the Bill and Melinda Gates Foundation in Seattle; World Bank headquarters in Washington, DC).

This book is not about the biomedical aspects of the disease nor the intricacies of controlling oncho in the field. These are areas where I have limited expertise and experience. Rather, this book recounts the oncho-control history from a macro perspective. That perspective was based in part on the World Bank's role as the lead sponsoring agency and "fiscal agent" for the control effort, and on my own responsibilities as the Bank's Oncho Manager for 20 years and as the Chair of the Committee of Sponsoring Agencies during 1991–2004, which oversaw the completion of OCP and the scale-up of APOC. The primary focus is on the oncho partnership, including how it was assembled, widened, and sustained over decades to control, and pursue eventual elimination of, the disease throughout Africa. An important constituency of that partnership was the broad-based donor community, which remained intact and committed to addressing the problem for more than 35 years—unprecedented in the history of development assistance.

As anticipated in the 2005 concept note, governance, coalition building, private–public sector collaboration, and community empowerment turned out to be important themes in the book. Other themes emerged during the research phase. These included transformational decisions taken by individuals in positions of authority, operational research that enhanced control operations and lay the groundwork for expansion of the effort to all of Africa, and the role of compassion at the individual and institutional levels that deepened commitment to controlling the disease. This last theme surfaced somewhat unexpectedly during the course of interviewing key players in the oncho story.

It is hoped that the international community will benefit from this account of the near-half-century effort to control and eliminate onchocerciasis throughout Africa. The lessons learned and best practices culled from this experience, as set out in chapter 9, are intended as guides in designing and bringing to scale new multilateral efforts to address global problems. Many of the principles and processes embodied in the oncho-control/elimination effort that helped yield success are applicable to large-scale partnerships regardless of sector and the nature of the problem to be tackled.

Acknowledgments

Support from a number of organizations and individuals was critical in producing this book. Financing for much of my travel for research was provided by the Mectizan Donation Program, the Kuwait Fund, Philanthropist John Moores, Sightsavers International, the George & Angelina Owusu Foundation, and the Izumi Foundation. That funding enabled me to undertake trips for interviews and document collection to Africa, Europe, the United Kingdom, Kuwait, and around the United States during 2014–2017. Most of the 114 interviews for the book were conducted with individuals either working or retired and living in close proximity to the World Health Organization, Geneva; the Ouagadougou headquarters of the African Program for Onchocerciasis Control (APOC); Merck's New Jersey headquarters; various nongovernmental development organization (NGDO) offices in Europe, the UK, and the US; the Atlanta-based Task Force for Global Health; the Kuwait Fund in Kuwait City; and the World Bank in Washington, DC.

I am particularly indebted to Jan (Hans) Remme, former manager of the Tropical Disease Research Program (TDR) Task Force on Onchocerciasis Operational Research, and David Addiss, director of the Focus Area for Compassion and Ethics at the Task Force for Global Health, for their advice during many hours of discussions throughout the manuscript-preparation process. Both read through several manuscript iterations and recommended adjustments that greatly improved the final product. Remme assisted in locating graphics to facilitate the reader's understanding of the disease and its transmission. He was also a key source for maps, based on empirical survey data and projections from model simulations, that reveal declining oncho prevalence levels throughout sub-Saharan Africa resulting from effective control operations.

As my editor during the three-year writing phase, Mojie Crigler provided invaluable advice regarding the book's overall structure and clarity of presentation throughout. I was extremely fortunate to have her editorial guidance. She is an experienced editor and writer who has authored two books on health, one of which covered neglected tropical diseases (NTDs). Her familiarity with onchocerciasis,

OCP and APOC, and key actors in the story was a major asset. She was also delightful to work with during the sometimes-tedious drafting process.

I am also appreciative of the editorial assistance provided by Ms. Delaney Fordell during the summer of 2018, through an internship set up through Kalamazoo College; and the opportunities to brainstorm on lessons learned and best practices through the OCP/APOC experience with graduate students (Gia Ferrara, Jenna Wozniak, and Kaitlin Kruger) in a reading-discussion course taught by David Addiss at the University of Notre Dame during the winter/spring of 2018. In addition, I wish to acknowledge the support of Andy Crump of Kitasato University in providing photos of oncho manifestations and the various aspects of controlling the disease. Many of the photos in the book were taken by him during the 1990s and 2000s in a variety of oncho-endemic African countries during the years he worked at the WHO/TDR.

This book would not have been possible without the extensive support of the organizations and individuals mentioned above, as well as 100+ interviewees who unselfishly contributed countless hours of their time during often lengthy interviews. However, any factual inaccuracies or deficiencies in presentation in this book must be attributed to me alone.

Riverblindness in Africa

Chapter 1

The Challenge

> Nakong is a place of horror. The people, a dying community, are losing the
> fight for survival against the tiny flies which multiply each breeding season
> in ideal conditions in the river. . . . The silence of this village of the blind
> was startling and oppressive. . . . The effect on the life of the community
> of this amount of blindness, and of the debilitating filariae is everywhere
> apparent. They lack even the energy to clear the bush or to protect their
> crops against the antelope. . . . The vicious spiral down which they are
> sliding is all too obvious: less energy—less land farmed—less food—even
> less energy.
> —Sir John Wilson on his visit to the Northern Gold Coast in 1950

An Opportunity

When I was offered the position of Riverblindness Coordinator in the Sahel
Country Division of the World Bank, I was only mildly interested. The year was
1985 and I had never heard of "riverblindness"—much less "onchocerciasis," the
scientific term for the disease. From the little I knew, it did not seem to be an
important health problem for Africa, certainly not on the order of malaria or the
emerging HIV/AIDS epidemic. The location of the Riverblindness Unit in the
World Bank's Sahel Country Division (covering Burkina Faso, Mali, and Niger)
suggested the disease was confined to a few countries in an arid, low-income
subregion of West Africa.

Also, I needed a mainstream position to continue my career at the World
Bank. "Coordinator" was not a mainstream position, like "economist" or "loan
officer." Hence, it was not transferable into other departments in Bank Operations. However, this job offer might be my last hope of remaining in the Bank.
My three-year, fixed-term assignment as a Bank Evaluation Officer was about to
end. So, I took the job, with the intention of performing well and moving at the
soonest opportunity. Instead, I wound up remaining in that position until I retired from the World Bank 20 years later, as "Manager" of an expanded portfolio
covering onchocerciasis control for all of sub-Saharan Africa.

What follows is the story of the onchocerciasis-control campaign based, in part, on my experience in managing the World Bank's responsibilities with respect to the control effort, and on research and interviews covering the 50-year span of the campaign. This book examines the two seminal decades prior to my involvement, the 20 years of my experience in the effort, and the subsequent 12 years of consolidating control and elimination of the disease after I retired. It covers the ups and downs of the campaign, the shift from the pursuit of control to elimination of the disease throughout Africa, and the emergence of related efforts to eliminate the other major neglected tropical diseases on the continent.

(In public health parlance, the term "elimination" refers to the disappearance of the source of the disease in a confined geographical area—as in, malaria has been eliminated in the United States. The term "eradication" refers to elimination of the source of the disease worldwide—as was achieved through the Smallpox Eradication Program. "Control" generally means bringing the incidence and prevalence of a disease down to levels where it is no longer a public health problem.)

In the concluding section, I attempt to draw lessons from this long-term experience, focusing on aspects that might be transferable to other large-scale efforts to address widespread diseases or similarly challenging global problems.

Upon taking my new position, I started learning about onchocerciasis and the program to control it. Members of the Bank's "oncho team" and staff based at Program headquarters in Ouagadougou, Burkina Faso, brought me up to speed. I found the etiology of onchocerciasis fascinating and the impact of the disease on the rural poor far more pervasive and devastating than I had realized. Oncho was unquestionably a serious health problem, infecting more than 60% of the rural inhabitants in many areas of savanna West Africa. The challenge of pursuing an effective and lasting control effort was daunting.

Disease Etiology and Its Human Impact

Onchocerciasis is transmitted by a small, stout-bodied, fiercely biting blackfly—the "vector" for the disease. The *Simulium damnosum* complex is the most pervasive species of the vector and transmits an estimated 95% of the oncho cases in sub-Saharan Africa.[1] The fly lays its eggs on partially submerged sticks, stones, and leaves in the rapids of rivers and streams throughout the region. Fast-flowing water is necessary to provide oxygen for the blackfly larva to gestate to the hatching stage and emerge as a fly.

The female blackfly seeks out human beings to take a meal of blood required for the maturation of her eggs (figure 1.1). She can travel up to 500 kilometers (km) with prevailing winds but tends to congregate within a 15-km radius of a river or stream to lay her eggs. If the person bitten by the fly is infected with onchocerciasis, one or two microscopic worms—known as microfilariae—are usually ingested in the blood meal. Once ingested, the microfilariae undergo a transformation within the fly which allows them to develop into adult worms. But they can only achieve adulthood after being deposited into the body of a second human host. That occurs when that same fly, after laying her eggs, takes a second blood meal a few days later. Female adult worms usually grow to 33–50 centimeters (cm) (13–20 inches) in length and live with smaller male worms encapsulated in stationary nodules beneath the skin, often surrounding the waist and upper chest of the human host, though nodules can also be found on the limbs and head. Each nodule contains one or more pairs of worms—male and female. The adult worms live in nodules and spawn microfilariae for up to 14 years.

Over its life span, the adult female worm produces millions of microfilariae, which migrate through the human body just beneath the surface of the skin, causing intense itching, depigmentation, unsightly skin lesions, and skin atrophy. The itching is unrelenting and often excruciating. It can lead to suicide. Some microfilariae migrate to the eyes, where they die off, forming ocular lesions, leading to tunnel vision, and eventually permanent blindness. The lifespan of the microfilariae in the human body is two years. If ingested by flies, those microfilariae continue their developmental cycle in the fly, reaching the infective stage (L-3), and then maturing into adult worms in the next human victim.

Onchocerciasis is usually contracted by children younger than 6 years of age, and infection worsens when they begin working in the fields, out in the open with fewer people around so that they are exposed to more frequent fly biting. The greatest risk is for those who work and live within a 15-km distance from a river or stream where the flies congregate. Troublesome itching begins shortly after becoming infected. Skin lesions appear in the early to late teens. Blindness occurs on average at 30 years of age. Hence, the disease advances over some 24 years. Progression of the disease can be forestalled by interrupting transmission through vector control, that is, targeting blackfly larvae in the rapids of rivers and streams with insecticides. If transmission is interrupted, a victim is protected from fly biting and continual reinfection, enabling symptoms to regress. Under these circumstances, the individual can eventually recover, even completely, unless permanent pathological changes, such as irreversible blindness, have occurred.

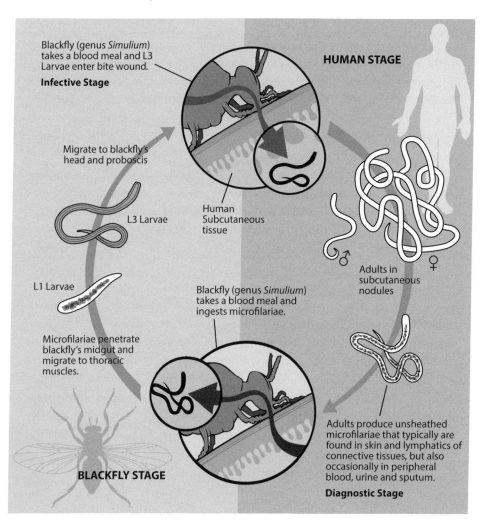

Blackfly (genus *Simulium*) takes a blood meal and L3 Larvae enter bite wound.
Infective Stage

HUMAN STAGE

Migrate to blackfly's head and proboscis

L3 Larvae

Human Subcutaneous tissue

L1 Larvae

Microfilariae penetrate blackfly's midgut and migrate to thoracic muscles.

Blackfly (genus *Simulium*) takes a blood meal and ingests microfilariae.

Adults in subcutaneous nodules

Adults produce unsheathed microfilariae that typically are found in skin and lymphatics of connective tissues, but also occasionally in peripheral blood, urine and sputum.

Diagnostic Stage

BLACKFLY STAGE

Figure 1.1. Riverblindness (Onchocerciasis) Life Cycle. *Source*: Basáñez, M-G., S.D.S. Pion, T.S. Churcher, L.P. Breitling, M.P. Little, and M. Boussinesq. "River Blindness: A Success Story under Threat?" *PLoS Med* 3, no. 9 (2006): e371. https://doi.org/10.1371/journal.pmed.0030371.

European Scientists Discover Onchocerciasis

While onchocerciasis is a centuries-old scourge, it was the last of the major tropical diseases in Africa to be discovered by European scientists.[2] Oncho was almost exclusively a rural disease impacting populations in hard-to-reach, remote areas.

Consequently, the pathology in victims was difficult to study. Furthermore, the principal symptoms of the disease—intense itching, skin depigmentation, and visual impairment—were frequently attributed to other, already-known diseases such as scabies, bacterial infections, trachoma, and cataracts.[3]

British naval surgeon John O'Neill first discovered onchocerciasis in 1875 by identifying microfilariae in the skin of colonial Gold Coast (later Ghana) patients as the cause of a severely itching skin disease, called "craw-craw" in the creole patois of neighboring Sierra Leone. In 1893, German zoologist Rudolf Leuckart discovered the adult worm in nodules excised from Gold Coast patients and named it *filaria volvulas*.[4] He suggested it might be the parental form of the microfilariae previously identified by O'Neill. In 1910, the French veterinary pathologist, Alcide Railliet, renamed the parasite *Onchocerca volvulus* when describing that same adult worm excised from a patient in Mauritania.[5] In so doing, Railliet placed it in a classification of parasites also found in veterinary animals, known as *Onchocerca*.

In 1915, Guatemalan Rodolfo Robles was the first scientist to make the connection between the parasite and blindness. He had been studying Guatemalans infected with the parasite, which almost certainly had been brought to the Americas via the slave trade. UNESCO data show that African slaves transported to the Americas during the 15th–18th centuries came primarily from areas that today constitute Senegal, Guinea, Ghana, Nigeria, the Democratic Republic of the Congo (DRC), the Republic of the Congo, and Angola.[6] These are the areas that have historically been heavily endemic with oncho. Robles discovered that the eyesight in patients improved after the adult worms were excised.[7] It took until the 1930s to confirm that the disease in the Americas, which was on a far more limited scale than in Africa, was essentially identical to the African version; and that the disease in Africa, too, was an important cause of blindness.

Scotsman Dr. Donald Blacklock succeeded in tracing the transmission cycle by which the parasite *Onchocerca volvulus* was passed from human to human (see figure 1.1). While working in Sierra Leone during 1922–1925, Blacklock noted a correlation between the high prevalence of nodules in the population in the Kono District and the presence of biting blackflies, which he identified as the species complex, *Simulium damnosum*.[8] His article, published in the *Annals of Tropical Medicine and Parasitology* in 1926, established the fly-parasite transmission cycle of onchocerciasis. This was the last of the important early steps in understanding the etiology of the disease.

In the early 1930s, Belgian ophthalmologist Jean Hissette reported that 20% of the villagers infected with onchocerciasis and living along the Sankuru River in the Belgian Congo were blind and that 50% had some loss of vision.[9] He discovered similar results among inhabitants living along the Uele River, also in the Belgian Congo. This was the first confirmation of very high levels of oncho blindness and impaired vision in Africa. Hissette's findings reaffirmed those of Robles 16 years earlier in Guatemala, on the causal link between the parasite and ocular impairment. In 1934, a Harvard African expedition accompanied Hissette back to the Belgian Congo to check out his findings and confirmed that they were correct.[10]

Hissette's discoveries raised a question later posed by Dr. Pierre Richet while working in Upper Volta (later Burkina Faso) in the late 1930s: why had it taken so long to discover that onchocerciasis was a serious cause of blindness in Africa? Robles had made the oncho connection to blindness in Guatemala 20 years earlier.[11] Richet, who would later become one of the most respected figures in French military medicine, was arguing that onchocerciasis was a much more serious disease in Africa than colonial studies indicated. In doing so, Richet was suggesting that oncho was a "neglected tropical disease" long before the term became popularized in global health. But, why was it neglected? Probably because onchocerciasis is almost exclusively found in rural areas and had little impact on colonial Europeans who lived predominantly in urban areas.

By World War II, the basic aspects of onchocerciasis had been investigated and were understood within the European scientific community. The extent of the disease and its severity, particularly in terms of blindness, were also beginning to be appreciated by Europeans working on tropical diseases in the British and French colonies. As the perceived magnitude of the problem grew, the question became how to contain the spread of the disease and alleviate its severity. The response took two tracks. The first involved raising awareness of the disease in Africa and in the developed world so that resources could be mobilized to tackle it. The second entailed developing a strategy to interrupt its transmission over a widespread area.

Raising Awareness

During the late 1940s and the 1950s, the work of John Wilson brought attention to onchocerciasis and its devastation in West Africa. Wilson had been blinded at the age of 12 by an accidental explosion during an experiment in a chemistry class at the Scarborough High School for Boys in Scarborough, North Yorkshire, UK, in 1931. After graduating from Worchester College for the Blind and receiving a law degree from Oxford University, he devoted his life to advocating for the blind, particularly in the British colonies. He traveled extensively in Africa in 1946–1947 and 1950–1951. Those travels instilled in him palpable compassion for the suffering of the blind "at the bottom of the pyramid who had to struggle to survive."[12] He was "appalled that blindness was something that you hid away in Africa. It was a disgrace to the family."[13] On those trips, Wilson developed what he termed "an amateur red rage"—a determination to do what he could to alleviate the misery of the visually impaired in the developing world.[14]

Wilson's 1946–1947 trip to Africa, as part of a British colonial office delegation to investigate blindness, was instrumental in driving him to establish, and subsequently lead, the British Empire Society for the Blind in 1950. After African independence, the Empire Society turned into the Royal Commonwealth Society for the Blind, and ultimately Sightsavers International through a name change in 1986. Wilson founded the International Agency for the Prevention of Blindness (IAPB) and became its first president in 1974. Each of these organizations under Wilson's leadership played important roles in raising awareness of onchocerciasis and in investigating its magnitude as well as methods for controlling it. "At the time, for many, onchocerciasis only existed in textbooks," his wife, Lady Jean Wilson, later remarked.[15]

During Wilson's 1947 trip to the Gold Coast, he learned of the "country of the blind" along rivers in the Northern Territories from reports of the British ophthalmologist Dr. Harold Ridley.[16] Ridley had been stationed in the Gold Coast in the Royal Army Medical Corps during World War II. In examining recruits for the war effort, he was struck by the high rates of blindness among candidates from the Northern Territories. He visited the Northern Territories in 1944 and spent two weeks in the remote village of Funsi. He examined 300 residents, about half of the village's population, and found "shocking" levels of blindness, with an overall rate of 7.3%, and 15.6% among villagers with oncho nodules.[17] Ridley's report provided the first recorded evidence of oncho-caused blindness in the Gold Coast.

Mindful of Ridley's report, Australian-born Dr. B. B. Waddy, medical officer of the Northern Territories, set out in 1948 to delve into the "sinister story of onchocerciasis" and its "diabolical vector."[18] He conducted studies in 14 smaller villages in the Sissili Valley with populations of 1,000 or less. Smaller villages enabled examining nearly all of the residents. His intent was to investigate the connection between oncho and blindness, and the disease as a cause of village depopulation. Waddy diagnosed oncho infection levels by taking snips of skin to sample the concentration of microfilariae in the skin of patients, a new method to measure infection levels at the time. He found prevalence levels to be upward of 70% in most villages, with average blindness rates of 10% across all the villages. His investigations revealed that 61% of blindness overall and 78% of the blindness among the men were caused by oncho.[19] Waddy also concluded that the disease was an important factor contributing to depopulation. The youth were watching their elders become blind and were moving away and not returning.[20]

Two aspects of Waddy's work were important in eventually developing an effective control strategy. First, though lacking any background in entomology, he homed in on the chief culprit in disease transmission: the blackfly, *Simulium damnosum*. Second, he concluded that any effective long-term approach to controlling the disease in the Gold Coast would have to include close coordination with the neighboring francophone countries—Upper Volta to the north, Côte d'Ivoire to the west, and Togo to the east. These two aspects were key to any effective, sustainable control strategy: (1) halting propagation of the blackfly vector, and (2) covering the known breeding sites of the blackfly throughout a multicountry area. Even though the Gold Coast's Ministry of Health did not publish Waddy's report, his findings appeared in his writings and influenced future efforts to control the disease in West Africa.

Wilson sought out Waddy during his second trip to the Gold Coast in 1950, meeting up with him in the hyperendemic Sisili and Kulpawn Rivers area in the Northern Territories.[21] Wilson had decided to visit areas where tax returns indicated that blindness was most severe (the blind were exempt from taxation). The governor of the Gold Coast arranged for the travel, and Wilson's wife, Jean, accompanied him. One of the first villages they visited was Nakong, on the bank of the Sisili River just south of the border with Upper Volta. Waddy had spent time in Nakong two years earlier, examining 90% of the roughly 1,000 villagers. He had found oncho infection levels of nearly 70% and a blindness rate of near 10%.[22] John and Jean Wilson stayed in Nakong for four days and nights, sleeping in a mud hut. Of all the villages they visited on that trip, Nakong made the greatest impression on John Wilson.[23]

He later described their visit to Nakong in his report back to the newly established Empire Society of the Blind:

> At Nakong 50 people met us on the muddy bank of the swollen river. They were like specimens from a medical museum and behind them their village lay silent as a cemetery. The clinical record showed that a 10th of the people in this village and a sixth of the adult males were totally blind. They showed us their houses with tiny entrances, probably a protection against animals. . . .

[A]s they shuffled along slowly behind us, it was difficult to believe that they had enough energy left to do so. We stood aside to allow two blind men to pass. They were walking one behind the other, both holding a long piece of bamboo at the front end of which a child was leading the way.[24]

Reflecting on their experience in Nakong, Jean Wilson later said,

We stayed there and talked to them and were told that every family had blind people. They accepted John because he was totally blind, but they couldn't accept that I could still see in my 20s. When they were told that I could, I was a phenomenon. It was such a dreary life in that village. They were not just blinded, but severely debilitated with lumps and bumps all over.[25]

John Wilson wrote in his diary, "As we left those villages, I felt sick and angry and was possessed with the urgent need to get something done about the situation."[26] He decided to raise funds for ophthalmic and entomological surveys of the Northern Territories through the Empire Society. The Wilsons estimated the surveys would cost £40,000—equivalent to $US 1.1 million in 2017 dollars according to my calculations. It was an overwhelming amount for a new organization that had been launched the year before, on a "wing and a prayer" and operating on a bare-bones budget with only three staff members, including the Wilsons.[27] Upon his return to London, John Wilson began radio-address appeals to raise the funding by describing what they had encountered in the "country of the blind."

During that trip to Nakong, the vehicle transporting the Wilsons got stuck and the driver set off to seek help. Jean Wilson described the situation in our 2015 interview:

We were stuck fast on a river bed in the middle of the day, sitting in the heat of the sun. John insisted that all the windows be up to prevent us being bitten. John said, 'I think Harold Ridley was right, this is onchocerciasis.' I said, 'John, onchocerciasis? I can't say it and I can't spell it. How am I going to raise funds for it?' And, as I watched these flies swarming up from the river, I said, 'John, let's call it river blindness.' This is how we got the name for it and it stuck.[28]

Jean Wilson's suggestion to call the disease "river blindness" was important in giving the nonscientific community a handle by which to recognize a serious public-health problem in sub-Saharan Africa. Though simplistic, the new name conveyed the basic features of the disease in layman's language in a way that the textbook term, onchocerciasis, could not. (When the World Bank began to address the disease in the early 1970s, the one-word term, "riverblindness," was used in Bank documentation. This is the nonscientific name for the disease that I have used throughout in this book. I prefer "riverblindness" to the two-word expression "river blindness" because the latter can be misconstrued as implying that rivers are the direct cause of oncho blindness.)

John Wilson was skilled at public relations. Publicizing the devastation of onchocerciasis in West Africa, notably in Ghana and Nigeria, enabled him to leverage support for his newly established British Empire Society for the Blind. By 1951, he had secured the participation of the Earl of Halifax as president, and Helen Keller as vice president, of the Empire Society. In the Gold Coast, he convinced the minister of commerce and industry to serve as deputy chairman of the Gold Coast Society for the Blind, which he established in 1951.[29] By 1953, £12,000 had been raised for ophthalmological and entomological surveys.

Wilson recruited Dr. Frederick Rodger to conduct the ophthalmological surveys. They were carried out in the Gold Coast, Nigeria, and the British Cameroons in the mid-1950s. Rodger compared the severity of various causes of blindness. His results showed that oncho was by far the largest cause in northern Gold Coast, followed by trachoma. In northern Nigeria, trachoma caused the greatest blindness, with oncho in third, behind cataracts. However, oncho exceeded all other causes in the hyperendemic areas in northern Nigeria.[30] Rodger also cited a high correlation between blindness and areas where blackfly breeding sites were the most numerous.[31] This finding led Wilson to conclude that an entomological survey was essential for a complete picture of the disease.

Wilson chose Dr. Geoffrey Crisp to conduct the entomological survey. Crisp found an average of 10 bites per person/per hour in most oncho-endemic areas, and as high as 100 bites per person/per hour in the heavily endemic areas.[32] His results showed that the fly infectivity rates with stage L-3 larvae, that enable the parasite to become an adult worm in the next human host, were extremely high in northern Gold Coast, with rates in one area exceeding 70%.[33] Crisp concluded that there was an "urgent need" for a blackfly control program in the Northern Territories. Without it, planned agricultural schemes in the area would probably fail.[34] Furthermore, he argued that the size of the Volta River basin, extending significantly into Sahelian French colonial West Africa, required French collaboration for a control effort to succeed.[35] But his inquiries with French authorities in 1953 were unsuccessful indicating that the French had little interest in a multicountry control effort at that time.[36]

The Outlines of a Multicountry Control Effort Emerge

Two oncho-control tools emerged after World War II: vector control and drug treatment. The insecticide DDT (dichlorodiphenyltrichloroethane) was used in the late 1940s to destroy blackfly larvae along rivers in Kenya, the Belgian Congo, and Uganda. The first important vector-control success was in Kenya where DDT was used along watercourses to eliminate the blackfly in the Kodera area, known as the "Valley of the Blind." It was, however, an unusual situation because the fly was a different species from *Simulium damnosum*. The East African species was *Simulium naevei*—a fly largely confined to that area that did not travel long distances and deposited larvae exclusively on the shells of East African river crabs. Vector control in Kenya, pursued by entomologists P. C. C. Garnham, director of the Division of Insect-borne Diseases at the Medical Research Laboratory in Nairobi, and a staff member, J. P. McMahon, eventually led to the elimination of *Simulium naevei* throughout the country and the cessation of oncho transmission countrywide by the mid-1950s.[37] That first vector eradication effort turned out to have lasting success because Kenya remains largely free from onchocerciasis despite being surrounded by oncho-endemic countries.

In Congo, Belgian medical doctor Marcel Jules Emile Marie Wanson focused on vector control with DDT along the Congo River adjacent to Leopoldville (later Kinshasa) in the late 1940s. Leopoldville was unique because both *Simulium damnosum* and the disease were prevalent in the city, whereas most African urban areas were free of oncho. Consequently, 45% of the city's European inhabitants were infected.[38] The impact on Europeans undoubtedly brought greater attention to the problem. Villages nearby were found to have infection rates of 100%.[39] The Congo River was so wide and turbulent that the only effective way to control the blackfly was concentrated aerial spraying with DDT. The approach involved spraying an aerosol that killed off both the blackflies and their larvae.[40] The positive results demonstrated for the first time that aerial spraying with insecticides could be effective over vast river systems.[41]

In Uganda, ground-based vector control with DDT along the Victorian Nile in the mid-1950s also wiped out the blackfly species, *Simulium naevei*. Again, vector control benefited from the isolation of the species, its short flight distance, and the location of blackfly larvae confined to the shells of East African river crabs. However, vector control pursued by George Barnley, an entomologist in the Uganda Medical Services, was not effective against *Simulium damnosum*.[42] This illustrated that vector control had to be expansive and comprehensive—covering vast areas of river systems including tributaries—if transmission of onchocerciasis by *Simulium damnosum* was to be interrupted effectively.

Two drugs became available after World War II; both were effective against the parasite, *Onchocerca volvulus*. However, both had serious side effects. Suramin was discovered and produced in Germany between the wars as a treatment for trypanosomiasis (sleeping sickness). Today, it remains the only fast-acting "macrofilaricide"—a drug that kills the adult oncho worm. However, suramin is only effective when administered via slow-intravenous injection.[43] Even then, it can be highly toxic and requires medical supervision during treatment. Consequently, it has never been considered as a possible "operational" drug for mass treatment.

Diethylcarbamazine (DEC) was discovered in 1947. It is effective against certain filarial diseases such as lymphatic filariasis, loiasis, and oncho, though it has little or no impact on the adult oncho worm. It is almost exclusively a "microfilaricide." When given orally, it kills nearly all of the oncho microfilariae in the body, which then build back up to previous levels within a year. However, the side effects of DEC can be severe, particularly when administered for the first time. The rapid destruction of thousands of infant worms often causes an immune reaction in the body, known as a Mazzotti reaction, which can result in blindness and even anaphylactic shock leading to death. DEC is, therefore, not a drug that can be used in mass-treatment campaigns to control oncho. The severity of the Mazzotti reaction led officials from the World Health Organization (WHO) to shy away from other microfilaricides to control onchocerciasis. Their default assumption appeared to be that other microfilaricides would have a mode of action similar to that of DEC.

Established in 1947, WHO was one of several organizations set up after World War II that eventually played important roles in the control of onchocerciasis. Its first technical meeting on onchocerciasis was convened in Leopoldville in 1954. By 1957, the WHO publication, *Bulletin of the World Health Organization* was opened to research articles on oncho. WHO convened a second conference on onchocerciasis in 1961 at the Regional Office for Africa (AFRO) in Brazzaville, in which both anglophone and francophone scientists participated. On the French side, the tropical disease research organization, Office de la Recherche Scientifique et Technique Outre-Mer (ORSTOM), which grew out of an earlier colonial research organization, was established in the late 1940s. In the early 1960s, ORSTOM began strengthening its entomological expertise with the recognition that DDT could be effective against a number of insect vectors that transmitted the most serious diseases in francophone Africa, notably malaria, sleeping sickness, and onchocerciasis.[44]

With independence, all the former French colonies, except Guinea, requested French support for the establishment of an intercountry facility to provide technical support, research, training, and coordination of control of the major infectious diseases. Those requests resulted in the establishment of the Organisation de Coordination et de Coopération pour la lutte contre les Grandes Endémies (OCCGE). The OCCGE took the place of the French colonial regional authority, Service Général d'Hygiène Mobile et de Prophylaxie (SGHMP), that had been established immediately after World War II to address sleeping sickness, malaria, leprosy, cerebro-spinal meningitis, and onchocerciasis. The director of the SGHMP, Dr. Pierre Richet, who had maintained that onchocerciasis was more serious in West Africa than research suggested, was chosen as the permanent secretary-general of the OCCGE. The United States joined France in funding the OCCGE, an important development that presaged future US involvement in oncho control.

The offices and laboratories of the SGHMP, known as Centre Muraz in Bobo-Dioulasso, Upper Volta, became the headquarters of the OCCGE in 1960. The location was tantamount to ground zero for onchocerciasis in West Africa. The OCCGE was instrumental in laying the groundwork for a possible future regional-control effort. Its scientists, largely ORSTOM-seconded French entomologists, succeeded in mapping onchocerciasis, as well as the extent of *Simulium damnosum* breeding sites, throughout a number of ex-French West African countries during the 1960s.[45]

Dr. Max Ovazza, head of the OCCGE's onchocerciasis section, and fellow entomologist René Le Berre launched the first experimental vector-control campaign in the upper parts of the Comoé, Black Volta, and Léraba River basins in Upper Volta in the early part of the decade. The project was financed by France's aid agencies, Fonds d'Investissement pour le Développement Economique et Social des Territoires d'Outre-mer (FIDES) and Fonds d'Aide et de Cooperation (FAC) over 1960–1965. It was clear by then that the principal method for controlling oncho in West Africa had to be vector control. No safe, operationally usable drug existed.

That experimental project in Upper Volta demonstrated that an effective vector-control operation had to be multicountry. Portions of at least seven countries in the Volta River basin were hyperendemic with savanna onchocerciasis that was transmitted by *Simulium damnosum*. *Simulium damnosum*, along with *Simulium sirbanum* that populated Sierra Leone and Eastern Guinea, were the two major species of blackfly in West Africa. Both traveled long distances and transmitted the savanna form of the disease throughout the region.

In 1966, the European Economic Community's aid agency, the European Development Fund (EDF), joined the oncho-control effort by financing a larger multicountry operation covering 60,000 km² of endemic areas in Upper Volta, Côte d'Ivoire, and Mali.[46] Even though the United States had joined France in establishing the OCCGE, it did not support this first multicountry effort. The US Agency for International Development (USAID) was reluctant out of concern that the scope of coverage was too limited, notably by leaving out northern Ghana.[47]

Nevertheless, the EDF-financed experiment was a bold attempt at multicountry control funded by external donors. The question was whether a regional oncho-control effort could be sufficiently large to be viable and receive adequate long-term donor support to be sustainable. The answer would depend upon the response of three key institutional players hitherto not directly involved—USAID, WHO, and the World Bank—as well as the interest and involvement of the other African countries in the Volta and Niger River basins that were impacted by the disease.

The Development Decade of the 1960s

Important changes in the 1960s made a large-scale regional program to control onchocerciasis in West Africa more likely. The first was increased United States involvement in Africa following independence of the former French and British colonies in the early 1960s. Independence opened up the continent to American efforts to exert influence that were seen as inappropriate during the colonial period. The Kennedy administration became far more active in Africa than the Eisenhower administration that preceded it. Africa was seen as an integral part of the Kennedy "New Frontier" programs, which included the Peace Corps and an ambitious effort to put man on the moon. Africa also became enmeshed in the Cold War. In the early- to mid-1960s, three West African countries— Ghana, Guinea, and Mali—were flirting with the Soviet Union and, to a lesser extent, Communist China. The nearly catastrophic Cuban missile crisis in 1962 reinforced the concern of US policymakers over Soviet expansion. The United States became intent on staving off communist inroads in Africa and was prepared to commit the resources to back up its strategic-security policy. American influence was manifested through the largest foreign-assistance program in the world, including an emerging USAID interest in oncho control.

In late 1966, two USAID public-health officers approached the World Bank about looking into what they perceived as a worsening onchocerciasis *cum* development problem.[48] The two officials—A. C. Curtis, chief of public health in USAID's Africa Bureau, and Z. Deutschman, a former WHO entomologist and consultant to USAID—asked Bank officials to investigate the negative impact of the disease on development. The major concerns were reduced human productivity in the rural sector due to blindness and losses in agricultural production due to the unavailability of fertile land near rivers where the disease ran rampant. The motivation of the USAID officials was to have the Bank—a well-respected, independent, development institution—conclude that the disease was an important development constraint in West Africa. Such a conclusion would better enable them to convince the higher levels in USAID to support a large-scale regional effort to control oncho.[49]

At that time, the ongoing control effort covering parts of Upper Volta, Côte d'Ivoire, and Mali was facing headwinds. Resources from France's FAC and the EEC's EDF were becoming constrained. USAID favored enlarging the ongoing effort to cover the perceived limits of the disease, notably by including northern Ghana, to strengthen the viability of the control effort. World Bank senior staff, however, were resistant to becoming involved. The health sector was considered the purview of WHO and, therefore, out of bounds for the Bank. This position was conveyed to WHO by Leonard Rist, who had been the World Bank's special advisor to the president since 1947. In doing so, however, Rist left the door slightly ajar by indicating the Bank's willingness to support bilateral donors interested in increasing their involvement in health. Rist communicated to Dr. N. Ansari, Chief of Parasitic Diseases at WHO, in 1967: "Under no circumstances could our Bank finance hygiene or public health programs, but we could maybe help certain American development agencies who, themselves, could eventually contribute to the fight against *Simulium damnosum* in Africa."[50]

USAID staff had brought to Rist's attention that some of the major Bank-financed hydroelectric dam projects may have been contributing to a worsening oncho problem in West Africa. These included the Kainji Dam in Nigeria and the Akosombo Dam on the Volta River in Ghana. That connection spurred Rist's interest in the disease.[51] The disease could not be ignored if it was implicated in Bank-funded projects.

By mid-1967, Rist had come to the view that "the project is worth supporting"—without specifying how.[52] Despite considerable communication within the Bank, with WHO, and with the EDF, no one in the Bank came up with persuasive data on the economic impact of the disease. Consequently, the World Bank was unable to provide USAID with the economic justification Curtis and Deutschman were seeking. The lack of economic justification made it far less likely that the World Bank would reverse its long-standing objection to financing health projects. In late 1969, the Bank's chief economist for the Western Africa Department, John de Wilde, suggested a compromise that, for the time being, satisfied the higher levels in the Bank. It was referred to as the "two-project" solution. The World Bank would not support the disease control effort. That would be left to WHO, with backing from bilateral donors such as USAID. But the Bank could support a development program in areas where the disease was brought under control provided such a program proved economically justifiable.[53]

The 1968 Tunis Conference on Technical Feasibility

In keeping with USAID's objective of establishing a regional oncho-control effort in West Africa, Curtis arranged for a technical meeting in Tunis in July 1968. The meeting was co-convened by WHO and the OCCGE. The presence and prestige of Pierre Richet, as OCCGE director-general, was important in generating attendance.[54] The World Bank sent an observer. The meeting brought together experts in parasitology, entomology, epidemiology, and ophthalmology to explore the feasibility of an intercountry program covering the savanna form of the disease throughout the Volta River basin.

Representatives from the seven affected countries attended: Dahomey (later Benin), Ghana, Côte d'Ivoire, Mali, Niger, Togo, and Upper Volta. The Volta River basin was selected because it was thought to have the highest rates of oncho blindness in Africa and, hence, in the world. The basin also had advantages because ORSTOM and the OCCGE had amassed operationally-important data throughout much of the area via disease mapping and pilot studies during the early- to mid-1960s. Furthermore, the area was considered to have good post-control development potential. Forest onchocerciasis farther south in several countries was excluded, in large part because it was deemed to be far less blinding. In any case, forest oncho would have been nearly impossible to address meaningfully due to the dense forest canopy that prevented large-scale aerial spraying.

There was general agreement in Tunis that a control program focusing on aerial spraying (defined as "non-residual" larviciding, i.e., no DDT for ecological reasons) of the heavily endemic savanna zones of the seven West African countries over a 10- to 15-year period would be technically feasible.[55] The aim would be to eliminate the parasite reservoir in the population in that seven-country area. The meeting stressed the importance of the socioeconomic benefits expected from successful control and encouraged the international organizations "mainly concerned with agricultural development in tropical countries," for example, the Food and Agriculture Organization (FAO) and the World Bank, to participate in the control effort.[56]

Finally, an "international study mission" was recommended to flesh out an inter-country oncho-control effort and to study the socioeconomic aspects of control.[57]

Several fallouts from the Tunis meeting were important.[58] First, the World Bank attendee, Loreto Dominguez, did not press for an economic justification for the proposed control effort, even though that had earlier been a sine qua non for any direct Bank involvement in a disease-control effort. In his back-to-office report, Dominguez wrote that the meeting "fully" confirmed that onchocerciasis is a "serious social problem," but that it is difficult to assess the economic impact "due to the extremely low standard of living prevailing among the affected population" and "in what measure, presently low standards are . . . a result of the debilitating conditions created by the disease."[59] Hence, he recommended that the World Bank work to ensure that any control operation be as cost-effective as possible rather than economically justifiable.

Second, while the Tunis conference enhanced the prospects for a regional oncho-control program, it also highlighted some key differences among participants and raised questions about going forward. In a meeting at the World Bank three months after the conference, a member of Ghana's Planning Commission commented that controlling onchocerciasis was less important to his country than to Upper Volta, because northern Ghana, where the disease was prevalent, was "sparsely populated." He said: "The Government of Ghana would therefore be more reluctant to put as much effort and money as might be required."[60] Dr. Ansari confided to Rist after the conference, that he worried "greatly" about leadership going forward and that he was "not in favor of entrusting it to the Brazzaville WHO office," that is, AFRO.[61] It was known that Ansari, at the time, had ambitions of leading the control operation through his office in Geneva.[62] This marked the beginning of an institutional cleavage within WHO between Geneva Headquarters and the African regional office in Brazzaville, over leadership of the oncho-control effort that would persist off and on well into the future.

Third, there was the larger question of the designation of leadership of the effort in all its political, disease-control, and development aspects. USAID had been an important player behind the scenes and could bridge the differences between the francophone and anglophone partners. However, it would be unusual for a bilateral donor to assume overall leadership; more appropriate would be for that responsibility to go to an apolitical international organization. WHO was a contender, though it would more likely assume a technical role. The OCCGE, under Pierre Richet, had provided leadership, but it was mostly a francophone organization, which could present difficulties in involving Ghana, which was already feeling isolated as the sole anglophone country in the proposed program. Leadership by the OCCGE would be even more problematic if oncho control were to expand eastward to cover Nigeria, one of the largest oncho-infected countries in Africa. Hence, the emerging oncho-control effort was in search of an institutional leader.

Blueprint for Regional Oncho Control—The Preparatory Assistance to Governments Mission

With overall leadership of the proposed West African program in question, the United Nations Development Programme (UNDP) stepped in to assume its traditional role of leading and financing a pre-investment study. The World Bank position, as of 1970–1971, was still John de Wilde's "two-project" proposal: the Bank would focus on the post-control development phase but would refrain from supporting disease-control operations. However, in a 1970 internal Bank memorandum, de Wilde suggested another role for the Bank: "The view has been repeatedly expressed that some international financial agency should eventually take the leadership in mobilizing multilateral and bilateral resources for financing the project. If indeed all the parties concerned agree that the Bank should play this role, I believe the Bank should be prepared to assume this responsibility."[63]

The initial plan was for the UNDP-financed Preparatory Assistance to Governments Mission (PAG) to begin in mid-1971 and complete its work in one year. The UNDP chose B. B. Waddy as the mission leader. The government of Upper Volta agreed to host the mission in Ouagadougou, given its central location in the proposed program area. The PAG terms of reference called for the collection of epidemiological and entomological data, the preparation of a phased control strategy, a blueprint for the structure and management of the program, and the identification of zones for potential development follow-up as well as feasibility studies for development projects in those zones.[64]

In accordance with the World Bank's earlier insistence on an economic evaluation of the control effort, one was designed into the PAG. At the request of Dr. Ansari, de Wilde promised to find an economist who could carry it out. After trying to find a suitable candidate for a month, de Wilde wrote back to Ansari, apologizing that he was unable to do so.[65] In the end, the PAG got underway without an economist to fill that role. And, post-control development planning was eventually assigned to the FAO to undertake separately from the PAG.

The McNamara Era and the Launch of the Onchocerciasis Control Program

In April 1968, Robert McNamara, former US secretary of defense, became president of the World Bank. McNamara was a highly controversial figure. He had been architect of the Vietnam War during the John F. Kennedy and Lyndon B. Johnson administrations. By the mid-1960s, it was becoming clear that that war had been a mistake. The huge cost in lives and societal divisions were becoming intolerable. Moreover, the war for the American side was proving to be unwinnable. By 1966, McNamara had recognized the mistake and recommended to President Johnson in 1967 a course of action involving winding down the war and gradually withdrawing US involvement.[66] Johnson rejected McNamara's recommendation, leading to McNamara's resignation in late 1967. The term of World Bank President George Woods was coming to an end in March 1968, and Woods had publicly recommended McNamara in 1967 to become his successor. McNamara was interested in working on economic development in the developing countries, and, at his request, Johnson nominated him to become World Bank president. The Bank's board of executive directors subsequently elected McNamara to become the World Bank's fifth president.

Upon assuming the Bank presidency, McNamara initiated several important development policy changes. Two of these were pertinent to the Bank's interest and involvement in oncho control: population control and poverty alleviation. In his first address to the World Bank's board of governors in 1968, McNamara stressed that the Bank would oppose rapid population growth as "one of the greatest barriers to the economic growth and social well-being of our member states."[67] Overpopulation in some areas of sub-Saharan Africa was beginning to be seen as a function of heavily endemic onchocerciasis because populations were moving away from infested river valleys onto overcrowded plateaus to escape the disease.

Sustained oncho control could alleviate overpopulation by allowing inhabitants to return to underpopulated river valleys without fear of contracting the disease. Resettlement of oncho-controlled areas could in turn lead to increased food production through the cultivation of more fertile land with ready access to water by farmers who would be more productive when free of the disease. Steps to address population growth, such as family planning, soon became part of an array of measures in a new sector in the McNamara Bank known as Population, Health, and Nutrition (PHN). Involvement in oncho control would be a step forward in this new direction.

Prioritizing poverty alleviation shifted the central objective under the Mc-Namara Bank from pursuing economic growth through large infrastructure projects to improving the well-being of the poorest segments of society through initiatives in smallholder agriculture and in the social sectors: health and education. The focus would be on project beneficiaries that included disadvantaged population groups as opposed to nation-states. Oncho control was centered around poverty alleviation. The disease was concentrated in rural sub-Saharan Africa, often in highly remote areas "at the end of the road." Freeing these areas from the disease by interrupting transmission would lead to improved health, productivity, and income levels of the rural poor.

An Historic Encounter

Shortly after assuming the World Bank presidency, McNamara chose Roger Chaufournier to become the director of the newly created Western Africa Department. As part of an earlier exercise under Bank President George Woods, Chaufournier had looked into possible activities to be financed by the recently established soft-loan window of the Bank, the International Development Association (IDA). The IDA provided concessional loans to the world's poorest developing countries, notably newly independent countries in Africa. One possible activity was support for health. An IDA Committee member, Luis de Azcarate, who had worked extensively on Africa, mentioned onchocerciasis. Chaufournier recalled, "[de Azcarate] described it as a disease which affects such a large part of the population in an area which is the most productive area of Africa, in the river valleys, so that people have to migrate to the plateau where they can eke a very meager livelihood. I was struck by that and got interested."[68] In the end, however, health got dropped out of the final IDA committee report.

After becoming responsible for West Africa, Chaufournier revisited the question of health, onchocerciasis, and development. He asked one of his staff, who worked on agriculture and was a medical doctor, to put together a think piece. Chaufournier recounted, "I said the only way we could move into health would be to demonstrate the clear link there was with development. And he [the staff member] put together a few ideas; for instance, that the working life of an African farmer was about half of the working life of a Latin American [farmer]."[69] As he continued to work on the idea, Chaufournier met with Marc Bazin, the Bank's division chief for the Sahel Countries. According to Chaufournier, Bazin said, "When we organize the next visit of Bob McNamara to Upper Volta, let's take him to these villages to get a visual perception of the problem. The head of the group who does research and started a small program of control is there and will take him to a village where the disease has been controlled. Let's listen to him for one hour."[70]

McNamara took that trip to Upper Volta in March 1972, accompanied by his wife, Margaret, and Chaufournier. Ostensibly the purpose was to survey the impact of a severe drought that was entering its fifth consecutive year. Starving Tuaregs, a nomadic population that occupied the arid parts of the Sahelian countries, were coming down into Upper Volta from northern Mali and Niger. There was concern that the drought could be leading to a full-blown humanitarian crisis in the Sahel sub-region of West Africa. The trip shifted attention to what McNamara perceived as an even more pernicious long-term threat to the well-being of Upper Volta's population and to the country's development—onchocerciasis. Addressing the disease might open up opportunities to counteract some of the impact of the drought. In our interview, Bernard Philippon, an entomologist involved in early preparations of a control effort, remarked: "The drought at that time strengthened support among the donors to take action to address onchocerciasis as a barrier to food production in riverine valleys contaminated by the disease."[71]

Regarding possible action to be taken, McNamara recalled years later,

We had heard, before and during the visit, about the terrible disease called riverblindness, and some had suggested that the Bank should play a role in doing something about it. We could hardly pronounce the name of the disease, much less spell onchocerciasis, but we were horrified by what we heard about it. Literally millions of people were at risk of a fate that could be worse than death in that society and time: becoming blind in the prime of life, thus maimed and unable to work and contribute to the society. The catch, though, was that we had only shadowy ideas about how to combat this disease. There was no good cure, and it covered a vast area of land, so any solution would need to be on a vast scale, in areas without real institutions and hardly any infrastructure.[72]

As the trip unfolded, McNamara became determined to learn all he could about the disease and, if possible, put together an action plan. He first sought to determine whether there was any realistic prospect of bringing this plague under control. McNamara was told that in Bobo-Dioulasso, 340 km southwest of Ouagadougou, French scientists, as well as the head of the UNDP-financed PAG, were studying oncho-control possibilities. He and his party chartered a plane to seek them out.

Once there, McNamara, Margaret, and Chaufournier met with René Le Berre and Jean-Jacques Piq, two ORSTOM scientists assigned to the OCCGE to work on the EDF-financed oncho-control operation launched in 1966. The results from that ongoing project were demonstrating that larviciding could be effective in reducing transmission of the disease. It was Le Berre and that project that Marc Bazin had recommended McNamara visit in his earlier discussion with Chaufournier at Bank headquarters. Le Berre, who led the discussion with the McNamara party, was an ebullient 40-year-old entomologist with an infectious enthusiasm for talking about onchocerciasis. He had received his PhD from the University of Paris-Sud on the blackfly, *Simulium damnosum*. Though he spoke halting English, he was able to convey through photographs, drawings and maps the details of the disease, including its transmission mode, and ideas for controlling it that were beginning to be developed under the UNDP-financed PAG.

Le Berre escorted the McNamara party to nearby villages along the Black Volta River where 75% of the population was infected and one out of seven villagers was blind. The party also saw small farming hamlets around the larger village of Samandeni, which had been deserted due to unrelenting blackfly biting and high rates of blindness. This affliction was particularly severe for remote villages "at the end of the road" as Le Berre termed them. Donald Easom, then the US ambassador to Upper Volta, later recalled the McNamara party's reaction: "[Mr McNamara] was struck, as was his wife, by the tremendous number of people who were blind, especially farmers who in their villages were being led around the place on a stick by a child. They were very moved by that."[73] The immense human suffering and the implications of abandoned land in the face of an extended drought presented strong justifications to McNamara for taking bold action quickly.

Le Berre's research for his PhD and subsequently for ORSTOM had concluded that the maximum flight distance for the female *Simulium damnosum* was 41 km.[74] However, investigations in the field by the ongoing PAG had led to a revision of that flight estimate upward to 100–150 km.[75] Consequently, any effective control effort could not be limited to ground-based larviciding but would require an aerial-based operation to spray the many remote, widely dispersed rivers and streams. Most experts, including Le Berre and those participating in the PAG, had concluded that the best hope for halting oncho transmission involved aerial larviciding, preferably via helicopter, of blackfly breeding sites in the widely dispersed rapids of fast-flowing rivers and streams. A successful control attempt would probably have to include the entire Volta River basin, covering portions of the seven-affected countries, a total area approximating the size of France, due to the blackfly's long flight distance. Furthermore, any sustainable effort would likely have to continue for 20 years because there were indications at the time that the adult worm could live in the human body for up to 18 years. Le Berre's presentation to the McNamara party included these basic parameters. McNamara's follow-on meeting in Bobo-Dioulasso with the mission leader of the PAG, B. B. Waddy, confirmed that this was the right approach for tackling the disease.

It had taken only a day, but the McNamara party headed back to Ouagadougou convinced of the importance of attacking the oncho problem and reasonably confident that they had found a way to go about it. McNamara had a reputation for seizing challenges and moving boldly to address them. What followed this Bobo-Dioulasso encounter was vintage McNamara. He later recounted, "Roger [Chaufournier] and I, then and there, determined that we *would* do something about the disease. We worked out a collaborative arrangement, letter-head and all, that brought together key partners, and we launched a campaign on the spot from Ouagadougou."[76]

The next day, the party traveled on to Bamako, Mali, where McNamara met with the Malian Minister of Production. The notes from that meeting indicate McNamara's thinking about the Bank's role in an oncho-control effort as well as the importance of such a program to Mali:

> Mr. McNamara said: While he had been encouraged by the results so far
> achieved by the study group [the PAG], he was seriously considering for the
> World Bank Group to take the lead in mobilizing an international effort to
> combat river blindness on a worldwide scale. . . . Mr. McNamara asked the
> Minister of Production whether river blindness was indeed a serious problem
> for Mali. The Minister [said] . . . the Government is placing great hopes in the
> regional study. He felt that a program to eradicate river blindness was not only
> crucial from a health and thus human point of view but would have extremely
> high economic returns. Virtually all of the areas affected by river blindness
> were among the most fertile ones in the country, some of which already had to
> be abandoned. Thus, with a relatively small investment, fertile land is
> reactivated and brought back under production.[77]

One month later, McNamara chaired a meeting in London with the heads of three UN agencies—the WHO, UNDP, and FAO, in addition to the World Bank—to form a coequal partnership of four cosponsoring agencies to launch a highly ambitious control operation. At McNamara's suggestion, each agency head agreed to appoint a representative to participate on a working committee to put together a detailed work plan for setting up the program. That committee became known as the Steering Committee and was the precursor to the Committee of Sponsoring

Agencies (CSA), which would guide the oncho-control effort throughout Africa over the next 40+ years. At its first meeting in July 1972, the Steering Committee recommended extending the UNDP-funded preparatory work for an additional year, through August 1973. It also agreed that the World Bank would establish a special fund (Trust Fund) to receive contributions to support operations implemented by WHO, known as the Onchocerciasis Control Program (OCP).

It was a bold, but risky, venture. It would be the World Bank's first foray into health. It would involve regionally coordinated operations across seven countries in the Sahel, several of which were barely on speaking terms, to cover an area of 660,000 km², slightly larger than France. The scope would be more than 10 times larger than the ongoing ground-based control effort financed by the EDF. It would require close collaboration among the four co-sponsoring agencies along with an eventual wide range of bilateral donors—a level of partnership that had never been attempted before for an operational program of that size.

It is ironic that, in the end, the most consequential push for a large-scale oncho-control effort came from the World Bank. As the preeminent international organization concerned with economic development, the Bank historically had had no interest or involvement in health and lacked the expertise to assess, much less oversee and lead, a disease-control effort. Moreover, despite its wealth of expertise and extensive experience in appraising projects from an economic standpoint, the World Bank could not come up with a solid economic justification for controlling onchocerciasis in West Africa. An important reason seemed to be that it lacked the methodology as well as the data for determining the economic return on a disease-control program. In the end, the humanitarian justification for pursuing the program prevailed.

Dr. Bjorn Thylefors, former director of the WHO's Prevention of Blindness Program, who was the OCP's first ophthalmologist in 1974, recalled: "McNamara saw the link between disease, environment, and economic development of that part of Africa. That's what WHO should have seen many years before, but WHO was still a very technical normative agency at the time, even though it had launched several large programs. The inspiration to create the oncho program has to be attributed to McNamara and his vision. He made it multi-dimensional by including FAO and UNDP, along with WHO as the technical agency. That was a fantastic thing that happened."[78]

Chapter 2

Launching and Scaling Up the Onchocerciasis Control Program

Clinical, entomological, parasitological, sociological, economic, and agronomic studies of the overall consequences of onchocerciasis in the programme area have shown not only that control of the vector, and hence of the disease, is feasible but that—in addition to the relief of suffering, which must be universally recognized as an end in itself—wide-ranging socioeconomic benefits would be made possible by the exploitation of lands that are now deserted although fertile.

—PAG Report, Geneva 1973

The Launch

In the spring of 1972, Dr. Jacques Hamon, a vector control specialist, replaced PAG Mission Leader B. B. Waddy. The change was made by WHO Director-General Marcolino Gomes Candau, following a call from Robert McNamara.[1] McNamara wanted more dynamic leadership for the PAG, which was not making much progress. The PAG had been underway since August 1971, but little had been achieved in developing a blueprint for the launch and implementation of the control effort, and the final PAG Report was due by the end of June 1972. McNamara strongly suggested that, without a change in leadership, the World Bank might assume full control over the preparation process.[2]

Hamon was, at the time, chair of the ORSTOM technical committee for Medical Entomology, Parasitology and Virology, and an ORSTOM-seconded scientist in the WHO Vector Biology and Control Unit in Geneva. Over the years, Hamon had worked extensively with most of the francophone ministers of health in the oncho-endemic countries and with the British entomologists working on onchocerciasis in northern Ghana. He had also been the supervisor of several highly reputable ORSTOM entomologists in his role as head of OCCGE Medical Entomology throughout the 1960s. Hamon recalled,

I felt inadequate when I took over because I had never worked on onchocerciasis or the oncho vector. And, the PAG Report was due in six weeks. But I knew well nearly all of the entomologists actively working on onchocerciasis in the proposed seven-country area. I had either been their supervisor at one point or they were close friends. Furthermore, I knew where all the relevant technical reports were located. So, I succeeded in producing an interim report to submit to UNDP to secure another year of funding for the PAG mission.[3]

The interim report coincided with the Steering Committee's decision in July 1972 to extend the PAG for an additional year, through to August 1973. As a result, Hamon became responsible for preparing the final PAG Report for submission to the UNDP, the World Bank, WHO, and the FAO, as well as to the governments of Côte d'Ivoire, Dahomey, Ghana, Mali, Niger, Togo, and Upper Volta. Extending the PAG allowed for additional time to complete an interim pilot project during 1972–1973 to test out the spraying equipment, refine the cost estimates, establish baseline data to measure progress in controlling the disease, and finalize the report.

The PAG was mandated with preparing a plan of operations to achieve "lasting control" of the disease throughout a "high priority area." Lasting control meant covering ecological zones "sufficiently large to obviate the need for continuous protection of the whole area against reinvasion by the blackfly vector."[4] The Volta River basin area was considered high priority because of the elevated prevalence of oncho infection and "the manifestly high rates of blindness."[5] It was also regarded as an important area of focus because progress had already been achieved in controlling the disease and data had been collected through pilot ground-based projects financed by the EDF in Côte d'Ivoire, Mali, and Upper Volta; and by the UNDP in Northern Ghana, Togo, and Upper Volta.

The availability of epidemiological and entomological data was central in selecting the boundaries of the OCP program area. Data had been accumulated over more than a decade by the Ministry of Health in Ghana and by ORSTOM/the OCCGE for the francophone countries. There were also ongoing entomological studies in northern Ghana, the Comoé-Léraba (now referred to as Cascades) region of Upper Volta, and as part of hydrological work on Lake Volta in Ghana. In the end, the seven-country area selected for vector-control operations covered 654,000 km². According to Hamon,

It was a rush to complete the PAG Report. There was good data from Ghana based on the work of B. B. Waddy and others. OCCGE had collected extensive data for all six of the francophone countries except Togo. But, since Togo was between Dahomey and Ghana, where we knew the location of the heavily endemic areas, we simply drew a line across Togo connecting the southernmost endemic zone in Dahomey with the southernmost endemic zone in Ghana. We didn't have the resources or the time to collect data in new areas. It would have taken several more years to do so properly.[6]

Another important consideration was "the determination of the interested Governments, supported by public opinion, to cooperate in a control programme."[7] It was recognized that the disease was endemic beyond the program area, to the west, particularly in Upper Guinea, and to the east in central and northern Nigeria. However, by the early 1970s, Nigeria had discovered oil and preferred its own national control program. Guinea's president, Sékou Touré, had become increasingly estranged from his neighbors and paranoid about external threats. It was likely that he would not accept a program involving radio communication linking all of the OCP participating countries, and helicopters flying in from neighboring Côte d'Ivoire or Mali to treat Guinea's rivers and streams.[8]

The PAG leadership was aware of the possibility of infective flies reinvading the area from outside. However, Hamon viewed the purpose of the program to halt transmission of the disease for at least a 10- to 15-year period, long enough to find an operationally effective drug and to give neighboring endemic countries time to press WHO and the World Bank to expand the program to cover them as well.[9] The PAG Report was explicit in its expectation of future expansion: "According this priority to the area of the Volta River Basin in no way precludes the future extension of control operations to neighboring onchocerciasis foci in the African savanna zone."[10] In fact, the OCP would be just the beginning of a far more ambitious campaign. According to the report, the program "would constitute the cornerstone of future coordinated action against onchocerciasis and for the associated economic development in Africa south of the Sahara."[11]

The PAG Report stipulated the duration of the program to be "about" 20 years and estimated the total cost to be $120 million. Hamon explained his reasoning for the 20-year timeframe:

> No one knew at the time the precise longevity of the adult worm. We knew from research in Kenya that it was at least 10–15 years. However, I found an article in a Scandinavian journal that reported on a man—I think he was Swedish—who still had the adult worm living in his body and had only been exposed to *Simulium* biting flies once, 18 years earlier. So, we decided that the

program should continue for at least 20 years to cover the maximum lifespan of the adult worm.[12]

It was unheard of, at the time, to propose an international program of such long duration. But the technical parameters of the control effort dictated it. Any duration short of 20 years risked concluding control before the parasite reservoir had died out in the population, possibly resulting in renewed transmission and recrudescence of the disease.

Aerial spraying had not been part of the earlier projects financed by the EDF and the UNDP. Hence, it was necessary to conduct a pilot aerial-spraying project during the last year of the PAG. Hamon arranged to procure a helicopter with spare parts from the US Department of Defense and the Ministry of Defense of the Federal Republic of Germany. The helicopter and spare parts were brought through Côte d'Ivoire up to the border with Upper Volta. However, the German pilot lacked the papers to bring the equipment into Upper Volta and to proceed on to the PAG office in Ouagadougou. When it became apparent that he would not be able to cross the border, he offered to give the Voltaic customs official a 20-minute ride in the helicopter to impress upon him the utility of the helicopter in pursuing smugglers. After the ride, the pilot was permitted to continue on to Ouagadougou. The WHO office in Ouagadougou succeeded in getting retroactive approval for the importation of the helicopter and spare parts.[13]

PAG leadership decided that the ongoing EDF-financed project, covering 60,000 km² of Upper Volta, Côte d'Ivoire, and Mali, would form the core of the OCP and constitute the first of three phases to be implemented during 1974–1976. However, that project consisted of ground-based larviciding with DDT; going forward, DDT would not be used. The environmental risks for a 20-year aerial-spraying effort covering major river systems throughout West Africa were unacceptable. Instead, PAG experts chose to test out and employ one of the most benign insecticides for the environment available at the time, temephos (brand name Abate). Temephos turned out to be one of the least expensive larvicides to purchase and employ. Tests showed that it would carry up to 30 km downriver when applied during higher water levels.

The PAG devised the program's initial organizational structure, which continued to be refined by the Steering Committee. At the heart of the structure was the Steering Committee itself (later the CSA) with authority over nearly all aspects of the OCP: policies, budgets, formal program agreements, independent evaluations, and membership on advisory groups.[14] The PAG Report referred to the Steering Committee as the "executive organ" of the program. It consisted of representatives of the four sponsoring agencies: the UNDP, the FAO, WHO, and the World Bank. The chair of the Steering Committee would rotate among the sponsoring agencies. However, WHO could not serve as chair. That would be a conflict of interest because WHO was also the Executing Agency, which both reported to the Steering Committee and was responsible for implementing the policies and budgets determined by that committee.

As Executing Agency, WHO would select the program director and his/her staff. The director would report to, and participate in, the meetings of the Steering Committee. The two principal implementation units underneath the director were Vector Control (VCU) and Epidemiology (EPI). The VCU would carry out all of the aerial spraying operations and be responsible for entomological surveillance, operational research, and training pertaining to vector control and transmission of onchocerciasis. The EPI would undertake epidemiological surveillance, operational research, and training associated with assessing the incidence, prevalence, and manifestations of the disease. All reports and recommendations of the ecological panel, the scientific advisory panel, and the economic development unit would go through the Steering Committee for any interim decisions required.

In 1974, WHO chose one of its existing staff, Dr. Jacques Pierre Ziegler, to become the first OCP Director. Ziegler was known for his role in helping to successfully eliminate smallpox in Zaire (later the DRC). By the accounts of some staff, he was a technically solid, dynamic director who quickly got the program up and running.[15] René Le Berre, who had worked on the EDF-financed, ground-based vector-control project and who had briefed Robert McNamara in 1972, was selected to be the chief of the VCU. Dr. André Prost, a French epidemiologist, became acting chief of the EPI in early 1975.

Virtually all of the early higher-level staff of the OCP were European. They were predominantly French and, to a lesser extent, British. Most of these Europeans had been involved in fieldwork over the previous 10–20 years. The British tended to be experienced entomologists who had been active in sleeping sickness (trypanosomiasis) campaigns, in exploring ways to control the tsetse fly. They brought to the control effort the capacity for, and knowledge of, continuous data collection and analysis—an important part of the entomological tradition. The strengths of the French tropical-disease professionals tended to be organizational and epidemiological. In the opinion of tropical-disease historian Jesse Bump, "The French colonial staff, then ex-colonial, then OCP staff were so well organized that they could build a massive army. And they were such good administrators that they could run it all. Terrific leadership. In many ways, it was a perfect invest-ment opportunity because all they needed was money."[16] The heavy reliance on European staff would change dramatically over the life of the OCP. African staff were trained within the program to take on more responsibilities. Fellowships for Africans in entomology and epidemiology were financed by Britain, France, WHO, and some of the African participating countries. There was an early rec-ognition that building capacity within those countries was essential to ensure long-term sustainability of the control effort.

Overarching the OCP structure was a governing board comprising all of the partners in the program: the participating African countries (hereafter, referred to as the Participating Countries, the legal term used in the Operations and Fund Agreements), the donors, and the sponsoring agencies, as well as chairs of the advisory groups as *ex officio* members. The PAG lacked the authority to establish the governing board. Instead, it was set up via a memorandum of understanding when the Onchocerciasis Fund Agreement was signed by the donors on May 7, 1975. The governing board was initially known as the Joint Coordinating Com-mittee (JCC), with the name changed in 1979 to Joint Program Committee (JPC) to reflect its increased authority for final approval of all interim decisions taken by the Steering Committee. The governing board would have an independent chairman and meet annually. WHO Director-General Candau became the first JCC chairman during 1976–1978, following his retirement from WHO in 1973.

There were important advantages to the OCP's structure. The delineation of responsibilities among the sponsoring agencies played to their comparative ad-vantages and promoted collaboration. The responsibilities tended not to overlap in any major way that might have triggered competition or disputes. WHO was given the mandate to formulate and implement the disease-control strategy. As the only agency with technical expertise in health, it was best suited to manage control of the disease. The World Bank was designated the "Fiscal Agent" in the program agreement. As such, it had statutory responsibilities for (1) mobilizing all donor funding for the program, (2) determining a prudent level for the con-tingency reserve to be maintained in the Bank-held Oncho Trust Fund for un-foreseen emergencies, (3) forecasting the OCP's funding needs, and (4) manag-ing the program's financial resources via the Oncho Trust Fund. These were appropriate responsibilities, given its banking expertise and its ongoing direct contacts with donor-country finance ministries. The UNDP would be a donor to the program and focus on its traditional role of financing pre-investment studies related to control of the disease, particularly in agriculture, rural development, and resettlement of areas brought under control. The FAO would provide technical assistance to agricultural projects initiated by Participating Countries that, in turn, might be eligible for World Bank loans or credits.

Each partner was given a "seat at the table." The partners with a direct managerial role were on the Steering Committee at the center of the structure. Those with the greatest stake in the outcome—the Participating Countries, the donors, and the four cosponsoring agencies—had seats on the governing board. Other partners, such as university research entities and technical experts, participated on the ecological or the scientific advisory panels, which played important roles in advising the Steering Committee and the JCC on program policies, and had *ex officio* representation on the JCC. Engaging the stakeholders through this participatory structure helped ensure buy-in, ownership, and long-term commitment to the effort, even as the control strategy later shifted and more partners joined the campaign. The two principles—complementary division of labor and a stake in decision-making—were adhered to over the long run and were hallmarks of the effort in progressing toward achievement of the program's objectives.

Following receipt of the PAG Report, representatives from the participating African governments and members of the Steering Committee met in Accra, Ghana, in October 1973, to sign the OCP Operations Agreement. By signing, they endorsed the role of the World Bank in mobilizing the financing required to implement the OCP, and that of WHO as the Executing Agency responsible for carrying out OCP operations. The agreement also set out the responsibilities and obligations of the Participating Countries. It called for the free flow of equipment, insecticides, and OCP staff throughout the multicountry area, including aerial flyover and landing rights, duty-free entry of all equipment and material required for control operations, and uninhibited passage of staff and vehicles across borders. With the agreement in place, the Steering Committee began consolidating the institutional framework of the new program. The Committee met in Paris in June 1974 and finalized the organizational structure of the OCP, with the exception of the JCC, which was introduced in 1975.

In signing the Operations Agreement, the Participating Countries agreed to establish National Onchocerciasis Committees (NOCs) to coordinate national-level decision-making and actions in alignment with OCP requirements. An important purpose of the NOCs was to ensure that domestic resources were available to support OCP-related activities at the country level. Those activities included government support for control operations, development projects (including resettlement of the oncho-controlled areas), and country-level actions required to maintain OCP achievements. The NOCs were assigned general liaison and domestic-information functions. They became the locus of authority at the national level for coordinating with OCP management and with the NOCs of other Participating Countries. They were tasked with developing and implementing "a large-scale campaign to inform the population of the existence, methods and aims of the Programme."[17] These NOC responsibilities remained relatively unchanged throughout the life of the OCP.

Lining Up Support

Before bilateral donors could be recruited into the program, it was necessary to secure approval from the World Bank's Board of Directors for the Bank's participation in the OCP. McNamara went to the Board on May 1, 1973, and presented his case for involving the World Bank in the effort:

> The proposal before you is something of an experiment—the Bank has never been involved in anything quite like it before. . . . The organization of the program is complex; the campaign will have to be conducted over an extended period in the territories of seven countries, and the activities in each country, both in controlling the vector and in trying to reduce the incidence of the disease itself, will have to be very carefully planned out and coordinated [and] may need to be modified or even radically changed in the light of results achieved and continuing . . . research. Nevertheless . . . we believe that the program for the control of river blindness is soundly based on the best expert advice available and soundly justifies the support of the Bank at this time. If successful, it could well serve as a model for similar campaigns elsewhere designed to reduce the incidence of river blindness or other debilitating diseases and thereby improve the conditions of life for some of the poorest people in the developing world.[18]

It was unclear during the board presentation how much the World Bank might contribute to finance OCP operations. The annual costs of the OCP had not yet been calculated. After the PAG Report was issued that fall, Peter Wright, the program director for West Africa assigned as World Bank task officer for the OCP, reported that McNamara was prepared to recommend to the Board that the Bank finance 10% of the required amount for the program.[19] Based on the estimated cost of $7.5 million for 1974, the Bank Board approved a World Bank contribution of $750,000 to the Oncho Trust Fund in January 1974. That initial tranche enabled the OCP to begin to set up operations. The 10% share was roughly the proportion that the World Bank would continue to contribute to the program for the first several years. World Bank support for the OCP had to be in the form of a grant, which came out of the profits of the Bank. Its usual form of financing, a loan or credit, was not available in this case. Under World Bank procedures, repayment of borrowings had to be guaranteed by a government, through a loan agreement with the Bank. The OCP was an institutional entity, not a government, and had no way of providing that guarantee. All donor support for the OCP would be in the form of grants, deposited and pooled in the Oncho Trust Fund.

McNamara reported back to WHO Director-General Candau that "the Executive Directors for Canada, France, Germany, the United Kingdom, and the United States were amongst those who gave it their full support."[20] This was an early indication from key bilateral donors that they were probably willing to join the effort and contribute financing through the Oncho Trust Fund. During the remainder of 1973 and throughout 1974, donors were recruited into the program by the Bank's Oncho Team, consisting of the senior staff responsible for West Africa: Roger Chaufournier, Peter Wright, and Marc Bazin.

During a meeting of potential donors at the World Bank office in Paris in June 1973, the UK delegate asked why the costs associated with agricultural development in the OCP areas had not been included in the estimated costs of the program. The World Bank response indicated how the Bank's priority had shifted to disease control: "the launching of the control program could not be delayed until the appraisal work on the agricultural projects had been completed."[21]

Peter Wright arranged for Jacques Hamon to visit the capitals of Canada, the United Kingdom, and the United States to persuade them to join the program. Each donor agreed to do so, with the support of USAID and the Canadian International Development Agency (CIDA) being particularly strong.[22] By February 1974, a sufficient number of donors had been recruited to provide two-thirds of the $7.5 million required to enable the OCP to be launched. Those donors signed the 1974 Agreement in March. That Fund Agreement, along with the appended Operations Agreement (signed by the African participating governments and WHO), provided the financial and legal bases for launching OCP operations in December of that year. The 1974 Fund Agreement was signed by five bilateral donors: Canada, France, the Netherlands, the United Kingdom, and the United States; and three international organizations: the UNDP, WHO, and the World Bank. WHO signed as Executing Agency, not as a donor, and did not begin contributing to the Oncho Trust Fund until Phase II of the OCP, beginning in 1980. The Fund Agreement specified how the Oncho Trust Fund would operate in terms of receiving contributions from donors and disbursing financing to the OCP via WHO.

There were ongoing differences between the World Bank and WHO over the procedures for financing the OCP. The Bank was adamant that there be no strings attached to any donor contributions. All OCP financing would have to go through the Oncho Trust Fund, and no earmarked contributions could be accepted. Non-tied funding was essential to optimize resource allocation efficiencies and ensure maximum flexibility for the OCP to focus expenditures on the most important activities and areas to achieve the Program's objectives. WHO, on the other hand, wanted to also allow for earmarked contributions to maximize funding for the OCP.

An internal memorandum from a World Bank delegate attending a meeting on the OCP, to Peter Wright, indicated how strongly the Bank was wedded to the position of non-earmarked contributions: "I put very strongly to [WHO] the point that you had performed near miracles in getting untied funds and that any relapse on this could endanger the whole structure. He seized the point, as if it were new . . . (This is just another sample of a matter that seems obvious to us but which we must be very careful to explain in ABC terms to a bunch of MDs not familiar with development finance)."[23] The principle of keeping the financing clean, simple, and flexible prevailed and endured throughout the life of the OCP. It became a hallmark of successful financing for a program supported by a widening array of heterogeneous donors with varying interests and motivations for backing oncho control.

A similar adherence to consistency applied to the objective of the OCP in the Operations Agreement signed by the African governments, as well as to the strategy for achieving it. The objective was to eliminate onchocerciasis as a public health problem and obstacle to socioeconomic development in the program area. That basic objective remained unchanged in all six OCP Agreements. It was straightforward and clear to all partners and one they could identify with and buy into. Furthermore, the strategy for achieving that objective remained largely unchanged throughout the life of the OCP. It was to interrupt transmission of onchocerciasis for a long-enough timeframe to eliminate the parasite reservoir in the population in the Program area. Keeping the objective and strategy consistent and clear over time was an important ingredient for success. The various partner groupings—Participating Countries, donors, sponsoring agencies, as well as contractors, research entities, and independent oncho experts—had the same understanding of where the Program was headed. That enabled them to pull in the same direction to support OCP operations for more than 25 years.

Solidifying and Diversifying the OCP Donor Community: The Case of Kuwait

Kuwait became a donor in 1974, the first year of the OCP, and, despite its smaller size, lower income level, and lack of historical ties to sub-Saharan Africa, turned out to be more steadfast in its support for oncho control than nearly all the other donors. The Kuwait Fund for Arab Economic Development (Kuwait Fund) had been established in 1961, a few months after the country gained independence. It was the first developing country to establish an aid program.[24]

McNamara's office contacted the Director-General of the Kuwait Fund, Abdlatif Y. Al-Hamad, in early 1974, inviting Kuwait to join the oncho donor community. Prior to becoming director-general in 1964, Al-Hamad had been the Director of the Kuwait Investment Company, and he made sure to take the World Bank portfolio with him to the Kuwait Fund. Al-Hamad became and remained widely respected among the nearly 500 staff and management of the Kuwait Fund. Long after he had moved on, he was known among them as the "Godfather of Development."[25] As Al-Hamad described the McNamara communication in our interview: "I looked at [the information McNamara's office sent in 1974] and was convinced that this was something Kuwait should be involved in. The effort to control river blindness is critical to poor people and for development. There's a humanitarian aspect, a health aspect, and a development aspect. It touched on all the right concerns."[26] The information from McNamara's office included a recently completed World-Bank-produced film about the disease, entitled *A Plague Upon the Land.*[27] Al-Hamad remarked, "I showed the film to both the Council of Ministers and my board. It was the film that clinched the deal for Kuwait. I can still see that scene of the man walking with the young child guiding him holding onto a stick, and the child in the film, as described in the dialogue, was destined to become blind himself. I was really struck by that."[28]

A Plague Upon the Land had been produced in 1973 by two Bank staff members, Thomas Blinkhorn and Jaime Martin, who had never made a film before. Blinkhorn had read about the Bank's nascent work on the oncho program and thought that producing a film on site showing the oncho blind being led around by young children would be a powerful way of raising awareness of the disease and possibly useful in mobilizing funding for the control effort.[29] The Bank's external relations office backed the idea and provided approximately $100,000 in financing.[30] The film was shot largely in Upper Volta and in Ghana.

Blinkhorn later said that, upon completion of the film, "McNamara insisted the entire [Bank] management team come to the Eugene R. Black Auditorium to see the first in-house Bank movie. And he loved it."[31] The premiere external showing was at the World Bank Annual Meeting in Nairobi in September 1973, where McNamara gave his historic speech announcing a major shift in Bank policy to focus on eliminating absolute poverty in rural areas, notably in Africa. The film was the first of several produced by agencies and donors involved in the OCP. Two of these, *Mara, the Lion's Stare* and *Eyes of Hope* produced in 1985 and 1997 respectively, with support from ORSTOM, France's Ministry of Cooperation, and WHO, received 18 awards combined. The films played important roles in showing the faces of the disease, heightening awareness of it, and building international support for the control effort.

There were two other important factors that influenced Al-Hamad in his push to have Kuwait become a donor to the OCP. One was the obligation to give to the poor as one of the five pillars of Islam. He explained,

> This is part of our heritage and social relationships. You should never allow your neighbor to die of hunger while your stomach is full. It's a principle to give 2.5% [Zakat] of your savings [Nissab] for the benefit of the poor. That's in the Koran. That's the reason Kuwait started the Kuwait Fund. We launched it in an empty shed in the desert. Kuwait did not have paved roads, hot water, or electricity everywhere at that time. Kuwait was extremely poor but developing after discovering oil. We said we cannot develop without helping others. Our country is in the middle of the desert with no rivers around and we would have never been threatened by this disease, but we were willing to help out people whom we had never seen before. If you had asked the people who made the decision [to donate to the Oncho Program] if they could point out Upper Volta on the map, they wouldn't have been able to. But they knew these were human beings suffering from a horrible disease that we could help eradicate. We felt strongly about making a commitment to help other human beings, whether they were Muslims or non-Muslims.[32]

The other important factor was Al-Hamad's admiration for, and trust in, McNamara. As he put it,

> I've known the World Bank presidents all the way back to the first, Eugene Black, up to the present. McNamara was at the top, in my view. McNamara moved [the Bank] from a financial institution to a development institution.

He had courage, vision, integrity, and leadership. The Oncho Program will go down in history as one of his legacies. He had the courage to talk about population and health and other topics no one else would touch. He wasn't a banker. He was a development practitioner.[33]

In several respects, Kuwait's entry into the OCP donor community strengthened the oncho-control effort and related African rural development. First, during the initial two financial phases of the OCP, 1974–1986, the Kuwait Fund contributed $12 million to the Oncho Trust Fund. This level of support equaled or exceeded the contributions of several of the larger European donor countries. All told, the Kuwait Fund would contribute approximately $25 million to the oncho programs through 2020.

Second, Kuwait's involvement in the OCP led to an expansion of the Kuwait Fund throughout much of sub-Saharan Africa. Up to 1974, Kuwait Fund support had been confined to neighboring Arab developing countries. After joining the OCP, the Kuwait Fund provided $572 million in low-interest loans for 63 agricultural development projects over the next 40 years in sub-Saharan Africa. Much of this assistance has been directed toward development opportunities that have opened up in the oncho-controlled areas.[34] Today, the Kuwait Fund provides its largest proportion of foreign assistance, outside the Middle East, to sub-Saharan Africa, and most of its projects in Africa are in the health sector.[35]

Kuwait became one of the more active oncho donors. It hosted the third annual JCC meeting in 1977 and the governing board (Joint Action Forum, or JAF) meeting of the OCP's successor, the African Program for Onchocerciasis Control (APOC), in 2011. It encouraged other potential donors in the Middle East to join the effort. After the Kuwaiti decision to support the OCP, several other Middle Eastern–based donors joined the effort, including Saudi Arabia, the Al-Sabah Foundation, and the OPEC Fund. It was apparent during my interviews of the Kuwait Fund management team in early 2016, that the Kuwaiti authorities were proud of their country's involvement in the oncho programs over the years. Each of them had in their office some form of the iconic oncho statue depicting a young child leading a blind adult by a stick.

The First Six-Year Phase

By the spring of 1975 the World Bank had recruited enough donors and mobilized sufficient financing to carry the Program through its first six-year financial phase, 1974–1979, at a cost of $56 million.[36] The 1975 Onchocerciasis Fund Agreement was signed that May by nine donor countries (Belgium, Canada, France, Germany, Japan, Kuwait, the Netherlands, United Kingdom, and United States) and three international organizations (African Development Bank [AfDB], World Bank, and the UNDP). All of these donors stayed the course through the second financial phase, 1980–1986, and were joined by two new donors, Switzerland and the OPEC Fund, in signing the 1979 Fund Agreement.

Aerial spraying operations got underway in February 1975, nearly one year later than originally planned. Implementation followed the PAG plan of controlling the seven-country OCP area in three sequential stages. The first stage encompassed the area of the pre-OCP, EDF-financed project in Upper Volta, Mali, and Côte d'Ivoire, where all the data necessary to begin operations were available. The second stage expanded the first stage area by covering the remainder of Upper Volta to the northeast and the northern third of Ghana. The third stage completed the seven-country area by adding the northern parts of Togo, Benin, western Niger, and parts of Mali and Côte d'Ivoire further to the west up to the border with Guinea.

Through international-competitive bidding, the aerial contract was awarded in 1974 to Evergreen Helicopters, Inc., based in McMinnville, Oregon. Evergreen had responsibility for control operations for the first two stages of the OCP during 1975–1976. The contract was then awarded to a Canadian firm, Viking Helicopters, Ltd., based in Ottawa, Ontario. Both contractors deployed a fleet of helicopters, as well as one or two fixed wing aircraft to spray the larger rivers. By 1977, Viking was spraying 18,000 km of rivers per week. It was a large operation—equivalent to twice the lengths of the Missouri, Mississippi, and Ohio Rivers combined, each week. At the beginning, aerial spraying employed exclusively the larvicide, temephos.

Theoretically, if interrupting transmission of the disease could be achieved over a long enough period—at least equal to or longer than the lifespan of the adult worm—the parasite reservoir would die out in the population throughout the control area. The fly could then return and continue biting, but there would be no parasite to transmit. It was similar in concept to malaria whereby the *Anopheles* mosquito still exists in southern Europe and in parts of the East Coast of the United States, where malaria once existed in the local population. That mosquito no longer presents a malaria threat in those areas because the parasite has disappeared.

The Program had to find a way to determine levels of transmission. Epidemiological measures, notably skin snip counts of microfilariae, were inadequate for two reasons. First, changes in disease prevalence occur slowly; annual changes might not be detectable through skin snips because the adult worm lives well over a decade and produces microfilariae throughout that period. Second, at least a year is needed, on average, for new infections to appear in skin snips following an infective blackfly bite. That long latency period meant that employing skin snips to measure changes in transmission was unreliable. Consequently, the Program adopted experimental work on entomological surveillance carried out by Roger and Peggy Crosskey, a British husband-and-wife team of entomologists, who worked on oncho in Nigeria in the mid-1950s.[37]

While working in the Abuja area of Nigeria, the Crosskeys modified an entomological surveillance method—the "fly round," previously used for trypanosomiasis and the tsetse fly—to measure changes in transmission of oncho via *Simulium damnosum*.[38] The method, which entailed catching flies regularly at defined catching points and dissecting their heads, provided a measure of vector-infectivity in a localized area: the proportion of flies carrying the infective stage of the parasite (L-3 stage) that enables the parasite to grow into an adult worm in the next human host.

During 1975–1978, the OCP set up 525 "catching points" throughout the seven-country area.[39] About 250 of these, depending on the season, were visited weekly by fly-catching teams, comprising two fly-catchers and a driver with an all-terrain vehicle. Some 70 teams throughout the area caught flies daily, usually on the bank of a river over an 11-hour period, dissected them, and recorded infectivity rates for each area.[40] At the end of the week, that information was radioed to the operations centers in Bobo-Dioulasso and Ouagadougou, where it was discussed in a strategy meeting on Monday mornings, and then used to establish larviciding schedules and flight plans according to changing vector densities and river discharges. On Monday afternoons, the pilots were briefed individually by the aerial operations staff who gave them their itineraries and dosage data for the remainder of the week.[41]

The linchpin of effective vector control was the helicopter pilot, in the view of John Davies, OCP entomologist and acting chief of the VCU in 1980. He comments, "The success of the spraying operation depended upon the diligence and honesty of 6–8 well-educated, skilled, and responsible helicopter pilots. In the event a problem arose, such as a failure to kill blackfly larvae in a particular area, one only had to look at the flight logs to know who might be responsible and what remedial action to take. The pilots worked in exhausting conditions, in temperatures often exceeding 40°C (104°F) under the Plexiglas domes of their cockpits. Each had to maneuver by himself 40-gallon drums of petrol and insecticide 5–6 times a day during refueling stops. And they often slept overnight in rough accommodations on their routes."[42] A number of the pilots had flown for the American side during the Vietnam War.

ORSTOM/OCCGE entomologist Dr. Bernard Philippon, who became chief of the VCU in 1981, had investigated two entomological surveillance measures during his PhD research in the late 1960s.[43] The two measures were the annual transmission potential (ATP) and the annual biting rate (ABR). The ATP, which Dr. Brian Duke also employed in his research in Cameroon in the 1960s, was the theoretical number of infective flies that would be caught by a fly-catcher sitting at the same catching point by a river for 11 hours every day for a year. The ABR was the theoretical number of fly bites that the fly-catcher would incur by sitting at that same catching point 11 hours a day for a year. The two concepts were officially accepted by the OCP following a WHO scientific working group review in June 1977.[44]

Dr. Bernard Philippon, along with OCP entomologist Frank Walsh, worked with the OCP's ophthalmologist, Bjorn Thylefors, to come up with an ATP threshold level below which there would be no threat to eyesight. They concluded that an ATP below 100 would not impact the optic nerve.[45] OCP staff further determined that an ABR under 1,000 would be highly unlikely to yield an ATP of 100 or more. Therefore, underpopulated areas with ABRs less than 1,000 would be safe to resettle.[46] Conversely, underpopulated areas with ABRs as high as 8,000 or greater would be dangerous to resettle and would generate hyperendemic onchocerciasis relatively quickly within a newly resettling community.

The first evaluation of the OCP was conducted by WHO in 1978. (This first evaluation was intended to be an evaluation of Phase I and was given the name "Evaluation Report 1974–1979.") It concluded, "Vector control has been highly successful over the whole area and the results obtained so far are in line with those predicted by the PAG Mission."[47] The evaluation showed that ATPs and ABRs were declining at all the catching points in areas where vector control had been carried out for two to three years.[48] This was the first concrete evidence that vector control for oncho was working and achieving the objective of reducing disease transmission. This evidence by itself, however, was not proof of an improving situation in the infected population.

A measure that quantified the intensity of infection in the population was constructed by the OCP in 1977 and began to be employed in the early 1980s. That measure—termed community microfilarial load (CMFL)—which was suggested by Dr. Ole Christensen, was the average number of microfilariae in skin snips in adults 20 years of age and above in a village. While skin snips were unreliable for determining levels of oncho transmission, they were an accurate measure of the presence of the disease in a community. Declining CMFLs indicated reduced disease levels, improving symptoms, and lessened risk of blindness. Continuing vector control, leading to declining ATPs and ABRs would, after some delay, result in falling CMFLs; the true measure of improving health in an at-risk population.

Although the CMFL was not yet an available indicator, the 1974–1979 evaluation detected signs of improvements in the at-risk population. Skin snips revealed that "where larviciding has been continuous for three years, [there is] a noticeable decline in the prevalence of the disease among young children."[49] Those results indicated that there were probably few, if any, new infections occurring in the broader population and that the numbers of infected were beginning to decline during 1975–1978. These encouraging prospects for the wider at-risk population could be inferred because children tend to be the first cohort to show improvement when overall prevalence starts declining.

Although this first evaluation of the OCP provided good news on the effectiveness of vector control in reducing oncho transmission and declining prevalence in children, there was also a warning: "The reinvasion phenomenon continues to affect the peripheral zone of the OCP area. Research has shown that most reinvading *Simulium* arrive in key areas in a gravid state. Many of these flies carry infective *O. volvulus*."[50] Reinvasion had been predicted by the PAG, but the scope and severity, including the size of the areas impacted and proportion of flies with infective larvae, were greater than anticipated.

The "reinvasion phenomenon" was first discovered along the Bandama River Valley in Côte d'Ivoire during the rainy season of 1975.[51] Three entomologists working with the OCP—Rolf Garms, Frank Walsh, and John Davies—carried out a detailed investigation of the problem during 1975–1978, and the results were factored into the 1974–1979 Evaluation and the 1980–1981 deliberations of the Independent Commission on the future of the OCP. Garms et al. conducted ground and aerial surveys to rule out any treatment failures as the cause of large numbers of older infective savanna flies (*Simulium damnosum* and *Simulium sirbanum* species) appearing along the riverine banks across sizable parts of Côte d'Ivoire, Mali, and Upper Volta during the rainy seasons of 1975–1978. They concluded that the flies were traveling 300 km or more in search of places to deposit their eggs after taking a blood meal—about twice the flight distance previously thought possible. These longer flight patterns were aided by the West African monsoon winds blowing up from the Gulf of Guinea in a northeasterly direction across the subregion.[52]

Reinvasion presented potentially severe problems for the future of the control effort. First, the Program could not achieve a lasting conclusion if infective flies continued to re-invade the seven-country area. Second, the populations living in the peripheral zones that were both sources and receiving areas of reinvading flies needed protection. At the 1977 JCC in Kuwait, the decision was taken to extend control operations into southern Côte d'Ivoire, the most prominent of these peripheral zones at the time. The Program began aerial spraying there in 1978. The 1974–1979 Evaluation concluded, "The extended treatment of rivers in southern Ivory Coast in 1978 has had a pronounced remedial effect on some of the worst affected sites."[53]

The third problem lay in the reinvading flies themselves and highlighted the importance of a broad-based regional approach. John Davies, an entomologist who had worked in Nigeria in the late 1950s and early 1960s before joining the OCP, discovered that localized vector control would not necessarily reduce the risk of oncho infection in the local population if that area was subject to reinvading infective blackflies. Davies, who had taken over responsibility for the Crosskeys' project in Nigeria in 1959, analyzed the Crosskeys' skin snipping data for 37 villages in the Abuja area that were subject to infective blackflies invading from outside sources.[54] Davies discovered, surprisingly, that larviciding that reduced significantly the number of biting blackflies, did not reduce infection levels in children. The data showed that "for boys, the mean earliest infection was not affected at all, and for girls, the earliest mean infection occurred at 5.7 years of age, a year earlier than before control."[55] Davies concluded that "although there were far fewer flies, the proportion of those carrying the parasite rose sharply, probably because the captured flies were older on average and had had more chances to ingest the parasite."[56] In the case of the OCP, flies coming from southern Côte d'Ivoire and probably from neighboring countries to the west of the seven-country area were older and more infective because they were traveling long distances from sources well outside the original area.

As Jesse Bump has pointed out, the Crosskeys-Davies project in Nigeria contributed importantly to the OCP strategy as it was modified and refined during the 1970s and 1980s. Bump writes,

> By testing the possibility of control in an area subject to reinvasion and demonstrating how the surviving flies' infectivity rose, the project showed that local fly control efforts were unlikely to offer a sufficient long-term public health solution. . . . [T]he Crosskey-Davies project was an important demonstration that overlapping transmission zones would have to be attacked simultaneously. The regional dimensions of transmission in West Africa had special consequences because it required supranational authority to manage an effective control program.[57]

One can conclude that the OCP was taking the right approach in establishing a regional supranational authority with the mandate to control the disease throughout a hyperendemic multicountry area. However, as the 1974–1979 Evaluation Report suggested, the program area selected in 1973–1974 was too small to cover the "overlapping transmission zones" in that part of West Africa. Research on the flight range of *Simulium damnosum* in the 1960s by René Le Berre had concluded that it traveled 41 km.[58] That distance was revised upwards by the PAG which, in 1972–1973, estimated a range of 100–150 km.[59] Both estimates fell far short of the blackfly flight range discovered later, in large part because they failed to take into account wind-assisted flight from southwest to northeast across the sub-region. Underestimates of the blackfly flight range were one factor, though not the sole factor, that led to the selection of an insufficiently large area under the OCP. The only long-term remedy was to expand the control effort, notably westward, to cover the limits of the blackfly's breeding sites in the West African oncho-endemic sub-region.

Consolidating the OCP and Assessing Its Long-Term Prospects

By the end of 1977, Program operations were covering the entire seven-country area and transmission indicators were improving. However, donor-related tension threatened to disrupt OCP operations. The German donor delegation, led by Professor Albert Knuttgen from the University of Hamburg, came to OCP headquarters in Ouagadougou and began questioning whether the disease was a serious cause of blindness in the OCP area and whether the ongoing vector-control strategy was the best approach for controlling the disease. Dr. Bjorn Thylefors, the OCP's first ophthalmologist, recalled, "They were coming into the EPI Unit asking for data and drawing invalid conclusions, partly because we didn't have much data at the time."[60]

The Canadian donor delegation sought permission to have Canadian journalists visit OCP headquarters and the program area. Director Ziegler refused to allow the visit because he thought it would be too disruptive to the control effort.[61] The OCP, as a novel, multicountry disease-control program, was attracting considerable interest from the donors and the press. "There was a big media push at that time to tell this fantastic story," recalled Thylefors.[62] "Pierre Ziegler was a dynamic operations guy, but he was not a public relations man, nor a diplomat."[63] Having to cater to the donors and the press was a source of frustration to Ziegler, because doing so took time and attention away from Program operations.[64]

At the time, Marc Bazin, the World Bank division chief responsible for the OCP, was traveling and meeting with the donors to brief them about progress and to reinforce their commitment to the Program. By 1977, Bank Director Chaufournier was becoming concerned: strong donor support was deemed vital to the overall effort. Consequently, Chaufournier arranged to have Bazin seconded to WHO to replace Ziegler as OCP director. Rosemary Villars, former program officer in the OCP director's office, recalled the need for new leadership:

> Ziegler was technically solid and had been successful in getting OCP operations off the ground. But the Program was entering a new phase and required a different set of skills in its leadership. Bazin was a skilled diplomat accustomed to dealing with the media and the donors. He already knew many of the donors and they had confidence in him. He understood the types of information the donors were interested in, which was not the case with OCP staff. While director, Bazin stabilized and expanded the donor base.[65]

Thylefors described the new director: "Marc Bazin was an impressive guy: an elegant intellectual and a clever politician, though he had very little interest in the medical side of the Program."[66] Villars described Bazin's style of management and how it dovetailed with the need to keep the donors informed and engaged:

> He organized and rehearsed what was jokingly referred to as the 'Oncho Circus' by the staff. It involved presenting the activities of the Program to visiting donors and potential new donors. The exercise helped sensitize the staff to the types of information that interested the donors. It also focused on training the second level of staff on how best to explain their work to the donors and respond to donor questions—rather than always having the Program's chiefs interact with the donors, as had previously been the case. The intent was to prepare the lower levels of OCP to take over when the chiefs moved on in a few years' time, which is precisely what began to happen by the early 1980s.[67]

Bazin consolidated OCP operations in one large compound in Ouagadougou. During 1974–1977, the OCP's various offices were spread around in five different villas in the city. Bringing together all of the program's offices in one headquarters was an important achievement, which improved the efficiency of OCP operations. The compound was large enough to accommodate the additional staff required to expand OCP operations from seven to 11 countries in the mid-1980s. With additions, it was large enough to house the staff of the APOC when that program was established in 1995. The compound, which was dedicated in 1978 by WHO Director-General Halfdan Mahler, remained the headquarters for control operations for all of oncho-endemic sub-Saharan Africa for the next 37 years.

Dr. Bernhard Liese, who joined the World Bank's oncho team in 1977, described the impact of Bazin on the Program: "He was in full control of nearly everything. The oncho office in the Bank was *de facto* nonexistent during the years Bazin was OCP director. The only time we got involved was when looking into studies of the flight distance of the blackfly and to review the Independent Commission Report on the future of the Program. Bazin succeeded in turning OCP into an independent program, basically autonomous from WHO-Geneva, WHO-AFRO, and even the Bank to some extent."[68] That autonomy, reinforced by strong donor support, turned out to be powerful in enabling the OCP to focus exclusively on controlling the disease and achieving the program's stated objectives. Autonomy allowed the OCP to be managed devoid of any heavy-handed pressure from high-level WHO officials at headquarters in Geneva and/or in Brazzaville (AFRO Office). Otherwise, those officials might have been tempted to take advantage of the financially well-endowed program to pursue objectives other than strictly oncho control.

A coup d'état took place in Ghana on June 4, 1979. The new Armed Forces Revolutionary Council, led by Ghanaian Air Force Flight Lieutenant Jerry Rawlings, closed down one of the two OCP aerial bases, in Tamale, out of concern that aircraft might be employed to reverse the coup. Closure of the base violated the 1973 Operations Agreement and resulted in the cessation of aerial spraying throughout the eastern half of the OCP area covering portions of five countries. The resulting stoppage posed the threat of a resumption of oncho transmission throughout an area of approximately 350,000 km² with a population of around six million inhabitants.

Le Berre had dispatched the Ouagadougou sector chief, Dr. Azodoga Sékétéli, to Tamale in early 1978 to resolve several messy political issues.[69] Now Sékétéli could not get the new Ghanaian regime to reopen the Tamale aerial base. However, he succeeded in convincing the Togolese government under President Gnassingbé Eyadéma to permit relocation of the Tamale aerial base to Kara, Togo. The OCP sent a mission to Eyadéma to describe the strategy of aerial spraying and how it could stop transmission of the disease. Eyadéma had family members who had been blinded by oncho, which they attributed to sorcerers.[70] The president, however, understood the science and welcomed the new base. Before the end of 1979, it became operational and aerial spraying had resumed.[71] The base would remain in Kara for the duration of the OCP.

Chapter 3

Expansion and Rescue

A 20-year commitment was needed—a long haul for many doubting
donors, but with the World Bank as nag, cheerleader, guardian of the
coffers, and kindly sergeant-major, they stayed the course.
—David Wigg, "And Then Forgot to Tell Us Why . . . A Look at the
Campaign against River Blindness in West Africa," 1993.

Recommendations from the Independent Commission

Toward the end of Phase I (1974–1979), several of the donors expressed interest in
having an expert group look at possible options for bringing the OCP to a lasting
conclusion within a reasonable period of time. One concern was the reinvasion phenomenon and how best to address it to avoid a prolonged vector-control campaign at
exorbitant cost. A second concern was whether and how the ongoing control strategy
might be concluded in a way that the beneficiary countries would be able to sustain
the achievements. And, a third was whether the OCP might be able to pursue other
approaches to complement vector control and thereby shorten the control effort.

In 1978, the Steering Committee worked with Marc Bazin, in consultation with
the donors, to set up the Independent Commission on the Long-Term Prospects of
the Onchocerciasis Control Program (the Commission), to study the above issues
and to make recommendations to the JPC in 1981. The Commission, chaired by
Dr. Gordon Smith, dean of the London School of Hygiene and Tropical Medicine,
consisted of nine experts, including Dr. Abdoulaye Diallo, the director-general for
Public Health in Mali; John de Wilde, former chief economist for the World Bank;
and Douglas Lindores, vice president of the Multilateral Division of CIDA.

The Commission's primary task was to determine "whether and how" the
OCP could be "brought to a successful conclusion in the long-term."[1] "Successful
conclusion" was defined by the Commission as bringing oncho down to a level
where it is "no longer a public health problem" in the seven-country area and where
it "can be maintained" by the participating African countries "largely within
their own resources, individual or collective."[2] Regarding progress achieved during the first six years, the Commission concluded that the Program was "bringing

substantial health benefits to the area," "removing one obstacle to economic development," and was having "a considerable potential catalytic role for health personnel and health systems development in the area."[3] It also articulated the "overriding justification" for oncho control as: "unlike many other diseases, it is feasible to control its transmission over a large area, and the Program has been successful in doing so."[4]

Regarding the future, the Commission concluded that (1) "maintenance of the present Program boundaries would be difficult or impossible in the long-term;" (2) "indefinite control" in the areas subject to reinvasion would eventually precipitate "multiple resistance to available and environmentally acceptable larvicides"; (3) the long-term cost of continued vector control in those areas would be unsustainable; and (4) "Long-term success of the Program, therefore, entails expansion to the west, the direction from which the principal reinvasion is occurring."[5] The JPC endorsed these conclusions and OCP management set in motion activities to implement the Commission's recommendations. The first of these consisted of collecting baseline data for the areas to the west that were sources of reinvasion—four additional countries, Guinea, Guinea-Bissau, Senegal, and Sierra Leone, along with southwestern Mali west of the Niger River (figure 3.1). Control

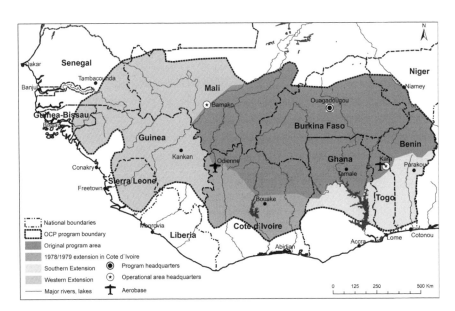

Figure 3.1. Onchocerciasis Control Program Areas, 1974–2002. *Source*: Hans Remme.

operations in these new areas, however, would have to await the available funding to carry them out.

The extension operations had to reach the westward limits of the breeding sites of oncho-transmitting flies to be effective. And, extending westward needed to be coupled with an extension of operations into the southern parts of Benin, Togo, and Ghana down to the forest zones. Full extension would nearly double the size of the program area and might save the entire control effort. But where would the additional financing come from?

The Commission recommendations were based on the premise that successful control could be confined to savanna onchocerciasis, thereby excluding the forest form of the disease. Evidence had shown that eye lesions and blindness resulted predominantly from savanna oncho.[6] However, the Commission acknowledged there remained unanswered questions regarding the possible interplay between savanna and forest onchocerciasis and their respective vectors.[7] For example, could forest flies ingest the savanna parasite and spread savanna oncho beyond the OCP-controlled savanna zones? Two forest fly species, *Simulium soubrense* and *Simulium sanctipauli* in Côte d'Ivoire, where the forest and savanna terrains overlapped, had shown signs of resistance to temephos. Would resistance spread to the savanna blackfly, *Simulium damnosum*? The Commission concluded that "a precondition for its [the OCP's] success is that there is a strong scientific staff and research program to answer [these] questions" and "ensure that operational and research activities are closely linked."[8]

The Commission identified important advantages to extending vector control westward to cover the "Senegal River Basin" (Guinea, Guinea-Bissau, Senegal, Sierra Leone, and western Mali). There would be cost savings because vector control covering the western extension area would halt the flow of infective flies back into western Côte d'Ivoire, southern Mali east of the Niger River, and southern Upper Volta (figure 3.1). Consequently, vector-control activities could be substantially curtailed, and possibly suspended in these zones by halting reinvasion. The Commission estimated that $3.3 million would have been saved in 1981 alone by reducing such activities.[9] Suspending vector control in those zones would also reduce the likelihood of savanna-blackfly resistance developing and spreading throughout the OCP area.

Most importantly, halting reinvasion would greatly enhance prospects for bringing the OCP to a successful and lasting conclusion. Some reinvasion would continue from Nigeria into Benin, but it would be minimized by the prevailing headwinds blowing from southwest to northeast. Reinvasion from the southeast would also be halted by extending vector-control operations into the southern parts of Benin, Togo, and Ghana. The Commission predicted that extending operations would reduce ATPs below 100 throughout the wider OCP area, with the possible exception of eastern Benin.[10] Furthermore, widening vector control to the west and the southeast would increase protection to approximately 30 million West Africans: 20 million inhabitants in the original area plus 10 million in the extension zones.

The Commission looked into employing existing or new drugs to complement vector control and accelerate elimination of the parasite reservoir in the population. The Commission discouraged use of either DEC or suramin, due to their severe side effects. The Scientific Working Group of WHO's Special Program for Research and Training in Tropical Diseases (TDR) had concluded in 1976 that the highest priority should be on discovering "new and non-toxic macrofilaricides" for onchocerciasis.[11] Consequently, the Commission recommended that the OCP, in collaboration with the TDR, establish a project with the goal of finding an operational macrofilaricide that would kill the adult worm. The recommendation called for project financing to "be provided to pharmaceutical companies for drug development and testing" to find the "highest-priority macrofilaricide."[12] The financing would come out of the Oncho Trust Fund and the project would be managed by the TDR under the supervision of a joint OCP/WHO committee. The financing required would likely be substantial because the resulting macrofilaricide would almost certainly not be sufficiently profitable to cover the associated research costs.

The Commission also recommended converting the OCP headquarters into a Multi-Disease Surveillance Center (MDSC) when the control effort was nearing completion. The MDSC would conduct surveillance throughout the OCP subregion. The proposed terms of reference called for detecting disease outbreaks and suppressing them before they spread, utilizing the Center's "fire-fighting" capacity.[13] The Commission suggested linking or merging the MDSC with the OCCGE, which would provide for coordinated laboratory facilities serving the entire West African region.

The Commission issued other recommendations, nearly all of which were eventually adopted, namely:

- Increasing capacity for data processing and analysis, including computer modeling
- Installing gauges to measure river flows and transmitting that data automatically via satellite to Program headquarters, where it could be relayed to pilots

- Transferring epidemiological ("human") surveillance responsibilities to national staffs (or village health workers) and paying them according to national pay scales
- Continuing research into new larvicides
- Training nationals in epidemiology and entomology to help sustain the OCP achievements following completion
- Experimenting with stopping vector control in localized areas where control had been established, to see if fly repopulation led to a resumption of oncho transmission
- Better synchronizing epidemiological surveillance data with entomological surveillance data, such as conducting human surveillance in villages near fly-catching points
- Better understanding the fecundity of the adult female worm
- Collecting baseline hydrobiological data in extension areas to monitor the impact of larviciding on fauna and flora of rivers and making adjustments to avoid adverse impact on local environments.

Adoption of the Commission's recommendations took place in the first half of the 1980s and set the stage for a major scale-up of the Program during the remainder of the decade and beyond. In anticipation of the extension's approval, OCP management began preparations shortly after release of the Report in August 1981. In accordance with the recommendation on drugs, the Onchocerciasis Chemotherapy Project (OCT) was established in 1983. Its stated purpose was "to accelerate the discovery and development of a safe, effective, low-cost, and easily administered drug for onchocerciasis . . . suitable for large-scale use and which . . . must kill or permanently sterilize the adult female worms of Onchocerca volvulus."[14] With the establishment of the OCT, the OCP began requesting $3.45 million per annum from the Oncho Trust Fund to finance OCT-supported research.[15] The recommendation for the westward extension was endorsed by the 1985 JPC in Geneva.

The additional activities resulting from the Commission's recommendations led to an escalation in the OCP budget and in required donor financing. The total cost of Phase II (1980–1985) came to $107 million, nearly double that of Phase I (1974–1979). And, the cost of Phase III (1986–1991) turned out to be $177 million—more than three times the cost of Phase I.[16] Even so, the cost of the OCP never exceeded $1 per-person-protected per annum; and the cost per-person-protected declined as the Program covered larger populations including the extension areas. The additional total financial requirements put pressure on the World Bank to find creative ways of securing greater funding from the existing donor community and to enlist new donors. However, emerging doubts among some donors during 1982–1983 regarding the viability of the vector-control strategy complicated fund-mobilization efforts. Those doubts arose due to signs of insecticide resistance and the perceived riskiness of the ambitious plan to extend operations westward nearly to the Atlantic Ocean and virtually double the size of the Program.[17]

The Economic Review Mission

To better understand the development implications of the disease and its control, the Steering Committee decided that the sponsoring agencies should carry out an economic review mission, covering all seven original OCP countries in preparation for the second six-year phase of the Program (Phase II, 1980–1985). The 10-member mission, including sociologists, agronomists, and ecologists from the FAO, the UNDP, and WHO, as well as World Bank country economists, led by Bank consultant, Elliott Berg, was carried out during 1978.

The mission's report concluded that the OCP would contribute to economic development to the subregion by increasing the quantity and quality of the two major factors of agricultural production in rural West Africa: labor and land.[18] On the labor side, there would be increased productivity from reduction in disability and blindness. The largest of the economic benefits would come from opening up new lands near rivers, with better soils than those in the departure areas. Bringing oncho under control would result in increased agricultural output in newly-available riverine valleys while simultaneously reducing erosion on "old lands" left by migrants when they resettled the new areas.

The report determined that the largest economic benefits would accrue to Upper Volta, which contained 49% of the population in the original seven-country OCP area. Upper Volta was characterized, more than the other OCP countries, by under-inhabited river valleys adjacent to overcrowded plateaus.[19] The mission argued that no one planning approach was appropriate for all seven countries to capitalize on the development dividend from successful oncho control because of the "varied needs of the countries concerned." The economic importance of the oncho-endemic areas and the role those areas played in national development strategies differed depending on the country.[20] Emphasizing settlement policies and migration into the oncho-freed areas was considered more relevant for Upper Volta, where the oncho zone covered 80% of the country, than for the other countries, notably the coastal states, Côte d'Ivoire, Ghana, Togo, and Benin.[21]

The mission estimated that the amount of "relatively-empty land" throughout the original OCP area, which was "suitable for agriculture," to be in the range of 134,000–154,000 km².[22] Another 21,920 km² were in the southeastern extension areas of Ghana, Togo, and Benin.[23] The Bank's Oncho Unit employed these estimates to extrapolate an estimate of under-inhabited, arable land in the wider 11-country OCP area of 250,000 km². This calculation was considered to be somewhat conservative because some of the largest tracts of moderately-productive, under-occupied land were known to be in the western extension zone—notably in Upper Guinea, western Mali, and eastern Senegal. That 250,000 km² estimate was subsequently confirmed in other studies.[24] The Oncho Unit also conducted an analysis showing that the sparsely-populated arable land had the potential to feed 17 million additional people per annum, based on existing technologies, cultural practices, and consumption patterns in the region.

The characteristics and potential of the landmass which includes the OCP area merit closer examination. There are three basic ecological zones in the wider subregion. The OCP area falls in the Sudano-Savanna zone (SSZ), which lies between the drier Sahelian zone and the forested zone along the coastal area adjacent to the Gulf of Guinea. The SSZ has been West Africa's largest source for food crop production, including cereals (millet, sorghum, and maize), fruits, and vegetables. It also became the largest livestock-rearing subregion after the droughts of 1969–1974 and 1983–1984, which forced pastoralists and their herds to migrate southward from the Sahelian zone.[25] The SSZ has also been a leading source for oilseeds (Sesame, Shea tree, groundnut), cashews, and cotton as a cash crop.[26] It was described in a 2008 study by the Economic Community of West African States (ECOWAS), as the "helpful agricultural region," due to oncho control and its attraction to rural migrants, given the "relative availability" of new farming land and pastures.[27] The SSZ is an ecologically fragile area owing to its relative aridity and soils subject to erosion. An important advantage to the SSZ is the wide availability of livestock and the potential for integrating herding with farming, thereby obviating the need for chemical fertilizers, which are expensive and potentially damaging to fragile soils.

Analyses have cited the OCP area within the SSZ as having greater agricultural-productive capacity than other areas in West Africa. The FAO classified 33% of the soils in the original OCP area as having an agricultural value in the "average" to "very good" range, compared with 16% elsewhere in West Africa.[28] Soils classified as "poor" in the original area made up a much smaller portion of the total than for West Africa as a whole.[29] In 1986, the average population density of the OCP area was on the low side, at 20.2 (inhabitants/km²).[30] The sparse population made it possible to set aside sizable amounts of land for protected forests and national parks as wildlife sanctuaries. Virtually all of the national parks of the OCP countries were in the OCP area as of the early 1990s and needed to be preserved as the area developed. With greater productive potential and low population density, the OCP area presented a convincing case for promoting environmentally sustainable settlement and rational land-use of the riverine valleys as the disease was brought under control.

It is unclear whether the under-inhabited valleys in the OCP area were abandoned or never fully occupied. The reasons for their under-population likely included factors in addition to onchocerciasis, such as other diseases, notably trypanosomiasis; colonial policies involving forced labor and military recruitment; and the dangers of wild animals. Nevertheless, the Economic Review Mission report concluded: "There is little doubt . . . that it [onchocerciasis] was widely present and that it is an important factor explaining the low rate of utilization of many riverine areas."[31] It noted that the empty villages in the oncho zones were closest to rivers where the impact of the disease was most severe: "This suggests that onchocerciasis was an important factor in the under-population and depopulation of many valleys and riverine areas."[32] In a 1989 publication, Remme and Zongo described repeated unsuccessful attempts by local populations during the 20th century prior to the OCP to establish villages in sparsely-populated valleys along the Red and White Volta Rivers, due to the disease. They wrote: "The river valleys were, therefore, not only virtually uninhabited by the year 1975, but they contained also the ruins of hundreds of villages as the evidence that many attempts at settlement had been made during this century but all of them had been doomed to failure."[33]

However, Berg's report stated: "The 'crowded plateaux-empty valleys' paradigm is not general in the OCP region . . . The OCP is an entomological unit, not an economic one. Few economic generalizations are fully applicable to the OCP zone of the seven participating OCP countries. Uniform approaches to development planning or economic policy are therefore unlikely to be equally suitable for all the countries in question."[34] On the face of it, the assessment that development constraints throughout the OCP area were varied and required different policies and plans depending upon the country, seemed relatively uncontroversial. Nevertheless, that assessment threw into question the basic economic rationale for launching the multicountry regional control effort—the presumed importance of the oncho-control/rural-development nexus throughout the seven-country area. That premise had been an important justification for donor support and for the active involvement of the UNDP, the FAO, and the World Bank.

Berg had been recruited to lead the economic assessment by Steve Denning, the World Bank division chief responsible for the Sahel countries and the OCP. Denning later commented, "Elliott should have been praised for asking the hard questions. Instead he was vilified by WHO and the donors."[35] The fallout from the Economic Review Mission led to a shift back to an emphasis on the health benefits of disease control and to the primacy of WHO in the control effort.

It is unclear whether that controversy had any impact on the decision, in 1980, to replace OCP Director Marc Bazin, an economist seconded by the World Bank, with Dr. Ebrahim Malik Samba, Director of Health Services in the Gambia. That decision was made by Dr. Comlan Quenum, WHO director of AFRO.[36] Quenum had just assumed direct responsibility for the OCP, knew the capable leaders in health at national levels in sub-Saharan Africa, and undoubtedly wanted an African in that position.

The changeover from Bazin to Samba took place at the JPC in Yamoussoukro, Côte d'Ivoire in December 1980. Bazin arrived with suitcases in hand and left immediately after to return to the World Bank in Washington, DC. There was no formal handover from Bazin to Samba, which disappointed some senior staff who had hoped for a smoother transition.[37] The two men came from very different backgrounds, which was reflected in their management styles. After working in the Bank for a short while, Bazin returned to his home country, Haiti, to be appointed minister of finance and economy under President Jean-Claude Duvalier and, later, prime minister and de facto president under a military government in 1991.

Samba had trained as a surgeon at the National University of Ireland and the University of Edinburgh. He supported himself through medical school through a fellowship from the Royal College of Surgeons and as an amateur boxer, earning £50 per fight.[38] After finishing medical school in 1963, he returned to the Gambia where he rose from a junior medical officer to the Director of Medical Services during 1964–1980.[39] He was a sturdy, energetic director with a forceful personality. He ran a tight ship with insistence on deadlines. His forcefulness seemed to intimidate OCP staff, at times. He was the first anglophone director, and the predominantly francophone staff were slow in accepting him as their new leader.[40]

Also, in early 1981, OCP management selected French entomologist, Dr. Bernard Philippon, to replace John Davies, who had been acting chief of the VCU for nine months in 1980–1981. Dr. Yankum Dadzie, an ophthalmologist from Ghana, was chosen to replace Bjorn Thylefors as the OCP's ophthalmologist. Thylefors was promoted by WHO to become the Director of the Prevention of Blindness Program in Geneva. The OCP established an office in Bamako, Mali, to collect data throughout the western extension area in preparation for launching operations there once the JPC approved the Plan of Operations (PLANOPS) for Phase III. Several OCP staff, including Bernard Philippon, were reassigned to the Bamako office to lead those preparations.

Upon assuming the directorship, Samba faced several major, pressing tasks, including: preparing for the extensions of the OCP, addressing emerging signs of resistance to temephos, and securing the additional financing to achieve these tasks. By the end of 1980, the OCP entomologists, Walsh, Davies, and Sékétéli, assisted by consultants Rolf Garms of the Bernhard-Nocht Institute (Hamburg, Germany) and Robert Cheke of the Natural Resources Institute (Chatham, UK), had concluded that the fly, *Simulium damnosum*, traveled at least 400 km with the wind currents.[41] The distance was nearly three times farther than thought five years earlier, and one-third longer than the 1974–1979 evaluation had concluded. This longer distance reinforced the importance of full coverage of the extension areas.

The push for the needed increase in financing began in 1982. Bilsel Alisbah, the World Bank's director of the Western Africa Department, established a special position in his department for a staff member to devote full time to the OCP. Jean-Paul Dailly, a Belgian, was selected for that position, as Onchocerciasis Coordinator, located in the department's Sahel Country Division. That year, Dailly and Samba went on the first of several series of Bank-led trips to meet with donors in capitals. Both were new to the Program and had not yet had extensive contact with donors. The objective was to shore up support for the expansion phase after eight years of reasonably effective operations confined to the original OCP area. There were beginning signs of donor fatigue, with some donors questioning of the way forward.[42] Dailly described his role and the purpose of these visits:

> I was hired for the oncho job to help strengthen donor support for OCP,
> which entailed considerable traveling to meet with the donors in capitals.
> I asked my Division Chief, Steve Denning, what my terms of reference were
> for the donor visits, and he responded "visit all the key donors but keep the
> Program off the front page of the *New York Times*." Dr. Samba and I saw the
> purpose of the trips as saving the Program during a time of growing skepticism
> among some donors. I tried to convince Dr. Samba that our most important
> task was to gain the confidence of the donors in him as a manager who
> could successfully tackle the reinvasion and blackfly resistance problems.
> Dr. Samba was masterful. He came across as a strong manager who both
> understood the problems and was developing solutions to overcome them.[43]

The trips succeeded in mollifying the more skeptical donors and resulted in recruiting three new European donors: Italy, Finland, and Norway.

Periodic oncho donor meetings were convened by the World Bank at its offices in Paris during the late 1970s. Beginning in the 1980s, these meetings became known as "Donor Seminars." The first such meeting took place during October 11–12, 1982, in Paris. The meeting was chaired by the vice president for West Africa, David Knox. In his opening statement, Knox laid out the parameters of the meeting: "We are not here to take decisions. The purpose of this seminar is to provide an opportunity for briefing, for the asking and answering of questions so that each of you can go back to your government or agency with a better appreciation of the issues and their financial implications."[44] The intention was to provide for an informal, low-key gathering of donors that would not offend the African countries by appearing to be taking important decisions in their absence.[45]

In his opening statement, Knox gave what he saw as the rationale for the donors to continue to support the OCP. He stated, "It [the Program] is of high priority because it addresses human suffering in the poorest part of the world . . . This does not mean that we should not ask ourselves questions about the costs and benefits . . . Nevertheless, I think we all recognize that we have a moral obligation to finish what we have started; and I think we can rightfully derive satisfaction from what we have achieved to date."[46]

An important purpose of the seminars was to give the donors an opportunity to indicate their levels of support for the Program via pledging. Information on financial commitments was essential for the Bank to plan out the fund-mobilization efforts required to sustain control operations. At the 1982 meeting, sufficient financing was ensured to complete the remainder of Phase II (1983–1985).

By the end of Phase II, 14 countries and four international organizations had joined the donor community and were contributing annually to the Oncho Trust Fund. The donor community contributed an average of $19 million per annum during Phase II to meet annual expenditures averaging $18 million. The surplus went into a "contingency reserve" to be held in the Trust Fund for unforeseen developments and emergencies. The World Bank invested idle contributions, including the reserve, in short-term securities pending disbursements to WHO to meet OCP expenditures. The interest derived from those investments assisted in building up the reserve. The Bank's oncho team decided that a prudent level for the reserve would be the equivalent of six months of OCP operations. Consequently, the initial aim was to build up the reserve to $9 million. That was achieved by the end of Phase II.

Increasing Needs, Rising Tensions

The Independent Commission had recommended the preparation of a long-term strategy (LTS) for bringing the OCP to a successful conclusion. At the 1984 JPC meeting in Niamey, Niger, the governing board discussed the draft LTS prepared by Samba and his management team. Bernhard Liese, the Bank's principal tropical disease specialist, described that discussion:

> Dr. Samba's presentation contained tentative cost figures for completing Phase III, in excess of US$200 million. Those estimates were not based on any meaningful evidence, that we could tell, and we felt they were excessive. We needed more realistic and precise estimates before we could approve the LTS. Bilsel [Alisbah] discussed with some of the donors what to do over the coffee break. There was no time to work it out with Samba and his team. After the break, Bilsel proposed that the OCP commit to preparing a Plan of Operations for Phase III [PLANOPS] with detailed cost estimates, as a condition for the JPC approving the LTS. The donors weighed in backing the Bank's proposal. Samba was livid. We had signaled we wouldn't accept his higher cost figures and we were asking him for more preparation after he and his team had worked hard to complete the LTS. Samba couldn't take his anger out on Bilsel, so he came directly for Jean-Paul [Dailly] and me after the JPC approved the Bank proposal. I was careful to lie low and distance myself from the quarrel which ensued, because I could see how furious Samba was.[47]

As Dailly later explained, the Bank's goal at the JPC was to hold the budget for Phase III to under $150 million. It was feared that $200+ million would be unachievable. It was roughly double the expenditures for Phase II.[48]

Differences over the Phase III budget led to a falling-out between Dailly and Samba. When both met again several days later at OCP headquarters in Ouagadougou, the disagreement reached a breaking point. Samba accused Dailly of hindering the effort to secure the financing Samba thought was required to carry out the extension operations.[49] In the end, the cost estimates for the PLANOPS, when prepared in detail in the spring of 1985 by a World Bank team with the assistance of Samba and his chiefs, turned out to be considerably less than Samba had thought necessary. But the damage had been done. Samba telephoned Alisbah back at Bank Headquarters and laid down an ultimatum: "Dailly has become a hindrance to securing OCP financing. Either he goes or I go."[50]

The situation was discussed between Alisbah, Dailly, and Sahel country division chief, Larry Hinkle, when Dailly returned to the Bank. The conclusion was that the rupture would prevent Dailly from remaining effective as Onchocercia-sis Coordinator. It was decided, with Dailly's concurrence, that he would trans-fer within the division to become Loan Officer for Burkina Faso. Dailly later said he regretted the incident. He had enjoyed working on the OCP and had devel-oped many close friendships, including with Samba. Samba and Dailly met again several years later while Samba was attending a World Bank meeting. They em-braced and reminisced as old friends. After serving as Loan Officer for Burkina Faso, Dailly became the World Bank's resident representative for the Central Af-rican Republic. He commented during our interview that he had taken the on-cho position to transition into mainstream operations. Onchocerciasis Coordina-tor was not a fully mainstream position, but Loan Officer for Burkina Faso was. So, he wound up where he wanted to be, in the end.[51]

In February 1985, I was offered, and accepted, the Onchocerciasis Coordi-nator position and began learning about the disease. I had served a two-year stint as a US Peace Corps volunteer in Guinea from 1964 to 1966 and thought I understood the difficulties of living in that part of West Africa. Guinea was a country recognized in Peace Corps circles as extremely challenging for volun-teer service due to scarce food, lack of basic amenities, and a rampant black market.

Twenty years after that assignment, starting my new job, I learned that oncho was rampant—widespread and hyperendemic—for hundreds of kilometers around Kankan, Guinea's third-largest city, where I taught in 1965–1966. Looking back, I understand why I never heard of the disease while there. First, it impacted the poorest of the poor with whom I, a foreigner, rarely communicated. They lived in remote rural areas where I rarely went. It did not affect those in urban areas who were better-off and politically influential. Consequently, the disease was invisible to me and my fellow Peace Corps volunteers. None of us, to my knowledge, delved below the surface to discover the suffering endured by the rural poor impacted by the disease. Also, the families of the oncho-infected felt shame and kept the oncho blindness and skin disfigurement hidden, as best they could.

As Oncho Coordinator, I realized the importance of bringing the disease out of the shadows by raising awareness of it in the international community. Dur-ing trips to the rural areas of Burkina Faso and Mali, I witnessed the suffering. I saw lethargic, middle-aged oncho-blind sitting around in their villages in quiet desperation hoping for some relief—elders who in their society commanded re-spect, but lacked the energy and focus to act out, or even appreciate, their right-ful authoritative role. Later, when traveling down to Bobo-Dioulasso, Burkina

Faso, I walked around some of the abandoned villages in previously hyperendemic oncho areas to gain some appreciation for the power of the disease to decimate once thriving societies.

Securing the Financing for Phase III and a Major Expansion of the OCP

Dailly stayed on for an additional six months to help me transition into the job. This involved finalizing the PLANOPS with Samba and his team and an extensive donors' trip that fed into a major donors' meeting at the Bank's Paris office. We met with as many donors as possible in Western Europe and North America during that September–October trip in 1985. The objective was threefold: (1) introduce me; (2) convince each donor to increase its support for Phase III, including the PLANOPS, by at least 25%; and (3) encourage the donors to "frontload" their contributions to meet the higher expenditures required during the first half of Phase III to launch the extension operations. If control covered the western extension area by 1988, cost savings would begin accruing during 1989–1991. Vector control in the extension area would shield the original area from re-invading blackflies, thereby enabling cutbacks in operations in the original area.

The increase requested from the donors was based upon a detailed costing of the PLANOPS. At the request of Samba, Bernhard Liese and his colleague, Lina Domingo, had assisted the OCP management in completing the costing exercise several months after the Niamey JPC. As Liese described it:

> Lina and I spent a week with Dr. Samba and OCP staff in Dakar, Senegal, during the Program's annual retreat in the spring of 1985. Samba and the Program staff realized while completing the costing exercise that the PLANOPS was becoming a very useful document. They were grateful for having gone through the process because they understood much better the various activities required to complete the western extension, and, ultimately to bring OCP to a conclusion. We arrived at a budget of US$133 million. At last, we had a fully-prepared document with justified expenditures that provided a strong case for going forward with Phase III. It established a base for the donors to commit to, and build upon, for the remainder of OCP.[52]

Upon arriving in Paris for the October 1985 donors' meeting, I was nervous about how the meeting would play out. Fewer firm commitments than I had hoped were forthcoming during the one-on-one donor meetings in capitals. How would the donors react to my financing speech arguing for more than an additional $100 million? What would happen if the pledging fell short?

Bilsel Alisbah was in the chair the next morning as the meeting opened. He was soft-spoken and understated in his opening remarks. As the meeting unfolded, it was evident that the donors liked and respected him and would follow his lead as chairman. Up for discussion was the PLANOPS document that spelled out the steps involved in carrying out the western and southeastern extensions. Samba had mastered the details of the plan and was convincing in his presentation on the necessity for, and advantages of, implementing it. He argued that completing it was essential to bring the OCP to a successful, lasting conclusion by the target closing date, 1997. The donors posed questions and Samba gave spirited and articulate responses. He often turned to his senior staff to respond to the technical questions on vector control and predictive modeling.

One surprise was the interest among the donors in socioeconomic development (SED) of the river valleys where oncho was being brought under control. This topic had not been raised during the donor visits in capitals. However, USAID had just completed its impact evaluation of the OCP in August 1985. The evaluation had concluded that the "OCP, to date, must be considered one of the more successful multi-donor programs in the short history of development assistance."[53] But it cautioned that "unless a directed and coordinated initiative is undertaken in the near term it is unlikely that the goal of socioeconomic development will be realized in any way proportional to the successful accomplishment of vector control."[54] The renewed donor interest in the SED would result in a greater focus on development of the oncho-controlled areas during the next decade.

My financing speech outlined the strategy for funding the PLANOPS, based on the estimates of $133 million for Phase III (1986–1991). It reiterated the call for a 25% increase in donor support and frontloaded contributions. It stressed building up the trust fund's contingency reserve. Given the uncertainties in expanding vector control over vast new areas, there was greater likelihood of resorting to the reserve at some point. It would need to add $6 million to increase the reserve to $14 million, equivalent to six months of program operations under the new phase.

I soon learned, in subsequent donor meetings, to give a copy of the financing speech to the interpreters the night before. Doing so helped ensure clear and accurate simultaneous interpretation of the financing presentation into French for the francophone delegates. It was critical for all the donors to understand fully the justifications behind the Bank's requests for increased support.

The tail-end of my financing presentation led into donor pledging. Alisbah opened the floor to the 18 donor delegations, in addition to the Bank, sitting alphabetically around a long oval table. The donors, when ready, individually asked for the floor to announce their pledge. Some pledges were in US dollars while others were in national currencies. I later tried to stage-manage the pledging by privately asking two of the larger donors, such as the United States and the Netherlands, to lead off with their pledges. The intent was to generate momentum and enthusiasm at the outset of the pledging, and, hopefully, boost the overall outcome.

Directly after the pledging, I had to tabulate the pledges and report back to the plenary—not a straightforward exercise. Roughly half of the donors pledged in national currencies. Hence, the exercise entailed adding up apples and oranges to arrive at the total in US dollars. I quickly learned to schedule a coffee break in the agenda directly after the pledging to allow for time to calculate the dollar equivalents of all pledges, to arrive at and announce an accurate final tally. When the result was highly positive, as in 1985, it was a thrill to announce the outcome to the plenary, consisting of donor delegations, sponsoring agencies, and Program management.

The total pledging at the 1985 donors meeting came to $110 million—larger than expected—with three donors (Switzerland, Norway, and the World Bank) pledging frontloaded, multiyear support for Phase III.[55] It was an outcome to celebrate. More financing was assured in that session than for the entire six years of Phase II. We had secured 83% of the estimated required financing for the OCP through 1991. That funding would enable a near-doubling in the size of the OCP, coverage of four new countries, and protection for 10 million additional West Africans.

Immediately following the meeting, the Bank issued a press release that served as the basis for number of articles that appeared in the European press the next day. The expanded OCP would become the largest intercountry health program in the world, covering approximately 30 million people in 11 countries by the early 1990s. The total area contained an estimated 250,000 km² of arable land that was relatively underpopulated. With effective control and the right policies, that oncho-freed land could attract sustainable resettlement leading to increased agricultural production throughout the subregion.[56]

Several developments transpired prior to the donors meeting that boosted the pledging. The conclusions of USAID's August 1985 impact evaluation of the OCP were strongly positive with regard to the Program's cost-effectiveness and the impact of vector control in bringing the disease under control and benefiting millions in the region. That evaluation influenced USAID, and made it far more likely that USAID would increase its Phase III contribution.

Prior to the meeting, Alisbah secured agreement from the internal committee responsible for the World Bank's Development Grant Facility (DGF), for an
increase in the Bank's contribution to the Oncho Trust Fund to $2.5 million an-
nually for 1986–1987. That agreement provided for a 25% annual increase over
the Bank's contribution to Phase II. The increase enabled us to showcase the
Bank's commitment for greater support for Phase III—the same commitment
being asked of the other donors. Also, fortuitously, the Netherlands' contribution, pledged in Dutch guilders, which had been the largest among the European
donors for Phase II, increased substantially due, in part, to the decline of the US
dollar in relation to the Dutch guilder by nearly 45% during 1985–1986. We
would soon become painfully aware, however, that the decline in the US dollar
was a double-edged sword in its financial impact on the OCP.

Also contributing to the upbeat results were presentations predicting favorable
vector-control results based on the simulations of a new OCP computer model. Two
years prior, mathematician Jan "Hans" Remme, who had worked on infectious-
disease modeling at the University of Dar es Salaam, was brought into the OCP's
applied research unit as a biostatistician by Samba. With that hire, the locus of data
processing and computer analysis of the OCP's operational results shifted from a
small group of consultants in WHO-Geneva to Remme and his assistant at OCP
headquarters. The shift was facilitated by the coming-of-age of microcomputers during the first half of the 1980s.

En route to Ouagadougou from Dar es Salaam for his interviews with Samba
and senior OCP staff, Remme had to change planes in Abidjan, Côte d'Ivoire. Upon
arriving in Abidjan, he discovered that his flight to Ouagadougou had been can-
celed due to a coup d'état in Upper Volta. Remme spent three days and nights at
the Abidjan airport waiting for flights to Upper Volta to resume. During that time,
in preparation for his interviews, he put together a mathematical model of onchocerciasis infection with data on onchocerciasis in books that he had brought along
from the University of Dar es Salaam. He termed it a "simple force-of-infection
model for onchocerciasis."

Over the subsequent two years that basic model was used to analyze and predict trends in onchocerciasis infection levels in areas under vector control. By
the mid-1980s, vector control had been underway for eight years or more throughout the original area. Entomological surveillance data demonstrated that vector
control was having a significant impact on transmission. ATPs were declining
nearly everywhere in the seven-country area. However, epidemiological surveillance data showed little if any reduction in prevalence in the population. The

absence of any meaningful decline in prevalence was worrying to the Expert Advisory Committee (EAC) and to some donors.[57]

With the model, Remme concluded that the CMFL was a better measure of the success of vector control than prevalence indicators. The CMFL measured the intensity of oncho infection rather than its breadth in the population. In Remme's view, it was "a much more sensitive indicator of the level of endemicity and epidemiological changes after control."[58] That conclusion was an important recognition that the traditional indicators—"prevalence" and "incidence"—were not very meaningful for onchocerciasis. The model showed through the declining CMFL, that, by 1983–1984, "some 70%" of the adult worms had already died out in the population in the central OCP area.[59]

The model revealed an approximate 10-year lag between the decline in the CMFL and the decline in prevalence in the population. Consequently, it was expected that the dramatic fall in the intensity of infection would result in an even more dramatic decline in oncho prevalence in another 2–3 years, with all indicators converging to zero during the subsequent several years. Remme presented these results to the EAC in Bouaké, Côte d'Ivoire, and later at the 1985 Paris donors meeting. The EAC members were "tremendously relieved and excited" to see the results revealing why prevalence data had not yet shown improvements.[60]

At this time, the OCP started collaborating with scientists from Erasmus University of Rotterdam in developing a more detailed computer simulation model of onchocerciasis transmission and control. That model, called ONCHOSIM, predicted in 1986 a required duration of 14 years for vector control to eliminate the parasite reservoir in the population. After 14 years, the CMFL and prevalence would fall to insignificant levels, indicating that the adult worm reservoir had virtually disappeared in the population, enabling vector control to be safely stopped (figure 3.2). It was an important preliminary finding that implied that vector control could be stopped in most of the original seven-country area by the end of 1991 (final year of Phase III) without major risk of renewed transmission. Stopping control in the original area assumed the extension operations would succeed in halting reinvading infective flies from the west and southeast. The model predictions presented by Remme strengthened donor confidence in the vector-control strategy at an important juncture—halfway through the Program when donors were being asked to double down on the strategy in the extension areas. The predictions were also a strong indication that the Program was on track in pursuing its stated objective of "eliminating the disease as a public health problem" throughout the original seven-country area.

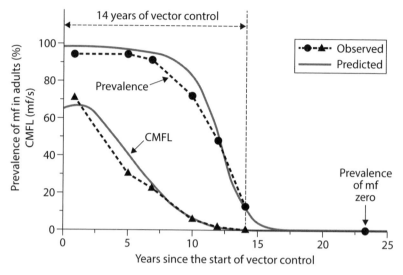

Figure 3.2. Predicted and Observed Decline in Infection Levels in a Hyperendemic Community in the Central OCP Area. *Source:* Hans Remme.

Solving a Crisis and Battling Resistance

The 1985 donors' meeting confirmed that support was strong as the OCP entered its most ambitious and expensive six-year phase. Program financing looked to be well-in-hand when the Onchocerciasis Fund Agreement for Phase III was signed by the donors in February 1986. However, two uncertainties were about to shake the oncho community's confidence in the long-term viability of the control effort: the decline of the US dollar and resistance to the Program's foremost insecticide, temephos.

The US dollar began declining in relation to other major international currencies in early 1985 and continued its slide during the remainder of the decade and beyond. That precipitous decline threatened the Program during 1986–1997—throughout Phase III and most of Phase IV. The problem was that the larger donor contributions, comprising 70% of all donor support, were denominated in US dollars, while most OCP expenditures were in non-dollar currencies. Contributions from the United States, the World Bank, Japan, Saudi Arabia, Switzerland, and the UNDP were pledged in US dollars.[61] Most OCP expenditures occurred in Japanese yen and Communauté financière d'Afrique (CFA) francs pegged to the French franc. Nearly 1,000 OCP staff were paid in CFA francs. Toyota vehicles and spare parts that made up the bulk of the OCP fleet were purchased in Japanese yen.

During 1986–1991, the dollar declined 40% in relation to the French franc and 51% in relation to the Japanese yen.[62] The impact was equivalent to an increase in the OCP's costs during Phase III of 15% or $20 million.[63] We quickly and unexpectedly found ourselves in a financial crisis and needed to somehow increase donor support even further after the Phase III pledges, while also working with Samba and his management team to reduce Program costs.

The financial situation deteriorated even further due to the increased costs entailed in battling blackfly resistance to temephos. Samba reported in 1986 that resistance had spread throughout original OCP area. Resistance should not have come as a surprise because it had shown up in two of the forest fly species several years earlier in Côte d'Ivoire. But this news was a blow to recent optimism that the OCP was on track in achieving its objective. My initial reaction was that our only control tool was rapidly becoming useless in the OCP original and extension areas. Loss of vector control might mean total collapse of the Program. Fortunately, unbeknownst to me, a working group had been researching oncho insecticide resistance at the ORSTOM Entomology Laboratory in Bondy, France, and at the OCP's Onchocerciasis Hydrological Research Center in Bouaké, Côte d'Ivoire, since 1977.[64] By the mid-1980s, that operational research had identified six additional larvicides that were effective in killing *Simulium damnosum* larvae.

The safest and most environmentally friendly of the additional larvicides—even safer than temephos—was *Bacillus thuringiensis* (*B.t.* H-14). *B.t.* H-14 is a biologic agent that produces a protein crystal that binds to receptors in the gut of the blackfly larvae, which results in their ceasing to consume the nutrients necessary to stay alive. The crystal is biodegradable and harmless to humans, invertebrates, and plants. *B.t.* H-14 was approved by the US Environmental Protection Agency in 1998 as a pesticide that "does not cause unreasonable risks or adverse effects to humans and the environment."[65]

B.t. H-14 cost more than any of the alternatives to purchase and apply because it had limited carry down-river and therefore required more flight hours to treat. The other insecticides found to be effective against blackfly larvae were, in order of increasing toxicity: chlophoxim, pyraclofos, etophenprox, permethrin, and carbosulfan.[66] The six larvicides, all of which were more expensive than temephos, could be rotated sequentially, with the last four restricted to use at heavier river-discharge levels that dilute their toxicity and minimize any negative effects on nontarget organisms.[67]

The Program adopted an insecticide-rotation strategy in 1986. It was a complex strategy that factored in river flows, toxicity to nontarget organisms, the costs of insecticide acquisition and application, and insecticide chemical structures. To avoid developing cross-resistance, insecticides with similar chemical structures could not be applied back-to-back. The strategy worked. By the early 1990s, resistance had been reversed for both of the organophosphates, temephos and chlophoxim, with no new resistance developing to the other five insecticides. Eventually temephos could be employed again in rotation with the other larvicides. The reversal was a breakthrough. No other vector-control operation, whether for disease control or for pest control in agriculture, had reversed insect resistance. However, this achievement came at a price. The cost of combating, and eventually overcoming, blackfly resistance exceeded $15 million.[68]

Sophisticated tele-transmission of hydrobiological data enabled the counter-resistance strategy to work. OCP staff set up beacons along the rivers throughout the OCP area, that measured river flows and automatically transmitted data via satellite back to OCP headquarters. Having accurate data in real-time allowed staff at headquarters to radio instructions to the pilots on where and how much to spray blackfly breeding sites with each of the six larvicides. This sophisticated setup meant that pilots became more precise in dosing, and even deferred spraying without the risk of renewed transmission when the data confirmed that stopping vector control in selected areas was feasible. The end result yielded important cost efficiencies within an otherwise expensive strategy to overcome resistance, while minimizing any adverse environmental impact from the more toxic insecticides employed in rotation.

The robust program of operational research within the OCP rescued the vector-control strategy in 1986–1987. From the beginning, roughly 8%–13% of the OCP budget was dedicated to operational, or applied, research. Apart from predictive modeling, much of this research focused on resolving issues related to aerial spraying during the first 15 years of the OCP, including environmental research and monitoring associated with the extensive use of larvicides. Whenever new larvicides were tested on their effectiveness in destroying blackfly larvae, they were also assessed for toxicity to nontarget organisms, notably aquatic insects, fish, and shellfish. Studies on the effectiveness of larvicides and on their potential environmental toxicity were carried out by the OCP's hydrobiology team at the program's hydrobiological laboratory in Côte d'Ivoire. The study results were then submitted to the Ecological Group (EG) for approval or rejection of the larvicide in question.

The Ecological Group was the brain of an environmental management program that actively safeguarded the aquatic environment throughout the OCP area. The EG consisted of only five independent ecologists, but it was backed up by the OCP's hydrobiology team in the VCU and the national hydrobiology teams in the Participating Countries. The OCP was unique, at the time, as a public-health intervention with an active program to protect the environment.[69] The Sponsoring Agencies (via the Steering Committee) had established the EG before OCP operations got underway in late 1974. The EG's terms of reference were threefold: (1) set up an environmental-monitoring program to continually assess the impact of larviciding on the aquatic fauna; (2) establish criteria for the selection of larvicides; and (3) appraise agricultural development changes and their impact on the local environment in the oncho-controlled areas.[70] The EG's larvicide selection criteria provided the basis for approval or rejection of larvicides in OCP operations.[71] The criteria stipulated that a larvicide could not (1) "reduce the number of invertebrate species or cause a marked shift in the relative abundance of species"; (2) have "a direct impact on fish" or the "lifecycle of fish species"; (3) lead to "bioaccumulation" or "biomagnification" in the interrelated food chains in the ecological community; or (4) impair human activities in the control area.[72]

Initially, environmental monitoring took place at 40 sites in the original OCP area. Over time some sites were closed as aerial spraying subsided in the original area, and new ones were established in the extension areas. By the early 1990s, the Program had settled on 20 sampling sites throughout the wider OCP area—10 for invertebrates and 10 for fish.[73] National hydrobiological teams were formed and trained by the OCP in monitoring methods in the eight Participating Countries subject to larviciding. These teams became active in monitoring, collecting data, and assessing results in annual meetings with the Ecological Group. Results for the fish populations showed, after 20 years of larviciding, "no evidence of a reduction in species richness" or loss of species.[74] For invertebrates, there was "an initial deleterious impact" after the application of temephos, chlorophoxim, and *B.t.* H-14, with "partial recovery" in the short-term. After several years, the studies showed that these larvicides "had little impact" on the environment. The more toxic insecticides (e.g. carbosulfan and permethrin) had greater effects on the invertebrate fauna, however "the ability" of the invertebrates "to recover was demonstrated, even if, at a slow rate."[75]

On the whole, the OCP's environmental program was comprehensive and consequential in protecting the far-reaching aquatic environment across the Volta and Niger River basins. The sponsoring agencies were foresighted in establishing the EG at the outset. Vector-control operations unconstrained by ecological considerations could have resulted in long-term environmental damage. Despite the high cost to purchase and apply, *B.t.* H-14 was employed the most after 1986 both because of its effectiveness and, in particular, its all-round safety for the environment.

The OCP's environmental program contributed greatly to the understanding of West Africa's aquatic environment. Massive amounts of data were collected and stored for the expansive river system in the OCP area, where little had existed previously. In addition to the collection of data, the OCP's environmental activities strengthened national capacities to carry out environmental assessments over the longer term. The database and strengthened national capacities could be employed by the Participating Countries for other sectors, such as monitoring and controlling use of pesticides and fertilizers in agriculture.

Bernhard Liese, chair of the Department of International Health at Georgetown University, argues that a key legacy of the oncho-control effort will be the program of operational research. He states,

> OCP set the standard for operational research involving ecological monitoring and adherence to environmental safeguards at a time when no other large development projects were giving attention to environmental impact. Those working on vector control understood the importance of applied research in resolving problems during implementation. They were acutely aware of the failure of the malaria eradication program just 10 years earlier. That program had no operational research in its budget and ultimately failed because it didn't develop backup insecticides. OCP staff were determined not to make the same mistake. Consequently, they worked closely with industry to develop new operationally-effective, environmentally-safe insecticides. And then they found ways to employ them rotationally to successfully reverse insecticide resistance for the first time ever—a method that became a model for other vector-control programs.[76]

Establishing a Proficient Process for Mobilizing Funds

It was becoming apparent by mid-1986 that the World Bank would have to redouble efforts to raise funding to overcome a budding financial crisis. I put together an informal fund-mobilization strategy to guide the Bank's oncho team. It involved three parts: (1) visit as many donors as possible in capitals to forewarn them of the difficult financing environment for carrying out the extension operations due to the declining dollar and the expense of battling larvicide resistance; (2) convene regular donor meetings to discuss the financial situation of the OCP along with policy changes and/or new initiatives; and (3) seek out potential new donors that could help reduce the burden on the existing donor community. Where new donors seemed promising, we would invite them to attend the donor meetings as observers.

I learned from the 1985 donors meeting that World Bank convening authority was a powerful tool. If we called a donors meeting, donor representatives would come from capitals rather than send attendees from local embassies, provided it was seen as a relatively high-level meeting. The earlier concept of the "donors' seminar" was insufficiently robust as a forum in addressing pressing issues needing urgent attention. The "seminar" notion was too informal and failed to attract high-level representation. So I changed the name to "Donors' Conferences."

Attracting higher-level donor attendance required that the meetings be chaired at a comparably-high level within the Bank—director, or preferably, higher. Arranging for higher-level World Bank chairmanship had the advantage of keeping senior Bank management involved in the Program on a fairly-regular basis. This was important because the OCP was not a mainstream Bank operation. Exposing senior Bank management to the Program's effectiveness and its multicountry impact helped retain their interest in, and support for, the control effort.

It was important to ensure that the donor meetings addressed substantive issues when setting agendas. The meetings could not be just pledging sessions. The donors needed to feel they were collectively addressing important issues. If they did, they would send higher-level representation, which, in turn, helped generate greater donor "ownership" of the Program. Greater ownership translated into more favorable donor disposition to increasing support when it seemed warranted.

There were other important criteria for the donor conferences. Attendance was limited to the donors, the sponsoring agencies, the OCP director and senior staff, and advisory groups to respond to technical questions. The meetings needed to be held at conveniently-located venues. Higher-level donor representatives would be less likely to attend if they had to travel long distances. Arranging for a donor country to host a donor conference had the advantage of increasing that country's ownership of the Program.

One-and-a-half days was the ideal duration—long enough to get into the detail of issues and make meaningful decisions, yet short enough to allow for the participation of high-level representatives. That duration allowed for corridor time during coffee breaks, a reception, and informal dinners following the first day's deliberations. These were essential in giving donors adequate opportunity to talk among themselves, as well as to the sponsoring agency representatives and OCP management. Scheduling informal get-togethers facilitated donor-to-donor communication and became a critical part of the process of keeping the donor community informed, engaged, and committed. When meetings focused on substantive policy or technical issues, arrangements were made for presentations by the OCP director and senior staff, who had the knowledge and expertise to generate and guide meaningful follow-on discussions. Outcomes were improved when the Bank chair summarized the collective-donor view following discussion of each agenda item.

In later meetings, we drafted and cleared a final communiqué with the donors in attendance. That communiqué was then placed on the agenda of the upcoming JPC as an information item. That process helped ensure that the JPC did not take decisions likely to face opposition from the donors. The Bank's presentation on financing, followed by donor pledging, were the final agenda items for every donor conference. It was important for the donors to have the opportunity to reflect upon each of the substantive issues on the agenda, as well as the overall required level of financing, before asking them to commit to a level of support.

The conferences became important opportunities for the donors to ask frank questions to the director and senior staff, and to the technical advisory chairs, without the Participating Countries present. The donors could probe without the risk of appearing obstructionist in front of the African governments. A key purpose was to elicit greater transparency than possible in the governing board sessions; and thereby, presumably, strengthen donor confidence in the Program. Another purpose was to provide an opportunity for the sponsoring agencies, technical advisors, and Program director plus senior staff, to listen to donor views on a variety of issues. In light of those views, proposals could be modified to elicit greater support from the donors prior to consideration in the governing-board session. The conferences were usually held in September or October prior to the governing-board meeting in December. The intention was to provide for adequate time to modify proposals to better align with donor positions before the JPC. This process helped ensure greater consensus around a proposal going into the governing-board approval stage.

For the financing agenda item, the Bank always presented its forecasts of program expenditures and the financing required to meet them, depending upon the multiyear phase in question. This agenda item was always scheduled at the end of the first day or beginning of the second day, just before donor pledging. The Bank's presentation sometimes generated donor questions and discussion of the financial needs of the Program. More often those questions were raised and answered during the Bank/OCP donor visits prior to the donor conference.

Donor pledging at the conferences served as dry runs for pledging at the JPC two-to-three months later. Donor pledging in front of the Participating Countries at the governing-board meeting was an essential part of the process. The Participating Countries benefited from knowing the commitment levels of each donor. That information helped them gauge which donors to approach to line-up bilateral funding for oncho-related initiatives at the national level, such as SED projects or control-maintenance activities. Pledging at the conferences enabled donors to revise their levels of support at the JPC in the light of other donor commitments and the indicative level of funding for the financial phase in question.

The donors' conferences formed the nucleus of a wider process to keep the donors informed and committed over the long-term. They were complemented by annual visits to the donors in capitals by the Program director and myself, in which we discussed that donor's proposed level of support, as well as specific concerns. Over time, the conferences became pivotal in mobilizing support for the oncho programs. Without them, backed by one-on-one donor visits, it would have been impossible to keep the donor representatives fully informed about these complex disease-control programs and adequately armed with the information to advocate effectively for continuing support within their own governments.

During my tenure, 10 oncho donors' conferences were convened during 1985–2004. The last of these was held at Bank headquarters in Washington, DC, and hosted by World Bank President James D. Wolfensohn. These meetings were critical in securing the $750 million required to implement the OCP and its successor, APOC, as they scaled up over a 20-year timeframe. By the end of the OCP in 2002, the donors' conferences had established a proven track record in ensuring the financial viability of the oncho-control effort. Unfortunately, the donors' conferences were discontinued by Bank staff after 2005 (see chapter 8).

During the 1985 donors' trip, Dailly introduced me to Suzanne Vervalcke, a recently retired director of the Multilateral Cooperation Division in the Belgian Ministry of Cooperation. I engaged Vervalcke's services as a consultant to assist in mobilizing financing for the OCP. Vervalcke had been a strong supporter of the OCP on behalf of Belgium. She knew firsthand most of the donor representatives and was familiar with the processes for requesting support from many of the European donors. She became extremely helpful in identifying and recruiting new donors.

Vervalcke had been shaped by harsh experience during World War II. Serving in the resistance movement in the early 1940s, she was arrested by the Nazis while taking messages back and forth between France and Belgium. She was condemned to death by a German court in January 1942. Hitler personally intervened to halt her execution, out of concern that executing a woman might turn her into a martyr and intensify resistance in occupied Belgium.[77] But she remained imprisoned by the Germans throughout the war.

Vervalcke and I, accompanied by Samba or the chief of the oncho liaison office in WHO-Geneva, Douglas Marr, visited the donors frequently during 1986–1989. She and I also sought out potential new donors. We focused on countries and foundations with connections to the OCP countries and/or to the oncho-donor countries. Our first big success was to recruit the European Commission via its development assistance program, the EDF, into the Program during 1987–1988. The EDF application process was unusually complicated because the OCP was a regional program. The process required statements of support from each of the European oncho donors to the European Commission, as well as written requests from each of the Participating Countries, as required under the Lomé IV Convention. Vervalcke was invaluable in navigating this complex process. Thanks to her efforts, we secured two substantial EDF contributions—equivalent to $8.8 million for Phase III and $9.9 million for Phase IV.[78] These contributions provided support when it was needed most to bridge the OCP funding gap in the late 1980s and early 1990s.

Vervalcke and I made several trips to Portugal, Luxembourg, and Denmark in pursuit of new donors. These were governments we identified as likely prospects either because of an historical connection to an African oncho country, as with Portugal, and/or as a close ally to a country in the oncho donor community. Luxembourg and Denmark also had track records of supporting humanitarian assistance. We succeeded with all three. During that recruiting effort, we also brought on board the Lisbon-based Calouste Gulbenkian Foundation, an NGO known for supporting health and education projects in lusophone Africa.

Thinking that South Korea might be similar to Kuwait, that is, a former-developing country that would identify with the endemic African countries, I traveled to Seoul several times to meet with Korea's Ministry of Finance. Those trips bore fruit when South Korea became an oncho donor at the end of Phase III. It helped in this case, as with other smaller donor countries, to present the oncho donor community as a collegial "Western club." The opportunity to join this "club" had considerable political and economic appeal to the smaller countries which lacked the resources to implement impactful bilateral aid programs on their own.

By becoming part of a coalition that included larger donors, they could leverage their contributions through the Oncho Trust Fund and have an important impact on a widespread, devastating disease. For these smaller donors, the size of their contribution was less important than being part of a multilateral effort.

At the 1988 JPC in Dakar, Senegal, we revised upward the expenditure estimates for Phase III (including the PLANOPS) to $175 million, an increase of $41 million or 30% over the 1985 projected budget of $133 million.[79] Half of that increase was attributed to the decline in the US dollar, and the remainder to the costs of combating blackfly resistance and financing clinical trials in the OCP countries of a new drug, ivermectin. Even though an additional $18 million had been secured to cover the first three years of Phase III, the Program faced a $23 million shortfall for the last three years, 1989–1991.[80]

The urgency of the remaining shortfall required a different approach. I developed a funding strategy focusing exclusively on the largest donors who had the resources to close the funding gap relatively quickly. Normally such a strategy would be discussed at a donor conference. However, none was scheduled in 1988. So, I had to pursue it bilaterally. The strategy entailed proposing that each of the 12 donors contributing at least $1 million per annum, increase their contributions during 1989–1991, by $500,000 per year.[81] If successful, the increases would bring in an additional $18 million. My thinking was that this proposal might be acceptable because these donors had a larger stake in the Program and a greater resource base than the other donors. If the strategy worked, we could raise the remaining $5 million through increases from smaller donors, recruiting new donors, and, if necessary, drawing down the contingency reserve.

I began pursuing this strategy with the two largest donors, the United States and the World Bank in early 1988. My request to the Bank's DGF Committee to increase the Bank's contribution by $500,000 per annum during 1989–1991 was approved. That increase placed the Bank in a stronger position to lobby for equivalent increases from the other larger donors during the lead-up to the 1988 Dakar JPC.

That spring, Samba came to Washington, DC, for a CSA meeting. We used that occasion to go to Capitol Hill and meet with the staffs of the Senate Foreign Relations and Appropriations Committees. Prior to joining the World Bank, I had been a Congressional Fellow on Capitol Hill and had worked with the Foreign Operations Subcommittee of the House Appropriations Committee to secure passage of US foreign aid legislation. That experience convinced me that we had a good chance of obtaining an increase for the OCP through an earmark in the appropriations legislation for USAID. Democrats controlled the House and the Senate at the time and were favorably disposed to increases in foreign assistance, particularly for humanitarian support for Africa. After listening to our pitch, the Senate committee staffs agreed to earmark $5 million for the OCP in the USAID appropriations bill for fiscal year 1989. Consequently, the USAID representative came to the Dakar JPC mandated to double the US contribution from $2.5 million to $5 million for 1989. That increase was timely in encouraging the other large donors to also commit to increases.

In the end, the strategy was only partially successful. At the 1988 Dakar JPC, eight of the 12 larger donors complied with the request. The result was an additional $9 million pledged in Dakar.[82] Even though a sizable shortfall of $14 million remained, it was eventually covered. The first contribution from the European Commission in 1989 brought the shortfall down to $5 million. By the end of Phase III, the trust fund's contingency reserve had been increased to $17 million, by investing idle contributions sitting in the fund. That reserve covered the remaining $5 million shortfall and enabled a healthy contingency reserve of $12 million to be carried over into Phase IV.

Chapter 4

The Game Changer—Ivermectin

There are few drugs that can seriously lay claim to the title of "Wonder drug," penicillin and aspirin being two that have perhaps had greatest beneficial impact on the health and wellbeing of Mankind. But ivermectin can also be considered alongside those worthy contenders, based on its versatility, safety and the beneficial impact that it has had, and continues to have, worldwide—especially on hundreds of millions of the world's poorest people.

> —Andy Crump and Satoshi Ōmura, *Proceedings of the Japan Academy, Series B. Physical and Biological Sciences*

The Search for a Breakthrough Antiparasitic Drug

In 1973, American pharmaceutical giant Merck and Company Inc. established a collaborative arrangement with the Japanese Kitasato Institute. Merck was searching for promising new antibiotics to enhance growth efficiency in livestock. At the time, Merck was setting up such arrangements with potential suppliers as part of an effort to secure promising compounds for product development. Merck sought out the Kitasato Institute because of the highly recognized expertise of Japanese scientists in the fields of microbiological research and natural product isolation.[1]

The agreement called for Merck to provide financial support to the Kitasato Institute for its ongoing research in exchange for the Institute delivering cultures that appeared novel, and hence candidates for further investigation into possible new antibiotics, to Merck Research Laboratories (MRL) in Rahway, New Jersey. Those cultures would be evaluated by Merck scientists and in the event that a new product was developed, approved, and marketed, Kitasato would share the royalties.

A year later, Merck management requested that the agreement with Kitasato be widened to include the selection and shipment of "unusual" nature-derived cultures to Merck to screen for bioactivity against parasites. Merck's screening of synthetic chemicals had been yielding diminishing returns by the mid-1970s. The objective was to discover new nature-derived chemical structures—not yet thought of by research chemists—which might prove useful in "unexpected ways."[2] That objective was also a function of Merck's interest, dating back to the early 1960s, in finding useful antiparasitic agents for the veterinary market. This focus was quite different from the original agreement with Kitasato to find growth-promoting antibiotics.

Merck's Animal Health Research Division had been pursuing animal anthelmintics—drugs effective against worm parasites inhabiting animal intestines. Merck's discovery of thiabendazole in 1961 was the first success in this area. By the mid-1970s, that interest was accelerating. A unique, proprietary, and closely protected screening process to discover anthelmintics was set up in MRL in late 1974. Merck animal health scientists saw this screening process, coupled with the unusual microbial cultures from Kitasato, as an opportunity to discover compounds with "novel modes of action" in hopes of achieving a "breakthrough" in chemotherapeutic activity against parasites.[3]

In March 1974, the Kitasato Institute sent a batch of 54 cultures to Merck. This batch followed some 1,900 compounds already received from the Institute for screening. The team of Kitasato researchers that identified and selected the cultures was led by Dr. Satoshi Ōmura, head of the antibiotics research group in the Institute. This latest batch consisted of microorganisms isolated from soil samples. The Kitasato team made its selection based upon a preliminary observation that the microorganisms might have promising bioactivity.

There was no indication which of the 54 cultures were most likely to be effective, nor any suggestion of the kind of disease the microorganisms might address, nor whether they might have antiparasitic activity.[4] Consequently, the cultures sat on shelves in Merck's Department of Microbiology for over a year. They were finally sent for screening in May 1975 to the Parasitology Department, where Dr. William Campbell worked as a Merck Senior Scientist.

Originally from Donegal, Ireland, Campbell did his undergraduate work at Trinity College where he studied Zoology as an honors student under a well-known parasitologist, J. Desmond Smyth. Campbell credits Smyth with having changed his life by developing in him a keen interest in parasitic worms.[5] Smyth encouraged Campbell to apply to a PhD program at the University of Wisconsin. Campbell describes himself as a shy, "diffident" 22-year-old.[6] Nevertheless, he succeeded in 1952 in pulling together the courage and the financing to make his way across the Atlantic to the University of Wisconsin, in Madison. He received his PhD from Wisconsin in 1957 in veterinary science and zoology with a minor in pathology.

In the final year of his studies, Campbell was preparing for a career in academia when his professor, Arlie Todd, brought to his attention a letter from Ashton Cuckler, who was actively looking to hire promising new PhDs to work in Merck's Parasitology Department. Todd encouraged Campbell to take up the offer of an interview, which Campbell did, but with a tinge of reluctance due to an anti-industry bias he had developed by then.[7]

The interview with Cuckler awakened an interest that Campbell had developed at Wisconsin in drug therapy (chemotherapy) to treat disease in animals. He left the interview thinking that the work at Merck might be more interesting than he expected. Soon after, Campbell received an offer letter from Cuckler. Having no other job offers, Campbell took the position of research associate in Cuckler's Parasitology Department at MRL in 1957.

Around this time, Campbell developed an interest in theater, which turned into a serious side-line of amateur acting in theater productions in the New Jersey area. He later took up writing poetry and painting subjects related to his work. Some of his colorful paintings were auctioned off to provide scholarship support for students pursuing studies in parasitology. Mark Siddall, president of the American Society of Parasitologists, referred to him as "a modest, selfless, humanitarian polymath."[8] In interviewing him over many hours, I was struck by the breadth of Campbell's interests and knowledge, along with his modesty and meticulous attention to detail. These qualities were undoubtedly important in leading a Merck research team to breakthrough findings in veterinary and human health during the 1970s.

The Discovery of a 'Miracle Molecule'

In the early 1970s, Merck scientists, led by Dr. John Egerton, developed the unique screening process which worked effectively in detecting potent anthelmintics. Initially employed in Merck's laboratories in Spain and installed in Merck's New Jersey labs in late 1974, the process was termed a "tandem assay" because it tested for effectiveness against both coccidian parasites, single-cell parasites that infect intestinal tracts; and nematodes, multicellular parasites, commonly known as roundworms. This screening process was highly valued by Merck management and every effort was made to keep it secret.

The tandem assay involved screening each microbial culture as it passed through a single mouse. Fermentation broths grown from an in vitro culture were fed to the mouse and the antiparasitic efficacy of the culture was gauged by the absence of worms in the intestine and/or absence of worm eggs in fecal pellets of the mouse. In Campbell's view, this assay was "absolutely critical" in discovering the highly potent antiparasitic agent that would prove effective against the microfilariae of the oncho parasite, *Onchocerca volvulus*.[9]

One culture in the batch of 54 sent by the Kitasato Institute proved to be strikingly effective. The finding was also extremely lucky. The detection of the highly potent molecule in the culture came close to being missed entirely. The only mouse used to screen that culture nearly died prematurely because of the toxic effects of an impurity in that particular screening.[10] If missed in that assay, it is quite possible that what became known as the "miracle molecule" would have never been found.

Follow-up testing showed the antiparasitic activity of that culture to be astonishingly powerful, even at the lowest doses. Campbell described his reaction when witnessing later testing, as "excitement that you knew you hadn't seen anything like this before."[11] The culture was identified as isolate #OS3153, a microorganism from a scoop of soil from a golf course near Ito, a small city 100 km south of Tokyo.

By January 1976, the microorganism had been tested on 10 different worm parasites in laboratory animals, as well as in sheep and dogs; and enough data had accumulated for Merck to hold its first formal interdisciplinary meeting on the compound. Campbell summarized the results known at that point: "We knew then that this new entity, without any molecular modification or formulation work, was the most potent anthelmintic known. It acted orally and parenterally. It had an unusually broad spectrum of activity. It apparently had a wide therapeutic index. And it probably had a novel mode of action."[12] Ironically, Merck management decided at the time not to pursue the compound for human health because testing indicated that it was less effective against hookworm and tapeworm, two of the more common helminths in humans.[13]

Campbell and Executive Director of Basic Animal Science Research Dr. Jerry Birnbaum concluded that the compound belonged to a new class of chemicals. Campbell suggested a name for the class—*avermecticins*. The name was shortened by Birnbaum to *avermectins*, which was accepted by the US Adopted Names Committee on New Drugs. Forty years later, on December 10, 2015, the Nobel Prize in Medicine was awarded jointly to Bill Campbell and Kitasato's Satoshi Ōmura for the discovery of avermectins, which, the Nobel Committee said, had provided "humankind with powerful new means" to improve human health and reduce suffering for hundreds of millions of people.

Merck chemists continued to work to refine the compound through chemical modification. But it was difficult to improve upon the avermectin formulation that had been found in nature. After extensive work, the chemists arrived at a slightly less toxic compound through hydrogenation. Merck scientists settled on the name, *ivermectin*, for the refined molecule. That basic molecule was a remarkable find— rare, potent, versatile, and safe. There has been no identical finding since—not among more than 100,000 cultures since tested in MRL; nowhere else on that Japanese golf course; and nowhere else across the globe.[14] There have been reports of similar molecules identified in Italy and in Australia, but nothing identical to that original find.[15]

The molecule was roughly 100 times more powerful than any other anthelmintic known at that time.[16] Even the smallest doses of ivermectin had antiparasitic activity. Its spectrum of activity was broader than any similar drug. It has since demonstrated effectiveness against a range of internal endoparasites, such as intestinal worms; and external ectoparasites, such as lice. It has been described in the literature as the first endectocide—an antiparasitic agent effective against both internal worms and external invertebrate insects.[17]

In February 1977, a Merck task force chose ivermectin for product development and eventual commercialization as a veterinary drug. Thereafter, Merck testing was widened and accelerated on a variety of parasites in a range of animals. This led to the important discovery in 1978 that ivermectin was effective against the pre-adult stage of the heartworm in dogs, but not lethal to the adult heartworm. This allowed the drug to be used as preventive treatment for heartworm disease without risking the life of the dog due to pulmonary embolism, a frequent occurrence when killing the adult heartworm.

Ivermectin was approved by the US Department of Agriculture in 1978 for an antiparasitic injection for cattle in the US market, under the brand name, Ivomec. Ivomec was registered in France and introduced in markets outside the United States in 1981. Ivermectin was approved for treatment of heartworm disease in dogs by the Food and Drug Administration (FDA) under the brand name Heartgard in 1987.

By the late 1980s, ivermectin had become a major veterinary commercial success for Merck, as the largest selling, most profitable drug in history for animal health, with approvals and sales in over 60 countries. The two largest formulations were Ivomec and Heartgard. By 1987, ivermectin had become the second-largest selling pharmaceutical product for Merck. Only Vasotec for congestive heart failure, and later, Zocor to control cholesterol, surpassed ivermectin in sales for Merck in the late 1980s and early 1990s.

Discovering Efficacy against Onchocerciasis

With Merck's decision to pursue product development and commercialization of ivermectin as a veterinary drug, John Egerton led Merck scientists in testing its impact on gastrointestinal parasites in horses. In April 1978, an assistant parasitologist, Lyndia Slayton Blair, suggested adding a test for the drug's efficacy on the microfilariae of *Onchocerca cervicalis*, a parasite in the skin of horses. *Onchocerca cervicalis* was widely prevalent in American horses, although it posed no significant health risk to them. The results of the test showed potent efficacy of ivermectin against that parasite.

Campbell quickly recognized the significance. The test results suggested a distinct possibility that ivermectin would be effective against *Onchocerca volvulus* in humans, because of the similarity to *Onchocerca cervicalis* in horses. Campbell had had a long-standing interest in the relationship between veterinary drugs and human formulations, and in onchocerciasis itself. He had worked on the human formulation spinoff of thiabendazole, released by Merck as Mintezol in 1964 to treat roundworms in humans.

Campbell had proposed setting up a drug screen in mice for *Onchocerca volvulus* in 1966. But that effort was stymied because *Onchocerca volvulus* would not take hold and survive in mice or in any other laboratory animal. Therefore, while the efficacy of ivermectin against *Onchocerca cervicalis* strongly suggested that ivermectin would be effective against *Onchocerca volvulus*, that hypothesis needed to be tested further by screening ivermectin's impact on similar surrogate species of that parasite employing different animal models.

Campbell remembered meeting Dr. Bruce Copeman, at an International Congress of Parasitology (ICOPA) meeting in Munich, Germany.[18] Copeman had been testing anti-parasitic formulations on another parasite in the *Onchocerca* family, *Onchocerca gutturosa*, utilizing a cattle screen, at James Cook University in Townsville, Australia. In July 1978, Campbell asked Copeman to research the efficacy of ivermectin against *Onchocerca gutturosa*. Campbell prepared the proposal calling for the testing of ivermectin throughout a range of doses. By November 1978, the results were in, showing efficacy of ivermectin against that parasite for all the proposed dosage levels. Copeman later reported to WHO his finding that ivermectin was effective in killing another cattle parasite in the *Onchocerca* family, *Onchocerca gibsoni*.

By December 1978, Campbell had concluded that there was enough evidence to bring to the attention of the higher levels in Merck the prospect of ivermectin's effectiveness against onchocerciasis. That December, Campbell wrote a memorandum to Birnbaum, his direct supervisor, expressing the view that the amalgam of recent results presented "a very exciting development."[19] Campbell recommended that Merck initiate discussions with WHO on the best way to proceed "from the medical, political and commercial points of view."[20] Birnbaum shared the excitement and passed Campbell's memo on to Dr. Roy Vagelos, president of MRL. Vagelos wrote a personal note back to Campbell strongly encouraging him to continue the research "in support of a possible evaluation of avermectins in human medicine."[21]

In March 1979, Campbell wrote to Dr. Brian Duke at WHO, an authority on onchocerciasis as that agency's Chief of Filariasis. Campbell informed Duke of the promising research results and invited him to come to Merck for further discussions on the prospects of ivermectin as a treatment for onchocerciasis. Duke accepted the invitation to visit Merck, but his response to the research results was lukewarm. Duke and others in the oncho scientific community had concluded—based in part on deliberations by the Independent Commission which was examining how best to successfully conclude the OCP—that a drug for onchocerciasis would need to kill the adult worm. Such a drug would address the root cause of the disease and possibly enable the OCP to eliminate oncho once and for all. While ivermectin had been shown to be potent against microfilariae, it had little noticeable impact on the adult female worm. Hence, ivermectin had promise as a microfilaricide, but not as the sought-after macrofilaricide.

The predominant interest within WHO and the wider scientific community in a macrofilaricide came out of the experience in controlling oncho up to then. Scientific advisors to the OCP, including WHO experts such as Duke, had been persuaded that the aerial spraying effort would be greatly enhanced if a macrofilaricide were found. That was the view of the TDR Scientific Working Group in 1976. The Independent Commission also took that position. One of the Commission's principal recommendations was the establishment of the OCT to support the development of an "operational macrofilaricide" (see chapter 3). The Commission downplayed the significance of a microfilaricide as of "limited usefulness" against onchocerciasis.[22]

The thinking was that if the reservoir of adult worms in the human population could be destroyed with a macrofilaricide, a permanent halt in transmission of the disease could be achieved relatively quickly. Then, the remaining microfilariae in the population would die out with minimal health risk to those infected. The lifespan of the microfilariae in the human body was only two years. It was unclear whether a drug, such as ivermectin, that was predominantly a microfilaricide would have any impact on oncho transmission. Interrupting transmission was critical to any successful long-term elimination effort. Otherwise, control would have to continue indefinitely, at mounting, and eventually exorbitant, cost.

There was also apprehension about the presumed side effects of a potent microfilaricide. DEC was a microfilaricide that had been used in the field during the previous 20 years, but often with a severe allergic reaction, the Mazzotti reaction, entailing extensive inflammation from the release of antigens when thousands of microscopic worms are killed off quickly. The reaction had sometimes led to blindness and even death by inducing anaphylactic shock. One hint, however, that ivermectin might be very different from DEC, came from Copeman's studies in Australia. Copeman informed Duke in 1979 that ivermectin had a slow microfilaricidal action. Duke subsequently told Campbell that he took "slow action" to be a promising sign for the drug's potential usefulness against onchocerciasis.[23] The potential for a Mazzotti reaction with ivermectin remained, but it was likely to be far less severe than with DEC because the inflammatory response to ivermectin treatment is greatly diminished.

During his visit to Merck, Duke expressed no willingness on the part of WHO to collaborate with Merck in further testing and developing ivermectin for human use. Apart from the experience with DEC, it is not entirely clear why WHO was reluctant. The microfilariae caused the debilitating itching, skin disfigurement, and blindness. Hence, there was a need for a safe microfilaricide that would alleviate the severest manifestations of the disease. And, perhaps ivermectin would turn out to have an entirely different mode of action that did not cause the dreaded Mazzotti reaction.

WHO experts were probably disinclined to favor further testing and development of ivermectin because they saw little usefulness for a microfilaricide in the OCP's vector control strategy. Furthermore, by the early 1980s, Duke had become the secretary of the OCT. Hence, at the time, he had a vested interest in the pursuit of a macrofilaricide.

There was no technical reason why a new microfilaricide could not be employed complementarily to enhance the OCP's vector control strategy and advance the West African effort toward elimination of oncho as a public health problem. The microfilaricide's usefulness was demonstrated 10 years later when the OCP delivered ivermectin in areas where vector control had not begun or was less effective. In fact, it became an essential add-on that enabled the OCP to be brought to a successful conclusion in 2002. By contrast, more than $25 million was invested in the OCT, and its successor, MACROFIL, over some 30 years without discovering an operational macrofilaricide. This investment was financing that, in retrospect, could have been employed by the TDR and the OCP to support research into more cost-effective methods of delivering ivermectin and support treatments in heavily-infected communities where suffering from oncho was most severe.

There also appears to have been reticence within WHO at that time to collaborating with a large pharmaceutical company. WHO apparently later rejected an offer by Merck to have the UN agency take responsibility for developing and managing delivery of ivermectin in oncho-endemic areas. Former director of the WHO Prevention of Blindness Program (WHO PBL), Bjorn Thylefors, reported seeing a letter sent to Merck in 1986 from WHO Assistant Director-General Warren Furth turning down the Merck offer on legal grounds. Thylefors later said, "I was struck and deeply disappointed in WHO's formalistic response to this offer from Merck."[24] WHO may have been uncomfortable with public-private collaboration in the late 1980s because it could be seen as favoring a specific pharmaceutical company in the development and use of its product. Such private sector collaboration was relatively uncharted waters for WHO at that time.

A further explanation for the lack of interest in WHO in ivermectin may have come from the top—Director-General Halfdan Mahler. Mahler, who led WHO during 1973–1988, was the chief architect behind the push to strengthen primary health care under Health for All by 2000, launched at the Conference of Alma Ata in 1978. The goal entailed strengthening health-care systems at the local level and a de-emphasis of "vertical" interventions. Attacking a single disease with a drug was a vertical program that Mahler was not interested in, according to Thylefors.[25] The reluctance to work with private pharmaceutical companies and incorporate drug donations into disease-control strategies would change dramatically over the next 20+ years. By 2012, WHO was actively collaborating with five major pharmaceutical companies on donation programs providing drugs for the largest neglected tropical diseases (NTDs) in Africa.

Ivermectin Clinical Trials—Merck Goes It Alone

Despite the tepid reaction from WHO in 1979, Merck management and staff were determined to press on with ivermectin. Researchers led by Campbell met in October of that year with three of Merck's tropical disease experts, who were medical doctors in the Clinical Development Department. Two of the three, Drs. Mohammed Aziz and Kenneth Brown, had worked in Africa and became actively involved in the ivermectin human clinical trials.

Brown was responsible for drug development for infectious diseases. He had previously worked in Ethiopia and was familiar with the treatment of oncho patients with DEC and Mazzotti reactions. He had witnessed deaths after DEC treatment.[26] Consequently, he was extremely cautious when preparing the protocol for the ivermectin human clinical trials. His priority was safety and he, along with Campbell, wanted to begin testing the drug's efficacy against hookworm, a parasite usually found in relatively healthy subjects.

Brown had been actively involved in recruiting Mohammed Aziz in 1976 to work in his office on infectious diseases. In our interview, Brown mentioned that Aziz was the first scientist he could ever recall being hired by Merck without a face-to-face interview. Aziz had outstanding academic credentials with an MD degree from Dacca Medical College, a PhD in clinical pathology from the University of Minnesota, an MPH from Johns Hopkins University, and a diploma in clinical medicine of the tropics from the London School of Hygiene and Tropical Medicine. He also had had well-respected mentors over the years.[27] Brown's office urgently needed scientists to work on infectious diseases. Furthermore, Merck was pushing at the time to diversify staff. All of the scientists working on infectious diseases were Caucasian. Mohammed Aziz was South Asian.

Aziz had been responsible for Sierra Leone, an oncho-endemic country, while working for WHO during 1975–1976. Consequently, he was familiar with the devastating impact of oncho. Having grown up in a small village in rural Bangladesh, he had retained a strong sense of empathy toward the rural poor. Campbell described him as "a deeply caring physician."[28] Aziz wanted to use oncho patients in the clinical trials, who would benefit directly from the testing.

Merck was considering two drugs for clinical development in 1979–1980. One was a nitroimidazole for Chagas disease and the other, ivermectin. Brown and Aziz agreed to flip a coin to determine who would take the lead with each drug. Based on the coin flip, Aziz assumed principal responsibility for ivermectin. He had only recently joined Merck and had not yet prepared a protocol for a clinical trial. So, Brown took the lead in drafting the protocol for the ivermectin Phase I trials.[29]

In January 1980, Merck's highest-level group of research executives, the Research Management Council (RMC), chaired by Vagelos, met to consider how to proceed with avermectins with respect to onchocerciasis in humans. Birnbaum and Campbell were flown by Merck helicopter from their MRL offices in Rahway, New Jersey, to the meeting in West Point, Pennsylvania, where they presented the case for developing ivermectin for onchocerciasis.

The meeting turned out to be a watershed in advancing ivermectin for human use. Vagelos expressed support for going forward with human trials in the meeting. He did so even though he was aware by then that the human formulation would not be a profit-making endeavor, given the low-income levels of the populations and the countries impacted by the disease.[30] Vagelos commented in a note to Birnbaum after the meeting that the Birnbaum-Campbell briefing was "one of the best organized and presented write-ups he had ever seen for a Research Management Council meeting."[31]

The RMC decided to proceed with a limited Phase I trial with very low doses of ivermectin, equivalent to one-twentieth of the "no-effect level" in the toxicology studies on laboratory animals.[32] They needed to be extra cautious because ivermectin involved a new class of molecules that had never been tested in humans. There was a possibility, however, that the drug might not demonstrate any efficacy at that low dose.

It was a momentous decision to proceed with human clinical trials. Embarking on such trials for a drug usually involved expenditures in the millions of dollars. It was clear there would be little or no financial advantage to Merck in pursuing the human formulation for onchocerciasis. But it was also apparent that there was a powerful need for a drug for onchocerciasis to alleviate immense suffering among tens of millions of Africans. There were other considerations favoring going forward. The already completed testing of ivermectin in animals would reduce somewhat the cost of testing and developing a human formulation. And, there were advantages in enhancing understanding among Merck researchers of this new class of molecules and their possible usefulness in human health.

Aziz was fervent and meticulous in organizing the Phase I trials. He sought a venue in Africa with quality facilities and clinical expertise, and selected the University of Dakar's Hôpital de Fann in Dakar, Senegal. He chose Professor Michel Larivière of the University of Paris and University of Dakar to lead the trial. Campbell later described the study: "It was (and should have been) a small trial; but it was hospital-based, well-controlled, conducted with meticulous attention to detail, and with extensive clinical support and follow-up."[33]

The 1981–1982 Dakar study involved 32 Senegalese males who were lightly infected. Aziz and Larivière refrained from selecting more heavily infected participants to avoid any Mazzotti-like reaction. It was a "crossover study" whereby low doses of ivermectin (5 µg–30 µg per kilogram) or matching placebos were given to two groups of patients. The patients were evaluated at close intervals over four weeks, with follow-up via skin snips at six weeks when they had returned to their villages. Ivermectin showed efficacy at all but the lowest doses, with complete elimination of microfilariae in the skin at the higher doses.[34]

Shortly after completion, Aziz, joined by Larivière and several other researchers in the study, wrote up the results. At Aziz's request, Campbell reviewed the draft prior to submission for publication. Campbell concluded that it had been written with "appropriate modesty and reserve."[35] The results were published in *The Lancet* on July 24, 1982.

Four months later, a letter to the editor appeared in the November 20 issue of *The Lancet* from a former OCP staff member. The letter was written by Dr. André Rougemont, a professor at the Faculty of Medicine, University of Geneva.[36] He said his views reflected his work on a technical paper recently completed with colleagues at WHO, Duke and Thylefors. The letter was highly negative on the prospects for ivermectin based on the Phase I results. Rougemont argued that the trial failed to assess the drug "in endemic zones where individual parasite densities are often very high and ocular lesions are frequent."[37] The trial showed that ivermectin only had "a moderately effective microfilaricidal action in very lightly infected patients free from ocular lesions."[38] He stated that it was "doubtful whether ivermectin has any advantages over diethylcarbamazine citrate . . ." (DEC).[39] He asserted that "the very nature of *Onchocerca volvulus* infection makes side effects inevitable if the drug used is a microfilaricide."[40] Rougemont argued that previous work showed that any "major advance" in the treatment of onchocerciasis "must be a macrofilaricide."[41] The letter concluded that ivermectin "brings no really new or interesting feature to the treatment of onchocerciasis, and the over-optimistic conclusions of Aziz and press reports of the drug's potential are not justified."[42] The letter implied that his views reflected those of WHO onchocerciasis experts, regarding the usefulness of ivermectin in the ongoing OCP control strategy.

According to Al Saah, a senior scientist who would represent Merck on the Mectizan Expert Committee for many years, ivermectin's novel mode of action consists of blocking nerve transmission in the parasite thereby paralyzing the muscles around the larynx and preventing the parasite from consuming the sustenance necessary to live. Ivermectin achieves this by targeting the glutamate-gated chloride channels in the nerve and muscle cells of the parasite. Importantly, the ivermectin molecule has no impact on the central nervous system in mammals and humans, because it is too large to cross the blood-brain barrier.[43]

Dismissal of the Phase I findings by experts who appeared to reflect the authority of WHO could have seriously stymied progress in assessing the potential of ivermectin. But the criticism had the opposite effect. It reinforced determination within Merck to pursue ivermectin studies to verify the Phase I results, along with the drug's potency and safety. Vagelos later said, "We then turned on one of the largest development programs in our history because we knew we were right, while recognizing full well that the disease afflicted the poorest people in the world who likely couldn't afford the drug."[44]

Aziz and Larivière followed up with skin snips of the participants in their villages 7–8 months after the last treatment in hospital. Surprisingly, the microfilariae had not returned. The longer than expected impact was an early hint, that would resurface several years later, that ivermectin might have a temporary impact on the fecundity of the adult female worm.

Aziz and Larivière set up a second Phase I trial in Paris in 1983, involving African immigrants. Again, the participants were lightly infected, but were given much higher doses of ivermectin, up to 200 µg/kg. All doses were effective, with greater efficacy at higher levels. The highest doses were well tolerated, suggesting that ivermectin was safe. A third Phase I trial was completed in 1984 at the WHO/TDR/OCP-supported Onchocerciasis Chemotherapy Research Centre (OCRC) in Tamale, Ghana, which had been set up to carry out drug trials for the OCT, under the leadership of Dr. K Awadzi. Various doses up to 200 µg/kg were compared for efficacy, in an open study. The results confirmed the findings in Paris. However, they were considered less reliable because there was no control group and the study population came from northern Ghana, an area that had benefited from nearly 10 years of vector control. Some patients in the Tamale study experienced a transient drop in blood pressure, or hypotension, and had to lie down, but that was largely the extent of side effects.[45]

Interest Grows in the New Drug

Based on the three-part Phase I results, *The Lancet* published an editorial in 1984 concluding that ivermectin was a "very promising drug." As a consequence, the views of the oncho experts in WHO began to shift from skepticism to budding fascination. A series of well-controlled, double-blind Phase II trials followed in Ghana, Liberia, Mali, and Senegal. In a change of heart, Duke took the lead in designing the protocol for the Phase II trials. He continued to design the protocols for the follow-on Phase III and Phase IV trials.[46] With the beginning of the

Phase II trials in 1983, the TDR and the OCP stepped up their involvement. Their interest was to assess the efficacy and safety of ivermectin in large field settings to determine its usefulness as a disease-control tool. The bulk of the financial support for the Phase II–III trials continued to come from Merck.

The Phase II trial assessed the efficacy of ivermectin compared to DEC, and addressed the ocular impact and safety of ivermectin. One finding was that a single dose of ivermectin was as effective as a large dose of DEC spread out over eight days, without the risk of a Mazzotti reaction. Moreover, the impact of ivermectin persisted in the skin for up to 12 months. The drug's longer-term efficacy was confirmed in each of the four Phase II trials. The follow-on Phase III trials showed that a single dose of ivermectin sustained a reduced level of microfilariae in the skin for up to 24 months. Excision of nodules from patients during Phase II showed that ivermectin did not kill the adult worm, but it delayed the release of new microfilariae from the adult female worm for at least three months. Hence, it was principally a microfilaricide with apparent limited macrofilaricidal action.

Dr. Awadzi, who led the trials at the OCRC, developed a scoring system for seven different clinical side effects, whereby the higher the composite score, the greater the number and intensity of side effects. The score was used to compare ivermectin with DEC and a placebo. The composite score for ivermectin was only slightly higher than for the placebo and was multiple times lower than for DEC, with patients in the DEC group often becoming sick and confined to bed by the second day of treatment.[47]

Extensive ocular examinations by ophthalmologists Taylor and Dadzie (who was released from the OCP by Samba to participate in the trials at the OCRC) in the Phase II and Phase III trials in Liberia and Ghana turned up particularly promising findings. None of the severe eye damage with DEC occurred in the ivermectin-treated patients. In previous experience with DEC treatment, there was rapid buildup of dead microfilariae in the cornea, leading to extensive allergic reactions and eye inflammation, sometimes resulting in total loss of vision. No such reaction occurred with ivermectin. Instead, ivermectin treatment resulted in a significant reduction of both live and dead microfilariae in the eye and no ocular complications. The Phase III trials showed that the long-term improvement in oncho-induced eye disease surpassed improvements in the skin. Ivermectin seemed to dramatically reduce the microfilariae in the eye, not by killing them but by drawing them out of the eye. One theory was that the ivermectin molecule is too large to penetrate the blood-retina barrier and therefore does not kill microfilariae in the eye. Instead, the live microfilariae leave the eye to fill the void surrounding the eye, created by the drug when killing off the microfilariae just outside the eye.[48] By contrast, the smaller DEC molecule penetrates the blood-retina barrier, quickly killing nearly all of the microfilariae in the eye and inducing a destructive inflammatory reaction.

Each of the Phase III trials (in Liberia, Ghana, Mali, Côte d'Ivoire, Togo, and Guatemala) tested the efficacy of ivermectin under three dose levels, 100, 150, and 200 µg/kg. The higher the dose during treatment, the greater the reduction of microfilariae in the skin during the first several days following treatment. However, by three, six, and twelve months, the impact at all three dose levels had evened out. The lower dose of 100 µg/kg was just as effective as twice that amount. In the end, these studies concluded that 150 µg/kg once yearly was the optimal dosage in terms of long-term effectiveness and minimal side effects.[49]

By late 1986–early 1987, the Phase III results were available. There was sufficient data for Merck to apply for regulatory approval in France for ivermectin to treat onchocerciasis. That approval process got underway during the first half of 1987, with France approving the drug for the treatment of oncho by October of that year—far sooner than expected.

There remained, however, the shared view within the wider oncho community, that further studies were needed to rule out the possibility of severe adverse events (SAEs) when ivermectin was used to treat far larger infected populations under a variety of field conditions. Also of interest was the effectiveness of the drug as a control tool on a large scale. To determine that, the drug had to be tested in mass campaigns in both savanna and forest oncho areas, and in a variety of oncho-endemic countries in sub-Saharan Africa and in the Americas.

Hence, it was decided to go forward with a series of Phase IV trials involving tens of thousands of oncho-infected subjects. These studies covered large communities in eight OCP countries (Ghana, Guinea, Benin, Burkina Faso, Mali, Côte d'Ivoire, Senegal, and Togo), three countries in earlier studies (Liberia, Guatemala, Malawi), and two countries where ivermectin had not yet been tested (Nigeria, Cameroon). The Phase IV trials in the OCP countries, involving a total of 50,000 people, were financed by the OCP, and the others by the TDR. Merck did not finance the Phase IV trials but one of the largest of those (in Liberia) was designed with input from Aziz.[50]

The central focus of the Phase IV trials was safety. One of the concerns in the Liberia study, conducted by a Johns Hopkins University team, was convulsions that had occurred in Collie dogs during testing in Merck laboratories. The team was looking to ensure that similar SAEs did not show up when treating large populations. None occurred. Under the Merck protocol, it was forbidden to treat children under five and pregnant women with ivermectin. Those implementing the Liberia study weeded out children under five by requiring each child to touch his/her ear by reaching over the head with the opposite arm—a method used by European bus drivers for determining which children could ride for free, which had proven quite accurate given the larger size of the head in proportion to the body in children under five. However, women who were pregnant were often unaware of their pregnancy or refused to reveal it. Consequently, the drug was given accidentally to women in the early stages of pregnancy. In those cases, no adverse effects were detected in the women or in the infants one year after delivery. These results were published in *The Lancet*.[51]

A parallel study in Liberia by the Johns Hopkins University team revealed slowing oncho transmission within a year when treating a high proportion of the infected population.[52] It was apparent that reducing transmission required the highest possible coverage with ivermectin in an area with a heavily infected population and intense blackfly biting. This was early evidence that ivermectin treatment, by itself, could reduce transmission. However, definitive conclusions about the long-term impact of ivermectin treatment on transmission and the important question of whether ivermectin by itself could eliminate onchocerciasis over time, would have to await the results of further studies over the next two decades.

Two additional large-scale community randomized studies on the impact of ivermectin on the optic nerve were carried out in Bo, Sierra Leone, and Kaduna, Nigeria. The studies found that there was no untoward impact on the optic nerve as had occurred with DEC.[53] Several outside foundations and academic institutions, including the Medical Research Council (MRC), the Edna McConnell Clark Foundation, blindness-related nongovernmental development organizations (NGDOs), and Johns Hopkins University, joined forces with the OCP and the TDR to support and carry out various Phase IV trials as well as the follow-on optic nerve studies. By the early 1990s, a broad partnership had come together to support Merck in testing the safety of ivermectin and exploring its effectiveness as an operational control tool.

Chapter 5

Getting Mectizan to Africa, Concluding the OCP

> We try to remember that medicine is for the patient. We try never to forget
> that medicine is for the people. It is not for the profits. The profits follow,
> and if we have remembered that, they have never failed to appear. The
> better we have remembered it, the larger they have been.
> —George W. Merck, Address to the Medical College of Virginia at
> Richmond, December 1, 1950

Merck Explores Options for Mectizan

With the discovery of ivermectin and the knowledge that the drug was effective and safe in treating onchocerciasis, the central consideration became how to get it to the populations afflicted with the disease. Merck management knew that those infected were extremely poor, living in rural areas. Selling the drug at a profit was not an option. Instead, the question was whether some of the production and delivery costs could be defrayed.

In 1984, Roy Vagelos was promoted to executive vice-president and assumed responsibility for the company's pharmaceutical, animal health, and specialty chemical divisions in addition to his duties as president of MRL. It was a clear sign that he was being groomed as Merck's next CEO. Within a year, the company's CEO, John Horan, retired and Vagelos became Merck's new CEO and chairman of the board. That promotion placed him in a solid position to pursue ivermectin for onchocerciasis.

The human formulation of ivermectin for oncho was trademarked "Mectizan," to distinguish it from the animal product. Merck's marketing department took on the task of trying to find an affordable price. A 6 mg dose of ivermectin in the veterinary market was priced at $3.50. So, in theory, a 6 mg tablet of Mectizan could also be priced at $3.50. But in practice, that was a nonstarter. That price was clearly out-of-reach for the oncho-infected populations in sub-Saharan Africa. The African health-care market was largely foreign to Merck. Most of its pharmaceutical products were geared toward the high-income, chronic-disease markets in the developed world. The largest selling products included statins for cardiovascular disease, Proscar for prostate enlargement, Pepcid for ulcers, and Vasotec for high blood pressure.

Charles Fettig, Merck's director of marketing for cardiovascular medications, was tasked in 1986 with coming up with an affordable price for Mectizan. Fettig initially came up with $1 per tablet. But that was deemed too high. Eventually Fettig proposed $0.10 per tablet to a high-level group that was meeting every Friday to come up with a plan for getting Mectizan out to the populations in need.[1] Even $0.10 was thought by some to be too high for a population for whom the per-capita health-care expenditure was roughly $1 per annum. Furthermore, Fettig's superiors in marketing questioned whether such a low price was worth the effort of developing a sales and marketing program.[2]

Among the most senior members of that group was Ed Scolnick, the new president of MRL. Scolnick, like Vagelos, was a physician by training. Scolnick became a strong proponent for donating Mectizan, arguing that Merck could afford it.[3] This carried particular weight coming from the head of MRL because some Merck researchers had been raising the concern that donating Mectizan could undermine future research into drugs for diseases concentrated in developing countries. Pharmaceutical companies, they argued, would be expected to follow the Merck precedent of donating new drugs for such diseases and forgoing financial returns to compensate for the R&D involved in producing those drugs.[4]

By the fall of 1987, the group had come to an understanding that the best course would be to donate Mectizan to the populations in need. But they had not yet developed a plan on how such a donation program would function. Before they could, word came from Paris that France's Directorate of Pharmacy and Drugs (DPD) was about to announce approval of Mectizan for human use to treat onchocerciasis. The timing was unexpected. Merck's experience had been that the French regulatory agency was among the slowest in approving drugs.[5] However, a French-national Merck employee, a parasitologist who had worked in Africa, Dr. Philippe Gaxotte, remained on top of the Mectizan-approval process in the DPD to urge it along. Moreover, France benefited from approving Mectizan quickly: West African immigrants infected with the disease living in and around Paris could be treated.

Throughout 1987, Vagelos tried to secure financial support to get the drug out to the affected countries and populations. He would devote most of his time over the next two years to Mectizan despite knowing that it would not be a money-maker for Merck—highly unusual for a CEO of one of the world's largest pharmaceutical companies that was actively producing and marketing several block-buster drugs. He visited the US Department of State and the White House, in an effort to secure $2 million to support ramping up Mectizan production in Merck's factory in Europe. How that amount was calculated is unclear, but it appears to have been an approximation of the first year's budget to scale up a Merck program to produce Mectizan and initiate delivery in Africa.[6]

At the State Department, Vagelos met with Deputy Secretary of State John Whitehead. Vagelos described onchocerciasis and its devastating impact on the infected populations, along with ivermectin's efficacy in treating the disease. Vagelos asked if the State Department could provide $2 million to cover the cost of initiating a Mectizan-donation program for Africa. He later described Whitehead's response: "That's great, we'll distribute the drug and plant the American flag all over Africa," as well as his own excitement, "Yeah, yeah, that's what we'll do!"[7] As Vagelos left the meeting, he was accompanied by one of Whitehead's assistants, and was told that the State Department did not have the $2 million available in its budget.

Vagelos subsequently met with Don Regan, chief of staff to President Ronald Reagan. A similar scenario unfolded: enthusiastic support, followed by cold reality delivered by an assistant. Merck staff also approached USAID with essentially the same result. USAID Administrator Peter McPherson later said that USAID had too much on its plate in 1987 to get involved in such a large drug-delivery program.[8]

Ironically, no one from Merck contacted the World Bank, which had statutory responsibility under the OCP Fund Agreement for mobilizing all financing for the oncho-control effort in Africa. In 1986–1987, I was actively engaged in securing the financing for the expansion of OCP from seven to eleven countries. There were eighteen countries, international agencies, and foundations contributing to the OCP, and donor support was as strong as ever. Almost certainly, I could have secured an additional $2 million from the donor community to begin incorporating Mectizan into the OCP control strategy. If not, $2 million could have been drawn down from the contingency reserve, which surpassed $10 million in 1987–1988. The reserve was designated for "emergencies and unforeseen developments" and the purchase of a newly-available drug at-cost would have been a justifiable expenditure.

In retrospect, it is fortunate that Merck did not approach the Bank. Had they done so, the result could have been a diversion of at least $2 million from ongoing operations during an ambitious, expensive, and uncertain period of OCP expansion. The OCP was far better off with the Merck donation program that subsequently unfolded, which provided for free Mectizan, thereby allowing for continued full-financial support for the program's other control-related activities.

Merck's Historic Decision

In the second week of October 1987, Merck management was informed by its Paris office that France's DPD was about to announce approval of Mectizan for onchocerciasis. The decision met Merck's internal requirement of having a drug approved by a "sophisticated regulatory agency."[9] Merck had not yet developed a plan, but the DPD's decision required a response. Vagelos called a press conference in Washington, DC, at the Russell Senate office building for the following Monday, October 21.

The press conference was attended by New Jersey Senators Bill Bradley and Frank Lautenberg, Massachusetts Senator Ted Kennedy, and WHO Director-General Halfdan Mahler. Vagelos opened by announcing the establishment of the Mectizan Donation Program (MDP), through which Merck would provide Mectizan free of charge to "all those who need it, for as long as it is needed." Kennedy commented that "Merck's gift . . . is more than a medical breakthrough—it is truly a triumph of the human spirit."[10] Mahler remarked that the announcement was a "symbol of industry-WHO cooperation through this marvelous cooperation we have had with Merck, which has led to today's breakthrough in making available a truly new remarkable drug, ivermectin."[11]

Mahler's statement was strange, given the tension and disagreement during the earlier stages of the human trials. Mahler had also been generally opposed to individual disease programs, such as the OCP, in his policy emphasis during the previous 10 years on strengthening primary health care in the developing world. That policy was critical of "vertical" single-disease control efforts as an uneconomic use of resources because they failed to address "universal" health needs. Mahler's policy emphasis may help explain the relative dispassion within WHO toward the OCP during the late 1970s and much of the 1980s; however, that detachment opened the door for the World Bank to take the lead on the OCP during those years.

Thylefors, the WHO official responsible for exploring ways to deliver Mectizan via NGDOs during the late 1980s, later said, "Delivering a pill for a single disease did not fit with Mahler's approach to health care and he was not interested."[12] Nevertheless, over time, the oncho programs succeeded in achieving the objectives important to Mahler. The quest for Health for All by 2000 under the Declaration of Alma Alta rested on the principles of "economic equity" and "social justice."[13] The OCP and the follow-on program, APOC, helped advance those principles by strengthening human productivity, and, particularly with the OCP, widening the availability of arable land, thereby raising income levels of the poor, subsistence-dependent segments of the population in much of sub-Saharan Africa.

The last-minute word of French approval and the rushed press conference resulted in Vagelos taking important decisions quickly and largely on his own. The language describing the donation—"for as long as it is needed, to as many who need it"—had been under consideration in the weeks and days leading up to the press conference. Ebrahim Samba, director of the OCP, had been urging Merck management to donate the drug. Charles Fettig recalls participating in a conference call at the time between Vagelos and Samba to discuss the language.[14]

The donation was deliberately unlimited in time and numbers of people treated. It is clear 30+ years later that the open-ended nature of the Merck commitment was essential to reassure the international community that the drug would be available free over the long term. Without that assurance, it is doubtful that the donors, international organizations, the NGDOs, and African governments would have made the substantial investments in the extensive multicountry delivery network that made it possible to eventually reach 100+ million rural inhabitants annually. Vagelos remarked later that he was aware that the commitment had to be open-ended for the donation program to be successful, despite the much larger financial stakes for Merck.[15]

He recalled in our interview the situation surrounding the decision:

Once we got the call from Paris that the drug was going to be approved, so many things were happening that I had no time to go to the board. I held the press conference without calling anyone on the board. But I knew I would convince the board. I based the decision on what I felt was right at the time. There was really no other decision to take. And, I knew I'd get support within the company because of the people we had there at the time. Later, when we had a board meeting and I was asked about the decision, I explained what happened and asked whether anyone would have done it differently. And, nobody raised an objection.[16]

What were Vagelos's considerations and motivations for taking this momentous decision? It was the largest drug donation in history by a pharmaceutical company at the time, and the first in the developing world. In his words:

When it was clear we had a drug that could affect millions of lives, there was no question that we were going to do it. I really did not care what the business people in the company [thought]—if they had any hesitations—I was going to push it through anyway because it was going to have a big impact on millions of people. So, in making the decision, we did it with the idea that it was the right thing to do.[17]

Vagelos regarded the financial implications as secondary: "We were coming out with so many important drugs at the time that were huge—important antibiotics, Hepatitis B vaccine, [drugs] for peptic ulcers, glaucoma, prostate enlargement, acid reflux, and the statins for cholesterol—so if a drug was going to lose money, I could care less."[18] Merck was doing so well that, as he put it, the cost implications would get "lost in the froth." However, he reflected, "Of course, I had no idea how huge and expensive the donation program would become 30 years later."[19] When I asked him whether establishing the MDP was among his proudest achievements as president of MRL and Merck CEO, he responded, "Considering the prospects of eliminating a major widespread disease and the numbers of people that would benefit, it has to be up there near the top."[20]

In a second interview with Vagelos, I presented him with my characterization of why he took the MDP decision, to see if he would agree. I said, "The physician in you—your care for the patient—rather than the businessman in you, prevailed. Your compassion for the patient led you to do what was in your power to alleviate widespread suffering that was devastating millions of people in the poorest parts of sub-Saharan Africa. So, you took the decision to provide the drug free of charge—a step within your power to alleviate widespread suffering." Vagelos responded: "You are absolutely right. I am truly a physician and a researcher. I was never a businessman—I just happened to be running Merck. I don't think anyone would have characterized me as a great businessman. That was foreign to me. I am basically a doctor."[21]

Impact and Aftermath

As Vagelos said, it was "a decision that stunned the world." Vagelos described the impact within Merck as "electric."

> People were so pleased and ecstatic that the company was going to go forward with a program that would have this big of an impact. It infiltrated the whole company. It was clear that people decades later who were being recruited—especially on the science side—came to Merck because Merck had made that sort of a decision. The impact on the company was huge and wonderful.[22]

Publicity was extensive and highly favorable for Merck. There were news reports and articles in health journals. "River Blindness: Conquering an Ancient Scourge" was the cover article of the *New York Times Magazine* on January 8, 1989.

Authored by Erik Eckholm, science and health editor of the *New York Times*, the piece included vivid photos of oncho-infected West Africans and covered the Merck decision as well as progress in controlling oncho via the OCP. Merck was selected in 1986 by CEOs and directors through a *Fortune* magazine survey as "America's Most-Admired Company" based on its success in developing new products and generating profits. After the Merck announcement, the company was selected for that top spot for each of the next six years, 1987–1992—longer than any American company since the survey began in the early 1960s. The MDP decision was undoubtedly important in that selection.

Following the MDP announcement, there were statements from Merck management, including Vagelos, that it was possible to "eradicate" onchocerciasis, as smallpox had been eradicated. It was an overly optimistic assertion. There were important unanswered questions about Mectizan's effectiveness as a disease-control tool over a widespread, populous area. The most salient was whether Mectizan could interrupt, or even diminish, oncho transmission. The answer was unclear—but critical. If there was little or no impact on transmission, it would not be possible to eliminate oncho in a confined geographical area, much less eradicate it worldwide. The answer with regard to its impact on transmission would not come for several years, after extensive field studies and oncho-transmission modeling simulations. The larger question on the prospects for eliminating oncho with Mectizan alone–that is, the long-term effectiveness of the drug in halting transmission—would not become known until 2012—25 years later.

Various studies would show that Mectizan's impact on transmission is a function of population coverage in a circumscribed area. The more extensively the drug is distributed within an infected population, the lower the parasite reservoir, and the greater the difficulty for a fly to ingest a parasite when taking a blood meal. Theoretically, if 100% of the infected population is treated with the drug, it would be virtually impossible for the fly to pick up and transmit the parasite within that confined area for at least six months, possibly up to a year. Transmission would be interrupted and longer-term elimination of the disease would be feasible, provided the infected population in that area continued to take Mectizan at least annually during the 14-year lifespan of the adult worm.

It followed that the Mectizan-delivery infrastructure and methodology were crucial because they would determine whether sufficiently high coverage levels for eliminating onchocerciasis could be achieved. Developing and implementing cost-effective infrastructure and efficient delivery systems were the next major challenge.

Getting the Drug Out

Merck management began setting up an important component of the delivery infrastructure: an expert group to review and approve applications for Mectizan. That group would also monitor Mectizan distribution and investigate any adverse reactions during treatment. Vagelos ruled out asking WHO to assume this responsibility. He felt that the UN agency was too bureaucratic for this purpose.[23] Moreover, there remained lingering mistrust from WHO's initial reluctance to collaborate on ivermectin and accept the Phase I trial results. That mistrust deepened when Vagelos saw a preprint of a WHO article on the Phase III trials that left off the names of Merck researchers involved. Vagelos complained to WHO, even threatening to write to the New York Times unless the names of the Merck scientists were added.[24] WHO revised the article, adding the names of the Merck scientists as co-authors. But the damage had been done. Vagelos later remarked, "I don't know who was making the decisions in the organization, but it indicated to me that they weren't trustworthy to get the drug out."[25]

From Merck staff involved in vaccine development and sales, Vagelos had heard about Dr. William Foege, the former CDC director who had helped spearhead smallpox eradication. Foege was chairing the Task Force on Child Survival and Development, based in Atlanta, Georgia and funded by the UNDP, World Bank, and WHO. He was also the executive director of The Carter Center. Foege was recommended as someone who could organize and manage an expert group to oversee an effective Mectizan-distribution program for Africa, in part due to his success in managing the Smallpox Eradication Program in Nigeria. Vagelos felt that Foege's leadership would provide much-needed credibility in West Africa, where distribution of Mectizan would be focused.[26] He had hesitations about Foege's ties to The Carter Center because he did not want the donation program implicated in politics.[27] But, as Vagelos later learned, connections with former President Jimmy Carter presented distinct advantages in getting commitment from African heads of state to support Mectizan distribution in their countries.

Merck sent two vice presidents to meet with Foege in Atlanta in 1987 to determine whether he would be interested in heading up an expert group to facilitate Mectizan distribution. Foege had three concerns.[28] First, how long would Merck continue to give the drug free of charge? Second, how could the donation program ensure that the infected populations would take the drug long enough to prevent the severest manifestations of the disease, such as blindness? And third, what would be the extent of side effects when the drug was distributed on a large-scale? He recalled thinking that even one death per 100,000 would mean 10 deaths per million, and that would be excessive for the program to thrive.[29]

The Merck vice presidents went into an adjacent office and called Merck Headquarters. They spoke to Vagelos and were given the answer that Merck would give the drug free for "as long as necessary to treat onchocerciasis." Based on these assurances, Foege agreed to head up the MDP and chair the Mectizan donation expert group. He did so despite warnings from colleagues not to get involved with a for-profit entity because it would eventually "pull the plug" on the donation when the company experienced pressure on its bottom line.[30] Foege later summed up the significance of the Merck commitment: "This promise is as important in the history of global health as the breaching of the Berlin Wall was to democracy."[31]

I asked Foege whether he had set certain conditions for overseeing the Merck program. He responded, "No, that's not in my nature. My instincts were to trust them based on their commitment. There was mutual trust and the longer we worked together the stronger the trust became. I learned over time that a number of those at Merck that I worked with had a strong sense of altruism, more so than some of the church groups I'd worked with over the years."[32]

Foege became chair of a new entity known as the Mectizan Expert Committee (MEC). It was an independent group of experts selected by Foege, with advice from WHO and housed in the Task Force on Child Survival and Development. The arrangement included a secretariat for the Mectizan Donation Program accountable to Foege within the task force. One objective was to establish a set of procedures within the MEC for requesting Mectizan that would shield top Merck management from constant requests for the drug, knowing that those could be expected, especially from OCP's forceful director, Ebrahim Samba.[33]

Incorporating Mectizan into OCP

Samba pushed to involve the OCP actively in the Phase IV trials to get answers to two critical questions in determining whether ivermectin could be incorporated into the ongoing control strategy: (1) the drug's safety in large-scale treatment campaigns, and (2) its effectiveness in reducing transmission. During 1987–1988, the OCP financed eight community trials in eight OCP countries, treating 50,929 people who were monitored for 72 hours after receiving ivermectin.[34] As Remme later described it, the exercise took on the tenor of a "military operation" to get answers fast.[35] The largest trials took place in the Asubende area, Ghana; the Kara region in Togo; and in the Comoé River valley in Côte d'Ivoire. Those three studies combined involved treating 40,351 people.[36] Asubende was the largest community trial ever undertaken up to that point, in one of the most heavily-endemic zones in the OCP area. Given its size and level of endemicity, the data coming out of Asubende were particularly important in reaching conclusions on safety and transmission.

The safety results from the community trials were heartening. Of more than 50,000 individuals treated over a 10-month period, 9% reported some form of adverse reaction. But only 0.24% experienced what could be termed as severe adverse events (SAEs), that entailed, in most cases, "severe symptomatic postural hypotension" (SSPH).[37] The 49 cases of SSPH involved a significant drop in blood pressure after treatment, resulting in some combination of dizziness, weakness, fainting, and confusion after standing up. Hence, the SAEs were infrequent and temporary. Their occurrence was correlated with infection intensities. More than 75% occurred in Asubende, which included the most heavily infected population of the community trials.[38]

Samba was interested in the prospects for ivermectin in enhancing the OCP control strategy. He also saw ivermectin as a major cost-saving advantage. The Merck donation was timely. The drug became available during the rapid-expansion, high-cost phase of the OCP (Phase III) and in parallel with the rapid decline in the US dollar that significantly increased program costs, when we at the World Bank were intensifying pressure on Samba to economize. Moreover, where the drug could substitute for aerial spraying, it could help avoid intensifying the spread of blackfly resistance.

In the Bank, Bernhard Liese and I were wary of any wholesale shift to Mectizan in the OCP. Liese warned that the track record for drug treatment in controlling widespread diseases had not been promising. He cited praziquantel for schistosomiasis in Egypt, where a large drug-delivery effort was launched after praziquantel was discovered in the mid-1970s. Praziquantel had proven to be highly potent in killing the flukes that cause schistosomiasis. However, a UNICEF assessment in 1989 concluded that "chemotherapy alone" had not reduced schistosomiasis prevalence in Egypt. Drug treatment needed to be combined with other interventions including health education and vector control.[39] Onchocerciasis was likely to be extremely difficult to control with Mectizan alone because the disease was concentrated in difficult-to-reach rural areas. Given Liese's warning, I concluded that it would be risky—even foolhardy—to replace vector control with Mectizan delivery, regardless of the magnitude of any cost savings.

Furthermore, Mectizan's potential in interrupting transmission was uncertain because the drug was thought to have little, if any, impact on the adult worm. Halting transmission with a drug that killed only microfilariae would require reaching a high percentage of the affected population on a continuous basis for many years. I doubted that would be possible: the disease was too widespread with a parasite transmitted over hundreds of kilometers. But I was eventually proven wrong—thankfully. I did not foresee the development and implementation of a community-based method of delivering the drug, which could reach a high percentage of the at-risk population on a sustained basis. And, I was unaware of the almost-immediate, salient impact of Mectizan on itching and on intestinal worms—strong inducements for taking the drug.

When Mectizan was later distributed in the forest regions, where itching was most severe and debilitating, the drug relieved oncho-induced itching in as little as three days. Those taking the drug would later speak of experiencing "silence" for the first time in memory. Mectizan also killed off roundworms that the patient evacuated shortly after treatment. And, the drug worked against ectoparasites, such as scabies and head lice. It was even rumored among men to enhance sexual interest and performance—probably partly due to its impact on a range of parasites. Consequently, those eligible would line up to take Mectizan. In 2015, while conducting research for this book, I, along with Dr. Laurent Yaméogo, former OCP chief of the VCU, met with the village of Linoghin, Burkina Faso, to discuss their experience with the drug. The village had ceased receiving Mectizan two to three years earlier because oncho and lymphatic filariasis (LF), the other disease for which Mectizan was eventually donated, had largely disappeared. However, the villagers who attended the meeting, all of whom were men, were outspoken in wanting the drug back, as it contributed importantly to overall well-being.

My other concern, during the advent of ivermectin, was the donors. I was fearful that their commitment to the vector-control effort might begin to wane with the sudden intense interest in this new, free drug. A drop-off in donor commitment could have disastrous implications for the ambitious plan underway of extending vector control to the west and southeast, and for ongoing aerial-spraying operations making major inroads on the parasite reservoir in the population in the original area. Consequently, Liese and I argued in the CSA for a gradual integration of Mectizan distribution into the Program's control activities as a complement to, not a replacement of, vector control.

OCP staff managing the vector control operations focused on how Mectizan could complement aerial spraying. Sékétéli, chief of entomological evaluation for the western extension, described his relief to have the new drug: "I was nervous about the vector-control results in the Gambia River Basin, Guinea, and Mali. They weren't as good as we had hoped. With ivermectin we had a solid backup, while before we only had DEC with its severe side effects. I was so relieved to have ivermectin available for the at-risk rural poor, particularly for the areas where we could not rely fully on vector control to protect them."[40]

During a visit to World Bank headquarters in 1989, Samba proposed shifting the OCP's control strategy away from vector control to primary reliance on Mectizan. The principal motive appeared to be cost savings. I was alarmed. The vector control results throughout the original seven-country area were the best they had been. The CMFLs, measuring the intensity of infection, were declining rapidly nearly everywhere. That decline was a strong indication that the adult worm reservoir in the population was aging and dying out. The results aligned closely with those predicted by the new model, ONCHOSIM.

From what we knew, the declining CMFLs were to be expected. Vector control had been underway in the original area for nearly 14 years. The maximum lifespan of the adult worm had been approximated at 14 years through ONCHOSIM, with the average lifespan estimated to be 11 years. Hence, if vector control was as effective as the indicators implied, most of the adult worms in the original area were dying off by 1988 (12–13 years after aerial spraying began). I thought it would be a major mistake to displace a proven method of control in favor of the drug, which had not yet demonstrated effectiveness in blocking transmission.

Moreover, the extent of the cost savings by relying on Mectizan was unclear. Delivering the drug via mobile teams, the method most commonly used, was costly—as was aerial spraying. Vector control was high-tech, involving helicopters, fixed-wing aircraft, and large purchases of insecticides. However, the high-tech aspect was misleading. The cost of OCP vector-control operations averaged less than $1 per person protected from the disease per year during 1986–1989, when OCP expenditures and the size of the effort peaked. More than 30 million at-risk West Africans were protected at an average annual cost of $28.6 million.[41] The Program was spraying 50,000 km of West African rivers and streams nearly weekly—twice the lengths of the Nile, Amazon, Mississippi/Missouri, and Congo Rivers combined. Other disease control efforts, such as for HIV-AIDS, were far costlier on a per-capita basis. I felt I had to continuously impress upon the donors the cost-effectiveness of vector control operations, given their scope. There seemed to be an ever-present risk that the donors might swing in favor of replacing vector control with Mectizan, in part because doing so would reduce required contributions.

Our World Bank team held to the position that Mectizan must be phased in gradually as a complement to—not a replacement of—vector control. Mectizan treatment should be concentrated in the extension areas where vector control either had not yet begun or had been less effective, such as along the fringe forest zones in the south of the program area. Some EAC members supported this position. Ultimately, vector control supplemented by Mectizan distribution became and remained the modified control strategy from 1989 through the OCP's closure in 2002.

The Search for a Cost-Effective, Sustainable Approach to Delivering Mectizan

The OCP began delivering Mectizan in 1988–1989 via mobile teams. It soon became clear that that approach was unsustainable, particularly for the West African governments when assuming responsibility for disease control. Mobile teams had been the traditional approach for the British and French West African administrations during the colonial period. But they were costly, often involving higher-paid health-care technicians, vehicles, and per diems. The search began in the late 1980s–early 1990s for more cost-effective and sustainable approaches to deliver the drug. The search was initiated by a small group of largely blindness-prevention NGDOs, that played a pioneering role in uncovering new methods of drug delivery.

The NGDOs involved in blindness prevention had begun working as a body a decade earlier. Sir John Wilson set up the International Agency for the Prevention of Blindness (IAPB) in 1975. The IAPB was an umbrella organization that served as a coordinating hub for various blindness-prevention agencies including the NGDOs. Wilson and the IAPB pushed for, and succeeded in, establishing the WHO/PBL in 1978. That program turned out to be an important vehicle for improved NGDO coordination, which, in turn, generated interest and greater involvement in onchocerciasis.

In 1980, Thylefors, principal OCP ophthalmologist, became the director of WHO/PBL in Geneva. Thylefors was by then a recognized expert in onchocerciasis, having joined OCP at its launch in 1974. As WHO/PBL director, Thylefors encouraged NGDO involvement in oncho. Once Mectizan became available, Thylefors reached an agreement with Samba and WHO Chief of Filariasis René Le Berre, that WHO/PBL would be the principal Mectizan delivery channel for WHO-Geneva. Thylefors set up the NGDO Coordination Group for Ivermectin Distribution (Coordination Group). That group became the mechanism for investigating more cost-effective approaches to Mectizan delivery and would later serve as the vehicle for NGDO participation in a wider oncho partnership under APOC beginning in late 1995.

Following the donation announcement, the NGDOs were able to procure supplies of the drug from Merck's Paris representative, Philippe Gaxotte, under Merck's "Humanitarian Program." This program got underway prior to setting up the MEC in Atlanta. Under the program, Gaxotte had the leeway to supply Mectizan tablets to approved NGDOs. As Allen Foster, former coordination group chair, described it, Gaxotte went to NGDO meetings in Africa with suitcases of Mectizan tablets from Merck's European production facilities to supply the NGDOs for their oncho treatment activities.[42] These supplies became an entrée for the NGDOs to experiment with cost-effective methods of Mectizan distribution.

With supplies of Mectizan, a pioneer group of five NGDOs—Sightsavers, Helen Keller International (HKI), International Eye Foundation (IEF), Africare, and Christoffel-Blindenmission (CBM)—commenced treatment, mostly in non-OCP countries, where they had invested in blindness rehabilitation activities. They relied on their own resources, but were also backed financially by a new NGDO, the River Blindness Foundation (RBF), established in Houston, Texas, by software executive and philanthropist John Moores. Moores first learned of oncho and Mectizan in January 1990 through an article in the *Houston Chronicle* that featured retiring Dean of the University of Houston College of Optometry, Dr. William Baldwin. In the article, Baldwin spoke of wanting to treat oncho-infected populations in the Americas. He intended to buy a van, fill it with Mectizan tablets, drive to Central America and deliver the drug to those in need.[43] Moores invited Baldwin to lunch and together they hatched a plan to establish RBF.[44] Moores initially bankrolled RBF with $25 million. Baldwin became the RBF's CEO and Brian Duke, recently retired as WHO Chief of Filariasis, was hired as the RBF's medical director.

The RBF's objective was to leverage Mectizan delivery through the NGDOs in the Coordination Group. The Foundation began providing grants totaling $1 million to the NGDOs in 1991. RBF also financed the NGDO Coordinator position in WHO/PBL, enabling Thylefors to hire Yankum Dadzie from the OCP to work with the NGDOs to strengthen their drug-distribution activities. Duke became the first chair of the Coordination Group. By 1994, the RBF had increased the funding to the NGDOs to $7 million enabling them to expand treatment to seven million people.[45] By the end of 1994, even with RBF support, the NGDOs had reached the limit of their financial and manpower resources to address the massive need for the drug in the non-OCP countries.[46] A larger organized effort was required.

The contributions of three NGDOs are noteworthy in developing more cost-effective and sustainable drug-delivery approaches. The IEF and Africare were among the first to get involved in Mectizan distribution. They launched a joint project in Kwara State in Eastern Nigeria. An IEF/Africare consultant, Dr. Bob Pond, developed the first set of guidelines on Mectizan delivery while working in the Kwara State Blindness Prevention Program. In so doing, he highlighted distinct advantages of a community-based approach: improved cost-effectiveness and higher coverage. The method he favored relied on village health workers (VHWs). Data in Pond's 1990 handbook on community treatment showed that relying on VHWs achieved a 20% higher coverage at a 40% lower cost than delivery via mobile teams.[47] Pond's seminal work set the stage for further exploration of community-based approaches.

In 1990, Sightsavers selected Dr. Michel Pacqué to head up its oncho-control efforts in Africa. Pacqué had previously been part of the Johns Hopkins University team under Hugh Taylor that conducted Phase IV trials in Liberia, and, before that, district medical officer in Zaire (later the DRC). In Zaire, he developed an appreciation for the ability of local communities to manage their own health care. In Mali, Pacqué established a practice of relying on health extension workers to distribute Mectizan. With Pacqué's encouragement, distribution devolved to the communities. Key to Pacqué's confidence in the communities assuming that responsibility was his conviction that Mectizan was extremely safe. Hence, delivery did not require health-worker oversight. He explained, "We learned during the Phase IV safety trials in Liberia that you couldn't kill anyone with ivermectin even if you tried. Overdosing wasn't an issue."[48]

Pacqué soon realized the community could deliver Mectizan more effectively than extension workers. When the extension worker arrived to deliver tablets, invariably some community members were absent—either traveling or working in the fields. Or, an otherwise treatment-eligible woman was pregnant or breast-feeding within the first week of delivery and forbidden under Merck protocol to take Mectizan. So, the extension worker would leave tablets with the community, frequently a primary-school teacher, to distribute to absentee villagers when they returned and to women after giving birth and having breastfed for a week. Villagers serving as community distributors had better information than the extension worker about returning absentees and women delivering and breast-feeding. Hence, Pacqué began promoting a new concept of community-based delivery, known as "community self-treatment."[49]

Dr. Azodoga Sékétéli, one of the OCP's leading entomologists, transferred to the OCP Bamako office in the early 1990s to become chief of entomological evaluation for the western extension operations. While in Bamako, he took an active interest in the work of Pacqué and became convinced that the community could assume full responsibility for Mectizan delivery, and, in so doing, achieve higher coverage of the at-risk population. His confidence in the local communities stemmed from his earlier experience as an agricultural entomologist working with local farmers in applying toxic insecticides in agriculture.[50]

Senior OCP staff, Yankum Dadzie and Boakye Boatin, had doubts about a community-led approach. They joked that turning over responsibilities to the local communities would be tantamount to "throwing ivermectin tablets into the sea."[51] They also had concerns that community-based distribution in the core OCP area could undermine research on the effectiveness of vector control. It would no longer be possible to determine whether aerial spraying or Mectizan treatment was causing the disappearance of parasites in the population. Moreover, they feared that the collection of data for ongoing research would be impeded if distribution responsibilities were turned over to the communities.[52]

To resolve the disagreement, Sékétéli arranged for Samba to visit villages in the Malian sub-district (arrondissement) of Baguinéda, near Bamako, in July 1992. Samba was interested in identifying concrete ways for the local communities to assume control responsibilities from OCP—a process known as "devolution," that was favored by the donors. Community self-treatment was underway in Baguinéda in 1992, among 32 villages with approximately 28,000 inhabitants. Community-selected volunteers were delivering Mectizan to treatment-eligible inhabitants. Samba met with local chiefs and spoke with community distributors in the villages of Gnogna and Tanima.[53] He was struck by the enthusiasm and capability of the volunteer distributors to undertake treatment activities. The visit convinced him that the method would work more effectively than mobile teams or relying on extension workers.

Samba subsequently met with his senior staff and, according to Sékétéli, reprimanded them: "You've been telling me nonsense; the community members are far more capable of delivering Mectizan than you think."[54] He ordered his staff to flesh out the new concept and have it adopted in OCP-backed distribution projects. This led to a brainstorming session between Pacqué and OCP senior staff at the Bamako OCP office to elaborate on the approach.[55] Prior to becoming OCP director, Samba had been responsible for primary health care in his home country, The Gambia, and had developed confidence in the communities taking charge of their basic health-care needs. Pacqué commented, "Dr. Samba was the strongest proponent of going through the communities among all of the OCP senior staff."[56]

Samba had taken a bold decision, but it seemed problematic to many. The communities would need to formulate drug-delivery strategies, abide by safety protocols, keep detailed records, store tablets for safekeeping, and select community volunteers to deliver Mectizan. Doubts about this working were widespread. Resistance cropped up from a variety of quarters. Members of the MEC expressed concerns about the implications for drug safety in relying on volunteer distributors.[57] Some OCP staff remained doubtful that the communities could fulfill the data collection responsibilities.[58] National staff and extension workers feared losing per diem if the communities took over. Even the Sightsavers' home office in Haywards Heath, UK, had reservations, given the substantial levels of financing already raised for the existing extension-worker method. Pacqué recalled: "The change was difficult for them [Sightsavers management] to accept because they felt that the ongoing approach was working well."[59]

Because it was less than 50 km from Bamako, Baguinéda became a convenient venue to showcase the new method and convince doubters. Nationals working on oncho in their home countries were brought to Baguinéda to demonstrate the effectiveness of the method.[60] Sightsavers arranged for visits from nationals involved in oncho projects in Nigeria and Uganda. One of the most important of these was Dr. Emmanuel Gemade, the principal responsible for onchocerciasis in the Nigerian Ministry of Health. Catherine Cross, former manager of international programs for Sightsavers, later remarked, "That visit was pivotal in convincing an admittedly-skeptical Gemade that a community approach to ivermectin distribution would be feasible and effective in the most heavily-endemic parts of Nigeria."[61] The OCP set up visits to Baguinéda for its own staff and nationals working in the OCP extension countries.

Samba sought out Hans Remme to conduct operational research on this new method to verify its superiority, address safety concerns within the oncho community, and develop it further into an approach that would function in a variety of rural African settings. Remme had moved in 1990 from the OCP to WHO-Geneva to manage the TDR task force on onchocerciasis operational research (OOR), set up by TDR director, Dr. Tore Godal. The hope was that the task force research, by fleshing out the concept and demonstrating that local communities could adhere responsibly to safety protocols, would convince the wider oncho community—the MEC, sponsoring agencies, donors, and African governments—of the potential of the approach to ensure high-treatment coverage throughout sub-Saharan Africa.

The resulting two-year study produced an ambitious body of research focusing on ivermectin delivery, the breadth of decisions that communities were capable of taking, and the longer-term impact of the approach across African regions. The research was led by the task force chair, Professor Oladele Olusiji Kale, from Nigeria's University of Ibadan, and Remme. It involved 26 investigators and facilitators from oncho endemic countries, the OCP, the APOC, the NGDOs, tropical disease research institutes, universities, the TDR, and the MDP; and was undertaken in close collaboration with the expert advisory committees of the oncho programs, the NGDO Coordination Group, and WHO/PBL. The evaluation took place across eight sites in five countries—two in the OCP (Mali, Ghana) and three elsewhere (Nigeria, Cameroon, Uganda).

Based on the research, the task force concluded that "community self-treatment" was misleading. Pacqué, one of the investigators, later recalled, "The term implied that Mectizan was available for community members to self-medicate, as with an over-the-counter drug—whereas there was a strict protocol for ivermectin treatment."[62] The MEC objected to the term because it gave the false impression that the safety protocols were not adhered to.[63] Midway in the study, the name was changed to "community-directed treatment" (ComDT), a term suggested by Dr. Ralph Henderson, WHO assistant director-general.[64] "Community-directed" more accurately conveyed the essence of the method: active community decision-taking and leadership.

A principal conclusion reached was that ComDT was "feasible and effective" across "a wide range of geographic and cultural settings in Africa." Consequently, it was "likely to be replicable in other endemic communities."[65] The study teams also concluded that "distribution systems designed by the communities themselves achieved better coverages than distribution systems designed for them by control programmes."[66] The decisions amenable to community decision-taking included, *inter alia*: how and when to distribute the drug, who should be responsible for distribution and record-keeping, and how the process should be monitored.[67] Another important conclusion was that distribution systems with active community involvement and entailing substantial community ownership, appeared "to have greater potential for sustainability."[68] These findings led to the final report's bottom-line recommendation that ComDT become "a principal method for onchocerciasis control in Africa."[69]

As Remme later recalled, "We thought a community-directed approach would work. African communities are very organized. Think of the example in Ghana of organizing the funeral of a chief. It's massively complicated. Take the issue of land ownership in Africa. Nothing is written down, but everything is known throughout generations. It is the community that keeps it organized. Taking responsibility for ivermectin treatment is easy for the communities. It's peanuts for them in comparison. So, that was our hypothesis before designing and carrying out the multicountry study on community-based treatment."[70] Foege later said,

> Many people thought this will never work because the village people won't keep good records. In fact, this program was so important to the villagers because they knew the price of the parasite. They were so careful about the records they were keeping, and it impressed me. So, it slowly morphed into yes, [the communities] can do this. You can go right up to the periphery and have villages keep the records. You don't have to do this out of a clinic. This was one of those things with the program that I did not expect would be that good. It's one of the nice lessons from Africa, where people oftentimes start out with the idea that nothing will work.[71]

The demonstration effect of the method in Baguinéda and the task force's research into, and elaboration of, ComDT, gradually resulted in its broader acceptance as the basic strategy for delivering Mectizan. Eventual widespread adoption of ComDT revolutionized the approach to drug delivery and treatment in rural areas in much of sub-Saharan Africa—not only for Mectizan but for other drugs and interventions for basic health-care needs.

A key question remained, however. Would ComDT increase population coverage sufficiently to interrupt transmission of onchocerciasis? The answer would determine whether Mectizan by itself could achieve elimination of the disease as a public health problem and, perhaps, rid it entirely from sub-Saharan Africa. If not, the impact of Mectizan would likely be confined to alleviating morbidity, notably itching, skin disfiguration, and blindness. In the event of the more limited impact, the disease could remain widespread in Africa. Getting answers to this question would require continuing field studies over 1990–2012.

However, Remme and his collaborators at Erasmus University in Rotterdam succeeded in deciphering one important unknown by factoring ivermectin treatment into the model, ONCHOSIM. A primary source of data for the model was the Asubende community trial which involved treating a holoendemic population of nearly 15,000 during 1987–1992. The Asubende study showed for the first time that ivermectin treatment "can significantly reduce onchocerciasis transmission."[72] Impacting transmission required reaching at least 65% of the total population in an endemic area. The Asubende study also led to the realization that ivermectin was having an impact on the fecundity of the adult female worm. That effect was inferred from successively lower "rebounds" of microfilariae in the skin over successive years.[73] Remme cautioned that 65% was not a magical threshold, but a floor below which Mectizan treatment would have little impact on disease transmission over time.[74] The important question thus became whether ComDT could reach at least 65% of the total population on a sustained basis.

Subsequent studies sponsored by the TDR during 1997–1999, involving ivermectin treatment for LF, showed ComDT reaching an average of 75%–88% of the rural populations across 80 communities in Ghana and Kenya. By contrast, delivery through the regular health services averaged "around" 45% of the populations in comparable communities in the two countries.[75] A cost-effective delivery approach capable of reaching a high proportion of the at-risk populations was an important missing piece in designing a drug-based strategy. Key to ComDT was its potential to interrupt transmission, which was essential for Mectizan to become an effective tool in eliminating onchocerciasis over the long run.

Operational research through the NGDO Coordination Group in collaboration with Nigeria's National Eye Centre in Kaduna also led to the development of a simple, cost-effective approach for determining accurate doses of Mectizan per individual in community-based treatment campaigns.[76] Early on, scales were used to decide on the number of tablets for an eligible patient based on weight. Scales were found to be impractical and sometimes inaccurate in calculating the number of tablets to avoid under- or overdosing. Analysis of weight and height data resulted in a recommendation and subsequent endorsement by the MEC in 1993 for community distributors to employ dosing poles to measure treatment-eligible individuals by height, as the most appropriate and consistently accurate technology at the community level for determining numbers of tablets per individual.[77] That simple method eventually became widespread in ComDT projects in sub-Saharan Africa, not only for Mectizan treatment but for other mass drug administration (MDA) programs as well.

Pursuing the OCP to a Conclusion

Former US Congressman Barber Conable, who was elected as the World Bank's seventh president in 1986, undertook a Bank reorganization in 1987. That reorganization resulted in the transfer of the Oncho Unit from a country operations division (responsible for country development strategies and projects) to a sector division (responsible for health, nutrition, and education projects). The new division chief, Florent Agueh, was a seasoned Bank professional from Benin who had previously been the World Bank resident representative to Upper Volta. Agueh took a keen interest in the oncho work and joined me in participating in OCP meetings during the remainder of the OCP's third, six-year phase (Phase III). The director above Agueh was Michael Gillette, who assigned a lower priority to the OCP than his predecessor, Alisbah. Gillette saw the OCP as a special program outside mainstream Bank operations and focused his attention on traditional Bank work: formulating country development strategies and preparing and implementing projects in the Sahelian countries.

By 1990, I had been the oncho coordinator for more than five years. The World Bank's personnel policy encouraged higher-level staff to rotate into new assignments, usually in a different sector and/or a different region, after five years. The policy seemed designed to develop staff into broad-gauged development practitioners and ultimately better managers with experience in a range of countries in different sectors in a variety of regions in the developing world. Given the amount of time I had been Onchocerciasis Coordinator, Gillette suggested I look for a new position in the Bank. I started the process and went through two interviews in an agriculture division. But it was more important to me to continue to work on oncho, where I felt I was making an important difference in the lives of the African rural poor, than to move up the World Bank career ladder.

I reached out to Robert McNamara for advice. He had retired from the World Bank nearly 10 years earlier but had an office within walking distance of Bank headquarters. I had been in touch with him off and on because of his continuing interest in the oncho-control effort. I presented my dilemma. He responded, "That's a silly Bank policy. Development is a long-term process that requires continuity and extended commitment. Stay where you are, if you can." That was the advice I needed to hear and it carried considerable weight, coming from him. Thus, I became determined to stay in the oncho position. The next year, Gillette moved on and was replaced by Katherine Marshall, who knew the history of the oncho-control effort and fully appreciated its importance for West Africa. After that, no one in the Bank suggested I look for another position. In 1991, I was elected chair of the CSA, a position I held for the next 13 years. In another three years, I was promoted to manager of the World Bank's Riverblindness Programs, that included the OCP and APOC, covering 30 sub-Saharan African countries.

By the end of Phase III in 1991, all indications were that the extension operations had succeeded in halting reinvasion. OCP management decided not to pursue vector control in the northern portion of the western extension, covering endemic parts of Senegal, Guinea-Bissau, and western Mali. These areas turned out not to be important sources of reinvasion principally because the wind currents carried the vector northeastward across the subregion into arid zones inhospitable to blackfly breeding and disease transmission. Consequently, the population in these areas could be treated exclusively with Mectizan.

Shutting down nearly all sources of reinvasion enabled aerial spraying to be stopped in 90% of the original OCP area during Phase IV (1992–1997). As a result, operations continued largely in the extension areas for the remainder of the OCP. The estimated cost for the Phase IV plan of operations was $176 million, slightly less than Phase III.[78] With the maximum 14-year lifespan of the adult worm determined by ONCHOSIM, the EAC recommended in 1994 that the OCP be extended from 1997 to 2002, to allow for a full 14 years of vector control in the extension areas. The 1994 JPC in Yamoussoukro, Côte d'Ivoire, endorsed that recommendation. The projected cost of extending the OCP for five years (Phase V, 1998–2002) was $74 million.[79]

Vector control operations got underway in Sierra Leone in 1989. Roughly 85% the country was heavily endemic with oncho. Extensive aerial spraying brought biting rates down from a pre-control level of 60 bites per person, per day, in 1988 to one bite per person, per day, by 1994; and reduced the CMFL in the population by over 90%.[80] However, these strikingly effective results could not be sustained. Civil conflict beginning in 1991 worsened and erupted into full-blown civil war engulfing the entire country by the mid-1990s. The OCP was forced to suspend aerial spraying throughout the country in 1996.[81] UN-sponsored peace talks in the late 1990s, followed by British intervention in 2000, eventually brought an end to the conflict in 2002, when the OCP was being concluded. By then, biting rates and CMFL measures of infection intensity had returned to pre-control levels.[82]

Consequently, Sierra Leone became the sole OCP country that failed to eliminate oncho as a public health problem by the end of the OCP in 2002 (figures 5.1 and 5.2). In 2003, the APOC began supporting Mectizan treatment throughout Sierra Leone, as part of the APOC's special intervention zone (SIZ) program for the former OCP countries. That program targeted zones where active remnants of the disease persisted. Sierra Leone was by far the largest of the SIZs. The others consisted of isolated foci mostly in the extension parts of Benin, Togo, Ghana, Mali, and Guinea (figure 5.2). Fortunately, prolonged endemicity in Sierra Leone did not result in a major reinvasion problem for the other OCP countries. Most of the vectors originating in Sierra Leone turned out to be forest blackflies that did not travel long distances. The postwar Mectizan treatment effort, financed in part through

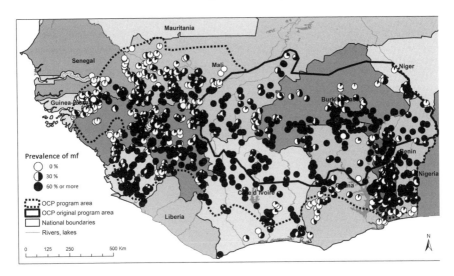

Figure 5.1. Prevalence of Onchocerciasis in the 11 OCP Countries in 1974. *Source:* Hans Remme.

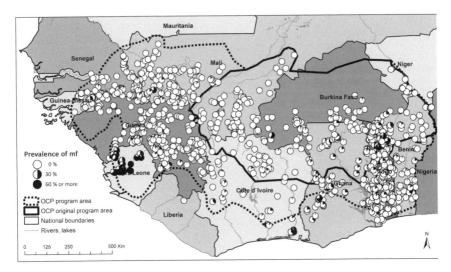

Figure 5.2. Prevalence of Onchocerciasis in the 11 OCP Countries in 2002. *Source:* Hans Remme.

the $6.4 million contingency reserve remaining in the OCP Trust Fund, reduced microfilarial levels in Sierra Leone's infected population and hence oncho transmission within the country and beyond its borders.

Once it became clear, by 1990, that the OCP was successfully halting reinvasion, Samba and I began traveling extensively to meet with donors in capitals to update them on control progress and line up support for Phase IV. We participated in one-on-one sessions in capitals with all of the donors—in East Asia, the Middle East, Western Europe, and North America. We reviewed with them the upbeat results in overcoming reinvasion and blackfly resistance. Samba explained how Mectizan was being integrated into the control strategy, i.e. focusing on the extension areas where vector control was unnecessary or infeasible and parts of the original area where vector control had been less than fully effective. He also highlighted the role that Mectizan could play in suppressing recrudescence anywhere in the OCP area once vector control stopped.

At first, I was wary of working closely with Samba given the fallout that had occurred between him and my predecessor. But, as we traveled and spent time together, we developed a mutual trust. He began referring to me as his "twin brother" in donor meetings. He sometimes recounted in jest the time that we wound up having to share a double bed in the only hotel room available in Karachi, while traveling from Bangkok to Riyadh. Our close collaboration, as the representatives of the two lead sponsoring agencies, WHO and the World Bank, became apparent to the donors. Some remarked that they valued highly that collaboration and saw it as an important asset to the control effort. It became a reason, in addition to the program's apparent success, for the donors to maintain their support during the post-expansion phase of the OCP.

Those trips, coupled with a 1991 donors conference chaired by Bank Director Katherine Marshall near Bonn, Germany, resulted in the donor community pledging $153.5 million in the Phase IV Fund Agreement, signed in 1992. That commitment covered 90% of the forecasted budget for the six-year phase.[83] The total cost of Phase IV came to $146 million—$30 million less than forecasted and $7.5 million less than the donors committed for the phase. The cost savings resulted primarily from forgoing aerial spraying in the northern half of the western extension and the use of Mectizan in place of vector control. All seemed well in hand to bring the OCP to a successful conclusion as we approached the end of Phase IV in 1997.

In 1994, Samba was elected to become director of the WHO Regional Office for Africa (AFRO). As CSA chair, I had a strong say in his replacement. Samba began openly advocating for Sékétéli, the OCP coordinator and second in command, to replace him. I did not know Sékétéli well. However, I had three concerns. First, from my limited observation he seemed somewhat heavy-handed in his management style, which might create friction with OCP staff. Second, he was an entomologist, which was not the priority expertise needed when Mectizan would be playing an increasingly important role in the OCP. Third, the OCP's autonomy had been instrumental in its success. It was a program flush with donor funding and there was concern that its ample resources might be diverted for purposes other than eliminating oncho. As OCP director, Samba had succeeded in minimizing interference from WHO-Geneva and WHO-AFRO, particularly the latter. I had observed the ongoing battles Samba waged to fend off influence from the AFRO director, Dr. Gottlieb Lobe Monekosso, who was Samba's superior, on paper. With Samba replacing Monekosso as AFRO director, I had a lingering concern that Samba might seek to control the OCP from AFRO via Sékétéli. As it turned out, none of my hesitations had merit. Although Sékétéli was not chosen as OCP director, he subsequently became a highly effective director of APOC and masterful in spearheading the scale-up of Mectizan treatment in Africa; and Samba respected fully the autonomy and independence of the OCP and APOC during his 10-year tenure as AFRO director.

With no obvious candidate from within the OCP, I thought it might work to second a highly qualified World Bank staff as OCP director, following the successful example of the directorship of Marc Bazin in the late 1970s. I had in mind Florent Agueh, my former division chief. I thought Agueh would provide strong leadership in winding the OCP down and transferring control maintenance responsibilities to the Participating Countries. He knew well the Program, the donors, and the ministries of health in the Participating Countries. He was francophone from Benin. Installing him as the OCP director would have the added advantage of helping to maintain strong World Bank support for the effort. Agueh agreed to take the position and he was acceptable to the other sponsoring agencies. Hence, it was decided that he would replace Samba. As a final step in the process, Agueh met with WHO Director-General Nakajima in Geneva. During that meeting, Agueh sensed that he would not have the full independence and authority required to be effective. Consequently, Agueh pulled out of the OCP director position just prior to taking up his post in Ouagadougou.

It seemed clear, by then, that the choice would need to be someone who was either working in the OCP or had otherwise been involved recently in program operations. After consulting around, I concluded that the best person would be Yankum Dadzie. Dadzie, a Ghanaian national, had been the OCP principal ophthalmologist for many years before becoming NGDO coordinator in WHO PBL. His participation in the Phases I–III ivermectin trials and recent involvement with the NGDOs in pursuing cost-effective, sustainable, community-based approaches for Mectizan delivery, were major assets. I knew Dadzie reasonably well and felt comfortable working with him. He was well liked, highly competent, and an effective collaborator, though his management skills were somewhat unknown. In the end, I offered the position to Dadzie, he accepted, and I communicated the selection to WHO, which, as executing agency, needed to formalize and announce the appointment.

Remme later recalled flying back home to Geneva with Dadzie from a ComDT workshop outside Kampala, Uganda in early 1995. For the first time ever, Remme decided to use the phone on the plane in business class to call his wife, Margaret. She relayed the news she had just seen on Swiss television that Dadzie had been appointed the new OCP Director. Up to then, the appointment had been kept secret in OCP circles. Remme was happily surprised to hear the news and ordered a bottle of champagne to celebrate with Dadzie on the return flight.

Dadzie thus became the fourth OCP director, starting in 1995 and continuing until his retirement in 1999. WHO selected Dr. Boakye Boatin, a Ghanaian epidemiologist working in the OCP under Dadzie, to serve as the last OCP director until the Program closed in 2002.

The Concluding Phase of the OCP

The December 1995 JPC was held in conjunction with the launch conference of APOC at World Bank headquarters in Washington, DC. As CSA chair, I gave the "CSA Reflections," an annual presentation at the opening of every JPC. The presentation was intended to summarize the views of the sponsoring agencies on the status of the control effort and future challenges. I wanted to set a tone of cautious optimism for the concluding phase of the OCP. I stressed that the basic elements were in place, "including an effective control strategy, steadfast donor support, close regional cooperation, and efficient management" to achieve the program objective of eliminating oncho as a public health problem in the West African subregion. However, we had to guard against "becoming overly complacent."[84] I saw potential danger in assuming that the war had been won and to thereby let up on the control effort during the seven years that remained.

The message was intended for the donors. They were being asked to double up their support—for both the concluding phase of the OCP and the opening phase of APOC. They would be tempted to turn full attention to APOC, a program benefiting several of the largest and most politically-influential countries in sub-Saharan Africa. I felt it was important to emphasize that any new focus on APOC must not come at the expense of reduced support for the OCP. Full control in the OCP area was not yet a done deal. In response to a question raised by a donor whether financial commitments made to APOC "might jeopardize funding for the OCP," I responded that "bringing the OCP to a timely and successful conclusion would be given the highest priority."[85]

As the entire OCP area came under control maintenance in the mid-1990s, vector control was phased out in most of the original area while Mectizan delivery was phased in. During this period, Mectizan played an important backup role in enabling the Program to stay on course and conclude as planned in 2002. Mobile teams remained the prevailing method of delivery into the mid-1990s.[86] But as it became clear that community-led distribution achieved higher sustained coverage, ComDT, with the strong backing of Dadzie, progressively replaced mobile teams.

In the later years of the OCP, Mectizan distribution reached 6.9 million people in 20,000 communities, roughly 18% of the at-risk population in the 11-country area.[87] Combining Mectizan treatment with vector control resulted in somewhat faster elimination of the parasite reservoir in the population, enabling vector control to be shortened by a year or two. Without Mectizan, it would have been necessary to extend the OCP and vector control operations somewhat beyond the 2002 closing date to achieve elimination of oncho as a public health problem in the 10-country OCP area (excepting Sierra Leone due to the civil war).

The OCP continued on its successful path during the last seven years under the highly capable leadership of Yankum Dadzie and Boakye Boatin. The final JPC took place at the OCP headquarters in Ouagadougou, in December 2002. The mood was celebratory. WHO Director-General Dr. Gro Harlem Brundtland gave the OCP "closure speech."[88] She recounted the OCP's achievements: preventing 600,000 cases of blindness; enabling 18 million children to grow up free of the disease; and opening up 250,000 km² of arable land near rivers, enough to feed 17 million people per annum. One achievement not mentioned was the OCP's protection of approximately 30 million people over at least 14 years, during which time the parasite reservoir largely died out in the population. Those years of protection prevented millions of noninfected, at-risk inhabitants from contracting onchocerciasis and spared millions of already infected victims from greater suffering caused by increasing infection levels that would have exacerbated itching and loss of vision.

Regarding the program's objective, Brundtland said, "We can all take pride in OCP. Its objective has been fully met. River-blindness has been eliminated as a public health problem in this part of Africa."[89] She added, "In reaching its ambitious goal of eliminating river-blindness, this Programme has been a forerunner in building partnerships and showing the way forward for health development. It is one of the earliest examples of a fruitful partnership with private industry."[90]

She singled out several partners for special thanks. They included: the World Bank "for having so successfully secured the funding of the Programme throughout its lifetime"; the donors for "the exceptional achievement" of retaining a donor community "practically unchanged for nearly 30 years"; the members of the CSA "for overseeing the operations of OCP, assuming responsibility for medium- and long-term planning and organizing external evaluation exercises"; and the African countries "ranging from high-level government officials to those who have sat patiently at riversides collecting black flies and those appointed by the communities to carry out ivermectin distribution."[91] Brundtland then thanked the only individual mentioned, "I cannot talk about OCP without pointing to one man who stands out. Without Dr. Ebrahim Samba, OCP would not have been what it is today. On behalf of everyone in this hall and millions of people in the region, I would like to thank you, Ebrahim, for your dedication and service to this cause."[92]

The director-general closed by saying, "The accomplishments of this Programme inspire all of us in public health to dream big dreams. It shows we can reach 'impossible' goals and lighten the burden of millions of the world's poorest people. When critics say the next proposal is too ambitious, that it will be too expensive, it will take too long, that funds will be wasted, that the job will be too complicated or dangerous—tell these critics to remember this day."[93]

Chapter 6

A Closer Look at Socioeconomic Development

> Apart from the great personal suffering it causes, onchocerciasis has a twofold destructive economic effect: not only is there reduction in the productive capacity of those afflicted by the disease, but the blind and near-blind become a charge on society; inhabitants of the fertile valleys flanking the rivers migrate to poorer lands that are over-cropped and, far from yielding marketable produce, do not provide an adequate means of subsistence.
>
> —PAG Report, Geneva 1973

Socioeconomic development (SED) was a primary driver behind the establishment of the OCP. It was a principal reason that Robert McNamara moved aggressively to establish a multi-country regional program to control onchocerciasis. The PAG Report in 1973 described onchocerciasis as "the most important single deterrent to human settlement and subsequent economic development of many fertile valleys, which lie uninhabited and unproductive. This situation inhibits the development of the vast savannah belt of the Volta River Basin area."[1] Considering the significance of the SED argument at the start of the OCP, a separate review and analysis is warranted, to trace the role of SED within the control effort and the impact of effective control on SED in oncho-endemic regions.

The Development—Onchocerciasis-Control Nexus under the OCP

Given the urgency in bringing the disease under control, it was decided not to incorporate rural development support activities in the program itself, but to encourage follow-on project support from the international organizations cosponsoring the control effort, such as the Bank, the UNDP, and the FAO; as well as from the bilateral donors funding the OCP. In the end, the OCP became and remained almost exclusively a disease-control effort. A SED unit was established in the OCP to collect data related to development of the oncho areas to facilitate development initiatives, but that unit only contained one professional who lacked the mandate to initiate SED proposals. It was intended for the FAO to lead on SED, but that agency failed to take an active role. In the end, support for SED in the oncho-controlled areas depended primarily on national governments, backed by the sponsoring agencies via the CSA.

The first initiative on SED, after the OCP was launched, was an Economic Review Mission in 1978 sponsored by the Steering Committee (later the CSA) to assess the disease as a development constraint and the potential of the oncho areas in terms of the arable land that could be utilized following successful control (see chapter 3). After that mission, there was a hiatus in oncho SED activity until the mid-1980s. Renewed donor interest was spurred in 1985, in part, by the conclusion of a highly positive USAID evaluation of the OCP that SED was not being given attention commensurate with the successful disease-control effort.[2] The implication was that the international community was missing out on an important development opportunity by failing to take advantage of the removal of a major constraint to economic activities in the rural sector in large parts of West Africa. In the October 1985 donors' meeting in Paris, the donors were near-unanimously vocal in urging the sponsoring agencies to step up their focus on SED.

In light of the renewed donor interest, I received strong support from Bank Director Alisbah, who had chaired the Paris meeting, to strengthen the SED capacity of the Bank's Oncho Unit. The unit's budget was increased and a new economist position was created to help prepare and implement a SED program. The first step under that program involved preparing terms of reference (TOR) for two regional studies to (1) conduct a development-potential inventory of the oncho zones in the 11 OCP countries, and (2) develop policy prescriptions for sustainable resettlement of oncho-freed areas. I also began leading Bank missions, that included representatives from other sponsoring agencies, to urge national authorities in selected OCP countries to consider interventions in oncho areas that might produce higher returns with removal of the disease as a development constraint. During 1986–1987, three such missions were completed in Ghana, Burkina Faso, and Guinea-Bissau. Unfortunately, the SED program experienced a setback in the 1987 World Bank reorganization, when the Oncho Unit was transferred from the Sahel Country Operations Division, which focused on country development strategies through a range of projects and sector programs, to a division confined largely to work on health and education projects. Nevertheless, preparations for the regional studies, that had gotten underway and were being coordinated through the CSA, continued.

The CSA agreed that the Bank would finance, and OCP management would oversee, implementation of the inventory study; and that the UNDP would finance, and the Bank's Oncho Unit would manage, the settlement study. Under international competitive bidding, Hunting Technical Services Ltd., was awarded the inventory study, which consisted of an assessment of physical and socioeconomic resources of the oncho areas with accompanying development proposals. That study was launched in 1987. The Institute for Development Anthropology was selected, also through competitive bidding, to carry out the settlement study, which entailed an assessment of settlement experience in the OCP countries coupled with policy recommendations to facilitate rational, environmentally-sound spontaneous settlement of oncho-freed areas. This study, referred to as the land settlement review (LSR), was conducted during 1988–1990. The two studies were financed by the World Bank and the UNDP at a total cost of $1.5 million. The results of the studies showed that the 11-country area consisted of one of the largest underutilized agricultural zones in Africa and that oncho control had already triggered spontaneous migration into riverine valleys, and, as a consequence agricultural production was increasing, in some cases rapidly.

The proposals that emerged from the inventory study did not easily translate into implementable development projects, however, when considered in the context of country development strategies. National economic planning often did not give priority to the region of the country containing the oncho area, even though the disease threat had been lifted. In the case of settlement, it was in the interest of the countries to adopt policies to promote sustainable, environmentally-sound settlement, given that substantial flows of migrants were already moving into controlled areas.

The LSR recommended a policy of "assisted spontaneous settlement" over government-planned settlement and laissez-faire spontaneous settlement. Assisted settlement involved governments, supported by donors and the NGOs, providing basic infrastructure and social services to facilitate and guide spontaneous resettlement, while allowing settlers to take basic decisions, including where to settle and what economic activities to pursue. It was also recommended that governments encourage security of land tenure, taking into account traditional tenure systems, and promote the development of markets in settlement areas. Security of tenure was considered to be a sine qua non for achieving sustainable settlement communities over the long-term. Vibrant markets were important as an outlet for production that encouraged local investment. They also promoted integration of the economic activities of host, settler, and pastoral populations, which was seen as critical for long-term settlement success.[3]

When the LSR results became available in 1992, I had begun chairing the CSA. That committee needed to decide how best to encourage the Participating

Countries to adopt the policy guidelines in the LSR report. There would need to be agreement among them to establish a consistent region-wide policy framework, as a prerequisite for rational settlement and development of the OCP area. Migration flows and settlement already underway implicated most of the sub-region. We concluded that the CSA should sponsor a high-level ministerial conference, involving all OCP countries, that would focus on sustainable settlement and development in the oncho-controlled areas. That appeared to be the best way to achieve buy-in at the appropriate levels within the 11 governments in support of a region-wide policy framework.

It was agreed in the CSA that the Bank's Oncho Unit would organize the meeting. Within the unit, we concluded that achieving the policy framework objective required involving heads of state, ministers, and representatives from ministries responsible for agriculture, rural development, and the environment, in addition to ministries of health. Bernhard Liese suggested enlisting the assistance of former WHO Assistant Director-General Warren Furth in organizing the conference. Furth had extensive high-level contacts in the Participating Countries. He agreed to take on the assignment as a Bank consultant and preparations got underway in 1993.

The Ministerial Meeting on Sustainable Settlement and Development of the OCP areas took place during April 12–14, 1994, at the World Bank office in Paris. The meeting had three main objectives: (1) to enhance awareness at the highest levels of the development potential of the oncho-controlled areas and the interconnection between spontaneous settlement of those areas and environmental risk; (2) to build a regional constituency in support of the policy framework to promote sustainable settlement of the oncho areas; and (3) to develop and reach agreement on a set of policy guidelines on sustainable settlement and development to be adopted by the Participating Countries. It was clear that attendance required high-level delegations that included heads of delegations with the authority to take and implement policy decisions. This was achieved as a result of the convening authority of the World Bank, with its influence and expertise in all of the sectors pertinent to settlement of the oncho areas.

Lambert Konan, minister of agriculture of Côte d'Ivoire, chaired the three-day session. Key participants in the opening session were: Abdou Diouf, president of Senegal; Blaise Comparé, president of Burkina Faso; and Paul V. Obeng, presidential advisor to Ghana's president, Jerry Rawlings. Ellen Johnson Sirleaf, assistant administrator and regional director of the UNDP's Africa region (and future president of Liberia and Nobel Peace Prize laureate), led the UNDP delegation. Edward Jaycox, vice president for the Africa region, headed the World

Bank delegation. All 11 Participating Countries sent ministerial-level delegations. Ten donor delegations participated, as did representatives from ORSTOM and the OECD's Club du Sahel, that had been involved in settlement and environment-related issues for many years.

Prior to the conference, the Oncho Unit prepared, for discussion, a set of guiding policy principles on sustainable settlement and development, that had emerged from the LSR. The principles, which covered issues ranging from land tenure, to transhumance, to the impact of settlement on women, generated spirited discussion during the three-day session. The result was greater awareness and appreciation of the complexity of land settlement in the oncho areas among participants. Following discussion, the principles were revised to reflect a consensus, and a final set of 15 guiding principles emerged as policy recommendations that were adopted by the 11 West African governments.[4] The key recommendations were

- Promote the social and economic integration of hosts, settlers, and pastoralists.
- Put in place a process of consultation and coordination to resolve regional issues, particularly problems associated with the movement of transhumant populations.
- Encourage "assisted spontaneous settlement" as the most appropriate for the OCP area, given the volume of migration and the financial and managerial capabilities of the governments.
- Support the formation of land management associations that involve hosts, settlers and pastoralists in land-use zoning for effective management of natural resources.
- Promote efficient markets in settlement areas.
- Put in place land-tenure regulations that take into account customary tenure systems, but also ensure secure land tenure and the access of women and youth to land and natural resources.
- Ensure that women's rights of access to, and control over, land are not lost in the settlement process.

The emphasis on gender issues arose out of the discussion and the realization that under systems involving individual tenure, women can be deprived of access to land by having to rely on tenure assigned to heads of households. Hence, it was recommended that women in new settlement communities be given explicit title to land.

The final document, including the recommendations endorsed by the ministers, as well as the rationale behind each recommendation, was distributed to all participants. That document concluded that (1) "successful settlement, the cornerstone of successful development in the OCP areas, requires a comprehensive set of policies"; and (2) "African governments and donor agencies must act immediately and decisively to adopt policies that will safeguard the unique opportunity provided by the control of onchocerciasis and ensure the sustainable settlement and development of the newly available lands."[5]

In the end, it was left that the 15 policy principles/recommendations would be addressed in the UNDP Roundtables and World Bank Consultative Groups where individual country development strategies are discussed with donors and development policies and projects are considered for support. The higher-level World Bank officials who participated in the Ministerial Meeting were pleased with the deliberations and the outcome. It was described by one, in her report on the meeting to World Bank staff, as "a resounding success."[6]

Demographic Changes

From the inception of OCP operations through the mid-1990s (when the disease had largely been eliminated as a public health problem), important demographic changes occurred in the West African oncho areas. Data on these changes was collected and analyzed in two regional studies supported by the sponsoring agencies. One was the LSR (discussed above). The other, entitled "Population Dynamics in Rural Areas Freed from Onchocerciasis in Western Africa," was organized by the FAO's land tenure service and carried out by the Committee for International Cooperation in National Research in Demography (CICRED), with financing from the FAO and the government of France.

The latter study, hereafter referred to as the FAO Demographic Study, was carried out during 1995–1996 following the Paris ministerial conference. It covered large parts of the oncho-controlled areas in nine OCP countries for which data were available; these areas were referred to as Onchocerciasis Reference Zones (ORZs). The study relied upon population censuses and historical demographic studies over a 30-year period to assess population changes that occurred following oncho control and the impact of those changes on economic activities. While a few of the ORZs were not as large as the entire oncho-controlled area in the individual country, they corresponded closely and were considered representative in terms of population changes and development impact. Both the LSR and the FAO demographic study gave particular focus to Burkina Faso as the country with the largest oncho-controlled area and the most active and consequential demographic changes.

The following sections examine the demographic changes that occurred in the oncho areas as the disease was brought under control. It draws upon the analyses and conclusions of the LSR, the FAO Demographic Study, and other related studies on SED in the oncho-controlled areas. The demographic changes were influenced by disease control, the economic potential of the oncho areas, and economic opportunities elsewhere in the individual country as well as in neighboring countries.

Upper Volta/Burkina Faso

At the center of the control-program design was Burkina Faso (Upper Volta was renamed Burkina Faso in 1984; for the sake of simplicity, I use Burkina Faso throughout this section). The disease was severe there, and the country had the largest tracts of underutilized land near rivers in the south. Moreover, it had the highest population densities in areas close by on the Mossi Plateau further to the north. Opening up new lands through vector control was seen as a way to ease population pressures through resettlement, increase agricultural production, correct population imbalances, and develop two major natural resources: land and water. The country was experiencing population pressures and land degradation in the more heavily populated plateau areas. Early reports justifying intervention argued that oncho control could make 41,000 km² of new lands, with an abundant supply of water for irrigated agriculture, available for resettlement and agricultural production.[7].

During the two to three years after the OCP operations began in 1975, vector control largely halted oncho transmission in Burkina Faso. As operations proceeded in three phases, from west to east across the country, the progressive disappearance of blackflies and incessant blackfly biting triggered spontaneous resettlement into the oncho-controlled areas. The 1976–1978 period marked the beginning of migration into the oncho areas in the lower 80% of the country, with zones to the southwest and southeast of Ouagadougou receiving the largest inflows.

By 1981–1982, four to five years after transmission had been interrupted, prevalence started to fall and declined for 10 consecutive years, to extremely low levels throughout most of the country by 1989—14 years after the launch of OCP operations. Epidemiological surveys undertaken in early 1989 in 55 villages in all of the oncho-endemic regions of the country demonstrated conclusively the rapid decline in oncho infection, as measured by the CMFL, and near elimination of the parasite reservoir in the population.[8] While reduction in the prevalence of infection would have given reassurance to would-be settlers that the oncho areas were safe, it was the earlier disappearance of blackflies and the halt in transmission that appeared to have been the strongest inducement to spontaneous resettlement.

According to censuses, the heaviest population movements into oncho-endemic areas took place during the late 1970s and early 1980s, followed by slower population inflows in the second half of the 1980s and into the 1990s. To the extent that onchocerciasis persisted after the late 1980s, it was not so severe to significantly inhibit resettlement and agricultural production. With the exception of one focus in the southwestern corner of the country, prevalence was below 5% everywhere by 2002. While, as of this writing, oncho has not yet been entirely eliminated in Burkina Faso, its persistence has not been a major barrier to economic activities.

Burkina Faso was the only OCP country to give national priority to development planning of the oncho river basins. With support from the UNDP and the French FAC, the Burkinabé government prepared in 1974 an elaborate plan for developing the country's oncho areas. It established the Volta Valley Authority (Autorité des Aménagements des Vallées des Volta), or the AVV. Under presidential decree, the AVV was given full control over 30,000 km² of land, roughly 10% of the country, in and around oncho river basins, to coordinate development planning and resettlement of areas under its authority.[9]

The AVV-designated zones were located to the south, southwest, and southeast of Ouagadougou. The AVV program during 1974–1988 resettled about 53,000 households into 412 villages in 12 planned settlements, most of which were to the east and southeast of Ouagadougou along the White Volta.[10] The estimated cost over that 15-year period turned out to be slightly less than $1,500 per household.[11] The program involved a top-down strategy that was relatively costly and encountered land-conflict difficulties by failing to incorporate the land rights of indigenous populations in settlement planning. The AVV continued in operation until the late 1980s, when it was reconfigured as an "assisted spontaneous settlement" program, officially designated as Office d'Aménagement des Territoires (ONAT).[12]

Lessons emerged from the AVV experience on the importance of integrating the needs and rights to land of host, settler, and pastoral populations. Security of tenure to land and water resources for all groups was found to be essential in designing and implementing successful settlement schemes. Traditional rights to land were held by indigenous heads of families under the authority of village chiefs.[13] Attempts to override or ignore these rights led to conflict and eventual failure of several AVV planned projects, as illustrated in case studies presented by the Club du Sahel at the 1994 ministerial meeting in Paris.

In an AVV project in Bourgouriba province in the southwest, near the border with Ghana, host populations led by a local chief fought attempts by migrant settlers to claim and farm the land, through a land-occupation strategy that resulted in failure of the settlement scheme.[14] During implementation of a project in Ganzourgou province, southeast of Ouagadougou, newly arriving settlers chased out the indigenous farmers by force of arms. In designing the project, the AVV Administration had failed to take account of the traditional land rights of the host population as agropastoralists. The end result was devastation of the natural-resource base in the area by the new settlers who, among other destructive activities, denuded the area of trees to sell wood in nearby Ouagadougou.[15]

The difficulties encountered under the AVV program eventually led to changes toward a community-based approach to resettlement. When ONAT assumed AVV responsibilities in 1990, an effort was undertaken to include the interests of indigenous populations in formulating land-tenure policies. The new approach was more participatory and consensus-based. The ONAT program also sought to address the issue of transhumance by identifying agreed-upon routes and informing herders where they could pass through a developed area without difficulty.[16] There was greater recognition that sustainable settlement required policies that promoted the social and economic integration of the rights and interests of hosts, settlers, and pastoralists.

One important impact of the AVV program was investment in basic infrastructure in oncho-controlled riverine valleys, such as roads, wells, dispensaries, and schools.[17] That investment helped attract spontaneous resettlement around the 12 planned settlements. By the late 1970s, it was evident that spontaneous resettlement was far outpacing planned settlement of Burkina's oncho-controlled river basins.[18] Studies by 1983 were showing that spontaneous settlement had resulted in more than 80% of the increase in cultivated land in the country.[19]

The FAO demographic study covered 10 provinces with a total area of 47,000 km^2 over 1975–1991.[20] The study area, or the ORZ, included most of the major river basins south of the 13th° 00' parallel and the principal valleys of the Black, Red and White Volta Rivers. All provinces in Burkina's ORZ experienced fairly rapid population growth, often higher than the national average of 2.9%, during the first decade of OCP operations, 1975–1984, with lower increases during 1985–1991. The province of Houet that includes Bobo-Dioulasso, almost doubled in population during that first decade, with an annual growth rate of 6.5%. Growth slowed to 3.7% per annum during 1985–1991. The province of Mouhoun adjacent to Mali experienced an annual growth rate of 3.7% during 1975–1985, that declined to 2.2% during 1985–1991. The faster population growth in the first decade can be partly explained by the rapid disappearance of blackflies during 1975–1977, signaling to would-be settlers that the disease threat had subsided.

Slower population growth after 1984 was probably due to reduced opportunities for resettlement resulting from the rapid in-migration earlier. By 1984, all the available lands had been developed in the Léraba valley in the southwest corner of the country.[21] In the Comoé basin next to the Léraba valley, village farmlands had doubled by 1984. And, in the Nazinon valley adjacent to Ghana's northeast border, 900 km² of lands had been cleared by then.[22] A 1985 OCP SED evaluation revealed that after 10 years of 10% average annual increases in cultivated land along the Red and White Volta Rivers in the south of the country, some areas were close to saturation levels.[23]

The provinces with large flows of in-migration and the highest population densities by 1991, were the provinces of Boulgou, Zoundweogo, and Ganzourgou, located in the center/southeast of the country, where the Red and White Volta Rivers begin to converge. These were areas where AVV projects had constructed roads and other agriculture-related infrastructure and were attracting spontaneous flows of new settlers during the 1980s. Demographic surveys showed that by 1985 the proportion of people born outside the ORZ ranged from 22% in Houet province to 75% in Boulgou province, whereas the proportion originating from elsewhere for provinces outside the ORZ was 5% or less.[24] This data was a strong indication that the oncho-controlled areas were magnets for inflows from other areas and were more attractive due to higher rainfall, the close proximity of rivers, AVV-sponsored infrastructure, or some combination of these.

Population inflows led to rapid expansion in the cultivation and utilization of available land. In 1985, the OCP conducted a large-scale evaluation (referenced above as the 1985 OCP SED evaluation) of the SED impact of oncho control in the Volta River basin after 10 years of vector-control operations. That evaluation involved comparing aerial photographs taken prior to control and 10 years later. They revealed dramatic increases in cultivated land of 9%–11% per annum along the Red and White Volta Rivers over the decade.[25] Similar increases had occurred elsewhere in the south of the country. Along the Black Volta River in the southwest, the percentage of cultivated land in the Samendéni region had increased from under 5% prior to control to 31.8% by 1985.[26]

Early in-migration attracted by the western provinces may have been partly due to faster control there under the OCP's first phase in 1975. There were strong flows of migration from the densely-populated provinces of Yatenga and Passoré

(50–100/km² in 1975) in the north on the Mossi plateau to the sparsely-populated cotton producing areas in the provinces of Mouhoun, Houet, Kossi, and Bougouriba (1–30/km² in 1975).[27] The highest in-migration occurred in the mid-to-late 1970s along the Black Volta which ran through three of those provinces.

Migration into Burkina's southwestern provinces was instrumental in the country's cotton boom that resulted in a near-steady increase of cotton production and exports during 1977–2005 by over 2100%.[28] The LSR reported a dramatic increase in cotton production in the isolated subsector of Niangoloko in Comoé province on the border with Côte d'Ivoire. Production surged from 50 tons in 1985–1986 to 500 tons in 1987–1988.[29] Settlement that contributed to this increase resulted primarily from Burkinabé migrants returning from Côte d'Ivoire.

The country's exports of cotton during 1976–1985 totaled $175 million and more than covered the government's investment in AVV settlement projects, estimated at $150 million over the decade.[30] The agriculture sector has historically been the important driver of economic growth for Burkina Faso, and, within that sector, cotton has been the most important cash crop and the most reliable and largest generator of export earnings, despite the vagaries of cotton prices on the world market.[31] Agriculture, and notably cotton, most of which has been produced in the oncho-freed areas, contributed to the country's impressive GDP growth during 1994–2014, which averaged 10.4% per annum.[32]

The FAO Demographic Study described an "inversion of migration" between the coastal countries and the countries in the SSZ. Following the inception of oncho control in the mid-1970s, there was population growth in the oncho-freed valleys reinforced by a reversal of population movements between Burkina Faso and Ghana and subsequently between Burkina Faso and Côte d'Ivoire. During 1960–1973, the population growth rate was less than 1% per annum in Burkina's central/southern provinces of Boulgou, Kouritenga, and Ganzourgou.[33] This low growth was primarily due to migration into Ghana and later into Côte d'Ivoire.

During the 1980s, this trend reversed. Burkinabé migrants returned from the early 1980s onward due to a crisis in the plantation economies of the coastal countries resulting from a downturn in cocoa and coffee prices, and political instability in Côte d'Ivoire. Migrants returned to urban centers such as Ouagadougou, as expected, but also to agricultural development poles in oncho-controlled areas that benefited from AVV-supported infrastructure, where they set up their own farms or engaged in cash-crop production. This was an important shift from earlier trends in which returning migrants settled almost exclusively in urban areas and refrained from agricultural activities. A 1991 national survey reported a population growth rate of over 3% per year in the receiving rural provinces of Boulgou, Kouritenga, and Ganzourgou.[34]

The challenge was to ensure that return-migrant settlements were sustainable over the longer-term rather than transient areas of exploitation. Doing so was more problematic with returning migrants from the coastal countries since many were young men without families. The FAO demographic study concluded that guaranteeing land and water rights was a precondition for sustainable settlement communities in the oncho-freed areas. Its authors argued for "clear rules regulating access to land in conformity with customary land rights that allow the native populations, migrants and livestock farmers to invest in the sustainable development of the land in order to ensure their subsistence without fear of losing this right one day."[35]

A study completed in 2014 by economists from Tufts University and the International Food Policy Research Institute (IFPRI) analyzed the impact of oncho control in Burkina Faso on demographic changes and resulting institutional development, independent of AVV support. The study, hereafter referred to as the IFPRI Study, relied on Burkina's decennial censuses of 1975, 1985, 1996, and 2006 as well as questionnaires for village elders regarding property rights and public services. Data was taken from 615 villages of which 60% were located in oncho-controlled areas.[36] The central hypothesis tested was that oncho control led to larger village populations with increased market-oriented property rights regarding land use.[37]

The findings of the IFPRI Study were that villages that benefited from oncho control increased in population by 25%–33%; were more likely to have market-oriented land transactions rather than land permits; and were "more closely served by rural amenities," such as markets, primary schooling, and telephone service. The study showed that disease control, at least in the case of onchocerciasis, leads to population changes that promote local institutional development, independent of government planning. The authors concluded, "Such demographic and institutional changes are clearly of great importance for Africa and other regions where endemic diseases are rooted in particular locations."[38]

Mali and Niger

Like Burkina Faso, the OCP areas of Mali and Niger contained some of the best agricultural land in terms of soil fertility and rainfall. However, unlike Burkina, the population densities of the ORZs of those countries by 1987 far exceeded the country average (approximately three times greater), given the large sparsely-populated parts of Mali and Niger that extend into the drier Sahelian zone. The total population of Mali's ORZ was 3.5 million (47% of Mali's total population) in 1987, and the population of Niger's ORZ was only 400,000 in 1988, reflecting the small geographic size of the oncho-controlled area.[39]

Population growth rates of the ORZs in both countries exceeded the country average for the 12 years following the launch of the OCP, particularly for Niger, where the ORZ population growth rate averaged 4.7% per annum during 1977–1988, and where the most heavily endemic Say Department had an annual population growth rate of 7.8%.[40] For both countries, the relatively high population growth of the ORZs resulted from in-migration based on the perceived high agricultural potential of the oncho areas. Mali's principal cotton producing regions, such as Koulikoro and Sikasso, are in the oncho-controlled areas and benefited from in-migration after 1975. Cotton production in Mali increased steadily after commencement of oncho control and doubled between 1977 and 1988 and doubled again during the 1990s. Mali was Africa's largest cotton producer and exporter during the 1980s and 1990s.

The OCP Coastal Countries

For Côte d'Ivoire, Ghana, Togo, and Benin, ORZ population densities, according to censuses 7–14 years after the launch of the OCP, remained below national averages, with a low of 11 km² in Côte d'Ivoire and a high of 37 km² in Togo. The lower densities reflected, in part, the existence of large urban areas outside the oncho areas in all four countries. ORZ population growth rates were highest in Benin (3.3%) and Côte d'Ivoire (3.3%). For Benin, the higher rate was attributed primarily to the Borgou Department, the country's second largest administrative unit with an area of 25,856 km² and a population exceeding 1.2 million (2013 estimate). Borgou, which includes the northern city of Parakou, had an annual population growth rate of 3.9% between censuses in 1979 and 1992.[41]

Côte d'Ivoire's ORZ population growth rate of 3.3% per annum during 1975–1988, was slightly below the national average of 3.8%. However, there were Departments in the northeast near borders with Burkina Faso, Ghana, and Mali with relatively high rates, notably the Départements of Ferkessédougou (5.1%), Bouna (4.4%), and Boundiali (4.8%). Two cities in the ORZ, Korthogo and Ferkessédougou, served as growth poles. The area surrounding Ferkessédougou is home to sugar and cotton plantations, and the city has sugar refineries established in the mid-1970s and acquired by a French company in 1997, that promote economic growth. Overall, the Ivoirian ORZ was a patchwork of sub-prefectures with population growth rates ranging from -1.1% to 12.2% throughout the northern 40% of the country.[42] Those with the highest rates were in the northeast relatively close to borders with Burkina Faso and Ghana. Higher population growth rates near international borders reflected a pattern in the wider OCP area in which populations settled along economically-active trading corridors.

The Ghanaian ORZ comprised three regions in the northern 40% of the country—Northern, Upper West, and Upper East. The Northern region covers 31% of the country, with ~8% of Ghana's population, a low density of 17/km² (1984), and a high annual population growth rate of 3.4% during 1970–1984, surpassing the national rate of 2.6%. The other two smaller regions to the north on the border with Burkina Faso, the Upper West and Upper East, had lower growth rates over the same 15-year intercensal timeframe. However, those regions had relatively-high population densities, reflecting the tendency of populations to congregate along trading routes near borders. The Upper East region, which includes the town of Bolgatanga near the Burkina Faso border, had the highest population density (87/km² in 1984) of any administrative region in an OCP coastal country.[43]

Togo's ORZ consisted of the Savanes Region, bordering Burkina Faso to the north, and the Kara Region. These regions had a combined population of 1.6 million, 25% of Togo's population in the 2010 census, moderate population growth of 2% during 1970–1981, and one of the higher population densities (37/km², 1981 estimate) in the coastal country ORZs. The density was greater than the numbers suggest because Togo's three national parks and protected forests cover sizable parts of the ORZ. Togo's ORZ experienced relatively-high emigration of primarily male, working-age population southward beyond the OCP area to employment opportunities, notably coffee and cocoa production, in the Plateaux Region.[44] The motivations reported by emigrants were overuse of farm lands, contributing to soil exhaustion in the ORZ, as well as economic opportunities in the receiving areas.[45]

The relatively low ORZ population growth rate of 2% is misleading, given the emigration and the population data that covered five years prior to the OCP. Parts of Togo's ORZ experienced substantial settlement and economic activity due to oncho control. One such area was the Mô River plain in the Kara region, around the town of Agbassa, where production of sorghum, rice, maize, and groundnuts surged tenfold during 1977–1988. Cotton production increased fivefold over the same timeframe in that area.[46]

THE WESTERN EXTENSION COUNTRIES—GUINEA AND SENEGAL

Following commencement of OCP operations in the western extension area in 1986–1987, the ORZs in Guinea and Senegal experienced population growth considerably lower than the other OCP countries. With time, however, population increases in the oncho-controlled areas in both countries accelerated, probably due to control. For Guinea, the population growth rate for the eight prefectures comprising the ORZ increased 0.8% during 1983–1990.[47] Those same prefectures experienced a growth rate of 3.4% during 1983–1996 based on the censuses of 1983 and 1996.[48] Consequently, the population density of the Guinean ORZ (regions of Faranah and Kankan in Upper Guinea) increased from 9.1/km² in 1990 to 14.9/km² in 1996.

The population growth rate for the ORZ in Senegal, covering seven arrondissements, was 2% during 1976–1988.[49] That rate could not be entirely attributed to oncho control because the data covered only two years of Mectizan treatment, 1987–1988. Data broken down by those seven arrondissements were not available for later years. However, the 2013 census showed that the population density of the two principal oncho regions, Kédougou and Tambacounda, which contained most of the arrondissements benefiting from treatment, was nearly three times higher, at 14.1/km², than the average density of 5.1/km² of the seven arrondissements in 1988. These data strongly suggest that the oncho area covering eastern Senegal experienced faster population growth during the 1990s and 2000s, probably due to Mectizan treatment and declining oncho transmission and morbidity.

There are potential advantages to increased population growth rates and densities in the oncho-controlled areas in protecting against recrudescence of the disease. The probability of an individual becoming seriously infected is a function of the number of flies and the corresponding number of human-beings available to be bitten. Hyperendemic areas are generally characterized by large numbers of flies and low population densities. Conversely, densely populated areas have low or nil infection rates, because fly-biting is diluted by high person/fly ratios. In his research in the late 1970s, French scholar of vector-borne diseases, J. P. Hervouet, concluded that oncho was unlikely to become a serious public health problem in villages where the density was greater than 35/km² and that it was rare to find serious blindness in areas exceeding 50/km².[50]

Cost-Benefit Analyses of the OCP

By 1990, most of the OCP cost data were available, including actual expenditures for 1974–1989 and estimates for 1990–2002. I concluded that it would be timely to conduct a cost-benefit analysis (C/B) of the Program. Doing so could strengthen donor support if credible results showed that investments in the control effort were yielding respectable economic returns. The C/B would enable donors to compare returns on the OCP with alternative projects. It was also important to calculate the OCP's economic impact for internal World Bank consumption. Prior to the OCP, there were questions within the institution about whether investing in a "soft sector" such as health could produce returns comparable to those in infrastructure, industry, or agriculture. The doubts led to resistance to the Bank becoming involved in oncho control. A properly designed C/B showing a satisfactory return on the OCP might dispel lingering doubts and strengthen support within the institution for future interventions in health.

Elizabeth Skinner, the Oncho Unit's research assistant, supported me in the exercise. We conducted a rudimentary analysis involving a calculation of the stream of economic benefits from preventing blindness and comparing them with OCP costs. We relied on data and analysis on the cost-effectiveness of OCP operations in Burkina Faso carried out by Bank staff (André Prost and Nicholas Prescott) in 1984.[51] They concluded that, on average, an oncho victim who becomes blind lives for eight additional years and dies 12 years prematurely relative to those who are not blinded by the disease. Consequently, the average oncho-blind victim loses 20 years of productive life (eight years while blind and 12 years due to premature death).

We derived the total blindness that the OCP would prevent over a 50-year period, based on the incidence of oncho blindness in Upper Volta prior to the OCP. We then estimated the value of the additional production that an individual who did not become blind would produce at the subsistence-income level of $150 per annum ($0.41 per day) and multiplied the value of that output times the cases of blindness prevented, to arrive at the stream of economic benefits over a 50-year timeframe. To factor in the better land in the oncho-freed valleys, we increased the value of subsistence income to $160 ($0.44 per day) for a portion of the population assumed to resettle those areas.

In comparing the stream of costs for the OCP with the value of the output produced by subsistence farmers protected from going blind, we calculated that the OCP had an economic rate of return (ERR) of 11%–13% per annum over the 50-year time horizon, 1974–2023.[52] It was a very basic analysis, but it gave an indication of the direction and magnitude of the economic return of the OCP. While previously working in the World Bank's Operations Evaluation Department (OED), I had conducted similar analyses for agriculture and transportation projects. By OED standards, a project with a 10% or higher ERR was considered successful. The C/B of the OCP was published in a journal of the University of Leiden in 1990.[53]

Five years later, it seemed opportune to undertake a more sophisticated C/B of the OCP. There were better up-to-date actual and projected cost figures. In fact, the actual plus estimated costs for the OCP for 1974–2002 of $556 million used in the C/B, turned out to be identical to the actual cost of the Program at its conclusion in 2002.[54] We also had data on resettlement of the oncho-freed areas from the LSR. By 1995, a new economist, Aehyung Kim, had joined the Oncho Unit. Together we carried out a more comprehensive C/B that took account of land- and labor-related benefits accruing through 2012. That analysis was published in a peer-reviewed World Bank technical paper in 1995.[55]

The analysis calculated the ERR for the OCP over the 29-year time horizon of the Program (1974–2002) plus 10 additional years, based on results from ONCHOSIM showing that protection for the at-risk population would continue for at least 10 years after cessation of control operations. On the labor benefit side, the analysis involved calculating the cases of blindness prevented by the OCP over 1974–2012, which came to 1,199,000.[56] That total was derived by multiplying the incidence of blindness prior to the OCP by the at-risk population and subtracting the cases of blindness that occurred during the OCP. Based on the 1984 Prost/Prescott analysis that preventing an oncho victim from going blind added 20 years of productive labor, we calculated that the OCP added 13,091,991 years of productive labor to the rural economies of the OCP countries over the 39-year time horizon.[57]

From that additional productive labor, we derived the additional agricultural production, assuming a labor-force participation rate of 85% and an output elasticity of labor of 0.66% (employing the Cobb-Douglas Production Function)—meaning that a 1% increase in labor results in a 0.66% increase in output. That output elasticity for labor was deemed appropriate for rural sub-Saharan Africa with only two factors of production, labor and land, and had been used in an earlier Bank study on the macroeconomic impact of HIV-AIDS. The end result, by comparing increased agricultural production from preventing blindness to total OCP costs in 1987 constant dollars, was an ERR of 6% based solely on labor-related benefits.[58]

The land-related benefits were calculated by employing the estimates of arable land by the 1978 Economic Review Mission in the original and southern extension areas and the estimates in the western extension area by the Bank's Oncho Unit.[59] Those estimates came to ~250,000 km² (150,000 km² in the original area, 49,000 km² in the southern extension zone, and 50,000 km² in the western extension zone).[60] Settlement and utilization of this land under the analysis took place during different time periods based on when OCP operations commenced in each of the three areas. It was assumed that utilization of the land began only after the incidence of the disease had declined to zero, which, based on an OCP study, occurred after eight years of vector control. Hence, utilization of the newly available land began in the original area in 1983 and in the extension zones in 1993–1995. Based on conclusions from the LSR, economic use of the land began slowly increasing in 1983, accelerated during the 1990s, and leveled off in the late 2000s, when most of the available land had been resettled.

The analysis assumed that the total land to be occupied and utilized would be 229,060 km² rather than the estimated 250,000 km², due to trends in urbanization and desertification. Based on the 39-year project horizon, 85% land utilization, and the output elasticity of land of 0.33 (a 1% increase in land results in a 0.33% increase in output), it was calculated that the land-related benefits, as measured by yearly agricultural production, compared to the stream of OCP costs, yielded an ERR of 18%.[61] This was consistent with an internal World Bank study in the Sahel countries in 1992, showing that increased production in the oncho-controlled areas was an important driver behind agricultural growth in those countries.[62] The analysis revealed that, while benefits derived from both land and labor were substantial, those accruing from the newly available land were roughly three times greater than those from improved labor.

Putting the land- and labor-related benefits together and comparing them against total OCP costs in constant 1987 dollars produced an ERR of 20% over the 39-year horizon.[63] This is a high ERR for any project regardless of sector and indicates a highly-successful project in economic terms. The analysis also showed the average cost of protecting an individual in the 11-country OCP area over the life of the Program to be $0.57 per annum in constant dollars.[64]

We tried to err on the conservative side in calculating the benefits. For labor, quality-of-life improvements were excluded as largely unmeasurable, as were productivity gains from reduced debility and disability by alleviating morbidity, notably troublesome itching and impaired vision. For land, the assumption of settlement and utilization of land after oncho incidence declines to zero, that is, eight years after vector control begins, was also conservative. The FAO demographic study, that took place after completion of the C/B, showed that spontaneous resettlement commenced in many areas two to five years after vector control started, with the disappearance of blackflies and interruption of oncho transmission.

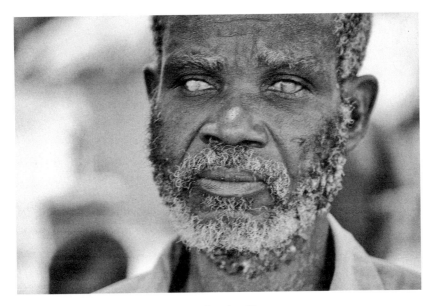

Plate 1. Man Blinded by Oncho in Asubende, Ghana, 2004.
Source: Kitasato Institute; Mark Edwards.

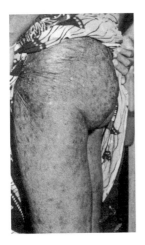

Plate 2. Agnes's Oncho Skin Lesions, Nigeria, 1990. *Source*: Uche Amazigo.

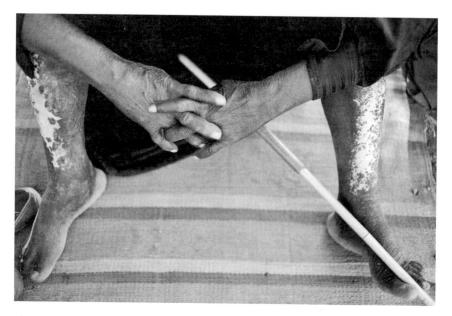

Plate 3. Oncho Victim with Leopardskin, in Shingbon, Taraba Region, Nigeria, 2010. *Source*: Mectizan Donation Program.

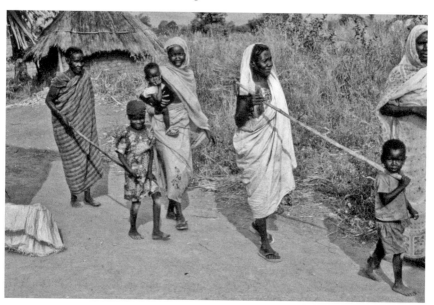

Plate 4. Children Leading Oncho-Blinded Women in South Sudan, 1997. Children in sub-Saharan Africa were often deprived of their childhood and education by having to take care of parents blinded in their prime by oncho. *Source*: Andy Crump (WHO TDR).

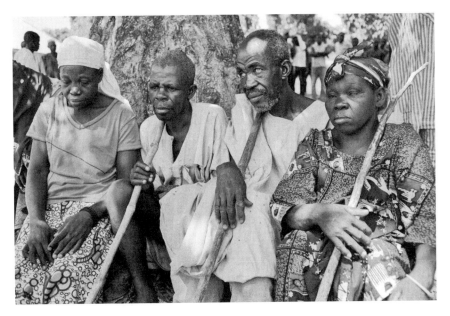

Plate 5. Two Oncho-Blinded Married Couples in Gangumi, Taraba Region, Nigeria, 2010. *Source*: Mectizan Donation Program.

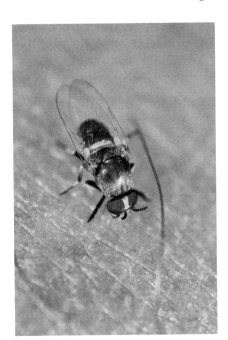

Plate 6. *Simulium damnosum*, the Most Common Oncho Vector in Africa. *Source*: Sinclair Stammers, Science Photo Library.

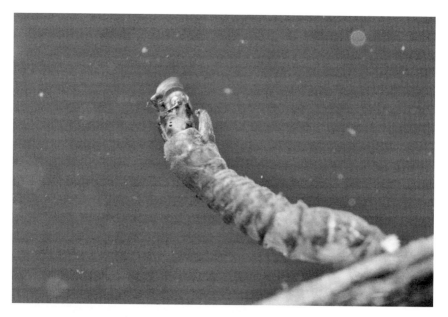

Plate 7. Feeding Blackfly Larva to Be Targeted by Vector Control. *Source*: Sinclair Stammers, Science Photo Library.

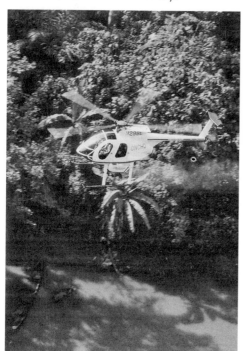

Plate 8. Aerial Spraying via Helicopter in Central OCP Area. *Source*: Onchocerciasis Control Program.

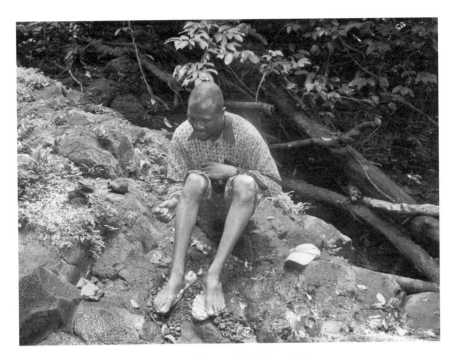

Plate 9. OCP Flycatcher. *Source*: Onchocerciasis Control Program.

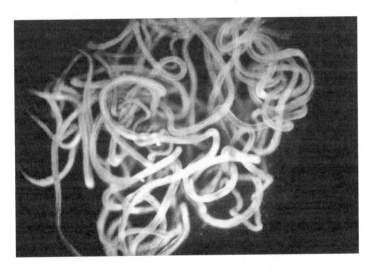

Plate 10. Photomicrograph of Adult Onchocerca Volvulus Worms in Nodule, Nigeria, 1992. *Source*: WHO Photo Library / WHO TDR.

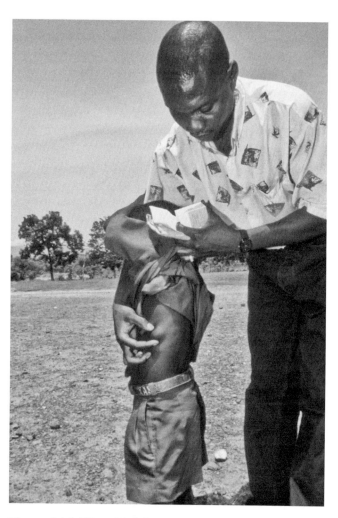

Plate 11. Adult Worm Nodule in Young Child, Nigeria, 1998.
Source: Andy Crump (WHO TDR).

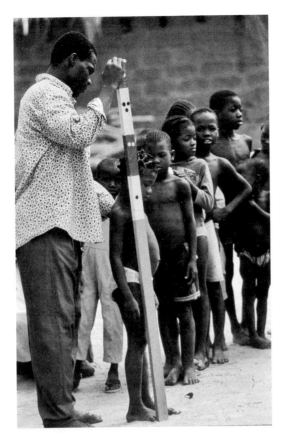

Plate 12. Measuring Height for Correct Dose of Mectizan in Nigeria, 2007. *Source*: Mectizan Donation Program.

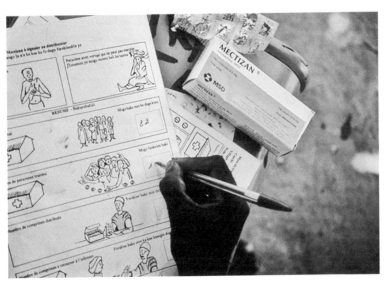

Plate 13. Community Distributor Recording Treatments, Mali, 1996. *Source*: Andy Crump (WHO TDR).

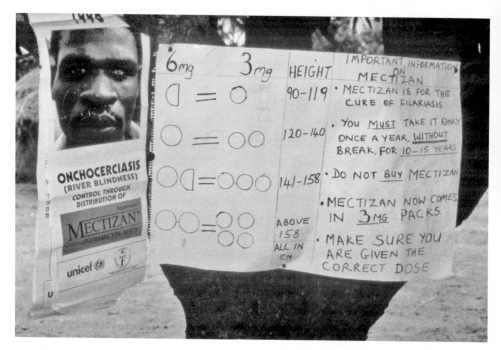

Plate 14. Poster in Nigeria Providing Information on Mectizan, 1998. *Source:* Andy Crump (WHO TDR).

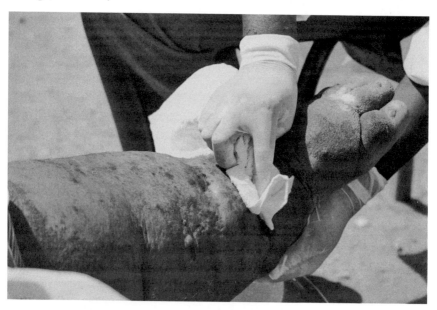

Plate 15. Treating LF (Elephantiasis) in Burkina Faso, 2007. *Source:* Mectizan Donation Program.

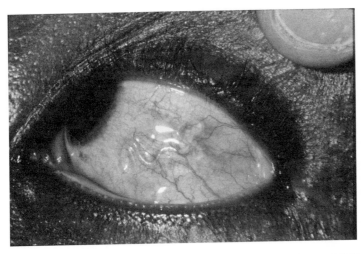

Plate 16. Photo of *Loa loa* Eyeworm Crossing the Eye, Used in RAPLOA Question-naire. *Source*: Robert Davidson.

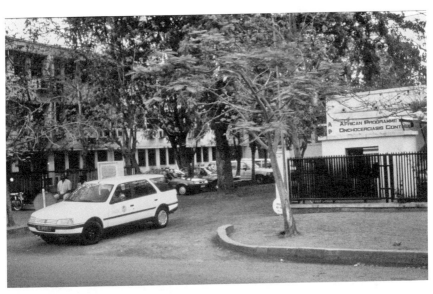

Plate 17. OCP/APOC Headquarters in Ouagadougou, Burkina Faso, 1999. *Source*: Andy Crump (WHO TDR).

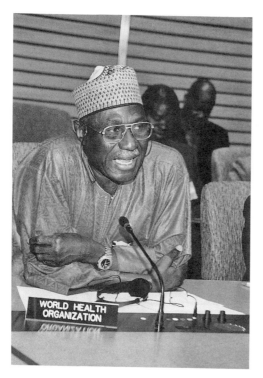

Plate 18. Ebrahim Samba Giving Presentation at 2004 Donors' Conference. *Source*: Bruce Benton.

Plate 19. 2015 Nobel Prize Ceremony in Stockholm. *Left to right*: William Campbell, Mary Campbell, Diana Vagelos, Roy Vagelos. *Source*: William Campbell.

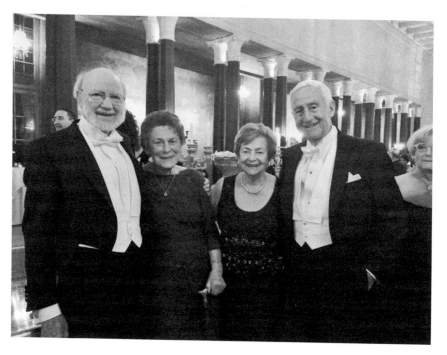

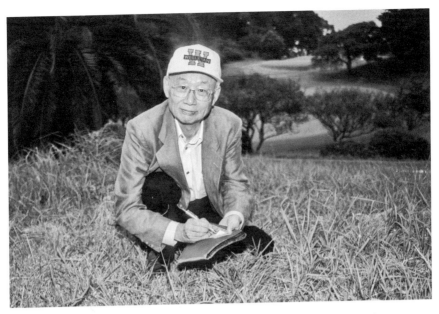

Plate 20. Satoshi Ōmura on a Golf Course in Ito, Japan. He is reenacting his 1973 retrieval of the soil sample containing the organism (*Streptomyces avermectinius*) that led to the discovery of *Avermectin* and the development of ivermectin by Merck, 2004. *Source*: Andy Crump.

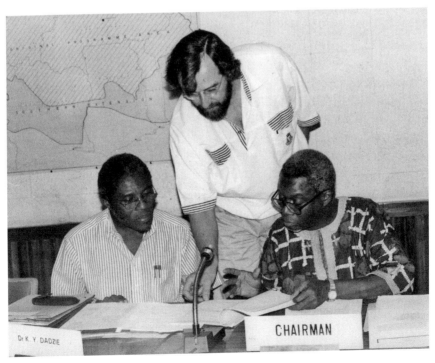

Plate 21. APOC TCC Meeting. *Left to right*: Yankum Dadzie, Hans Remme, and Chair Oladele Olusiji Kale, 1996. *Source*: Hans Remme.

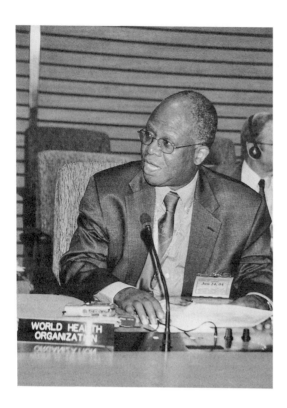

Plate 22. APOC Director Azodoga Sékétéli, APOC Donors Conference at World Bank Headquarters, 2004. *Source*: Bruce Benton.

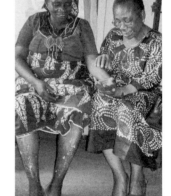

Plate 23. Uche Amazigo with Long-Term Patient Agnes, 2016. *Source*: Andy Crump.

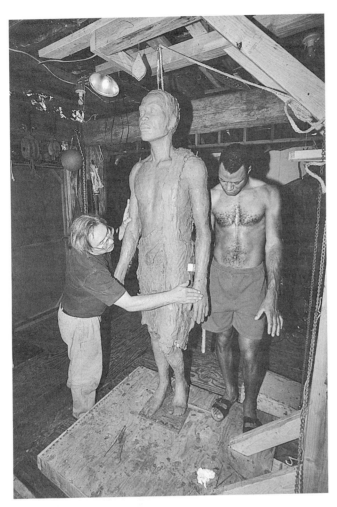

Plate 24. R.T. Wallen Sculpting *Riverblindness Statue* in His Studio, Juneau, Alaska, 1994. *Source*: R.T. Wallen.

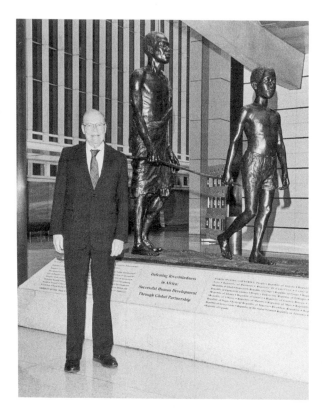

Plate 25. Robert McNamara in Front of *Riverblindness Statue* in the World Bank Atrium, 2001. *Source*: Bruce Benton.

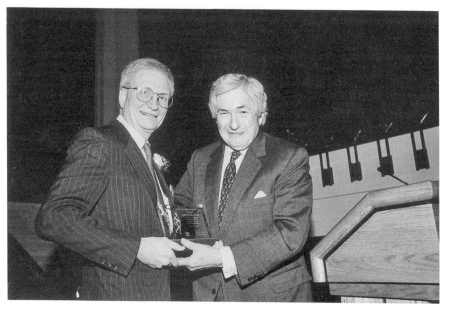

Plate 26. Author Receiving Special Presidential Award from World Bank President James D. Wolfensohn, 2000. *Source*: Bruce Benton.

Chapter 7

Widening the Effort to All of Africa

The Riverblindness Programs are the very essence of effective development partnership—results-oriented, comprehensive, widely representative, instilling ownership, capitalizing upon a diverse range of comparative advantages, and focusing on poverty-reduction. These programs demonstrate that effective partnership does not just involve an assemblage of individual partners. It requires active collaboration among them. We have seen it in the willingness of African neighbors to pool and share resources, in the mutually reinforcing steadfast support of the donor community, in achieving a broad consensus on a long-term strategy with a clear objective and a strict time-frame, and in providing a unique drug for the poorest without regard to profit.
—World Bank President James D. Wolfensohn, on the occasion of the 25th anniversary of the Riverblindness Programs and the unveiling of the riverblindness statue at WHO-Geneva, October 6, 1999.

Organizing for a Continent-Wide Battle

By the early 1990s, the OCP control strategy was well on track. With free Mectizan, a unique opportunity arose to address oncho in the rest of Africa. About 80% of the oncho at-risk population on the continent lived in non-OCP countries where vector control was not an option as the principal control strategy. Roughly half of the at-risk population in those countries lived in areas where the predominant form of the disease was forest onchocerciasis. Aerial spraying was infeasible in and around most of the forested areas due to the heavy canopy of the trees. Even if it had been feasible, employing a fleet of helicopters and fixed-wing aircraft to cover the non-OCP countries would have been prohibitively expensive due to the massive size of the area—roughly four times larger than the OCP area.

Non-OCP, oncho-endemic Africa consisted of 19 countries (20 with the independence of South Sudan in 2011) throughout parts of West, Central, East, and Southern Africa. It included an at-risk population approximately three times the 30+ million inhabitants covered by the OCP. Fortunately, free Mectizan offered the financial and technical feasibility of addressing the disease there. I was reasonably confident that the donor community would support another control effort, due to the evident success of the OCP and the size and political importance of a number of the non-OCP endemic countries. However, due to the population size, a second program would require developing a drug-treatment strategy at considerably lower per capita cost than the OCP's vector control–based strategy, to ensure adequate donor funding.

Pinpointing High-Risk Areas in Non-OCP Africa

In contrast to the extensive data on oncho in West Africa accumulated by the OCP over two decades, little was known about endemicity levels and the distribution of the disease elsewhere in Africa. Consultant work, NGDO activities, and prevalence surveys had shown that the disease existed in 19 non-OCP countries, with provisional estimates of an infected population of 14.7 million.[1] However, detailed information by country was lacking. For a Mectizan-based strategy to be effective, more data on oncho intensity and distribution were needed. Moreover, mapping oncho had to be relatively quick if drug-distribution activities were to begin and scale up under an accelerated timetable to benefit an at-risk population upwards of 100 million.

Dr. Adrian Hopkins, medical director of the CBM in Zaire (later the DRC) in 1991, described the situation:

> We wanted to treat a heavily infected village in one of the two Kasai Provinces. But in order to procure the Mectizan we had to prove to the Mectizan Expert Committee that the population warranted mass treatment. The Committee required a cluster-based survey before approving an allocation of Mectizan. We knew that there were many villages throughout that surrounding area that were also heavily infected. But we couldn't figure out a faster way to collect the data required by the Committee. The process was excessively labor-intensive and time-consuming. And, we lacked the financial resources to complete the surveys for the many villages nearby that desperately needed mass treatment.[2]

Around that time, WHO/PBL convened at WHO-Geneva a three-day conference, consisting of oncho experts and eight NGDOs to explore ways of giving guidance to NGDOs on where to focus their Mectizan-treatment activities. The conference took place in April 1991 and was led by the CBM's Allen Foster, who was chair of the NGDO Coordination Group. The participants reviewed possible rapid-assessment techniques to determine oncho prevalence levels based on manifestations such as worm nodules (encapsulated adult worms), leopard-skin, and blindness. They concluded that nodule prevalence ≥20% in males over 20 years of age was the equivalent of microfilariae prevalence in the skin ≥40% in a community, corresponding to meso-endemic or higher levels of endemicity. At that level, Mectizan treatment was deemed "highly desirable."[3] The next year, Drs. H. Taylor, B. Duke, and B. Munoz recommended a practical method for implementing the WHO/PBL-conference conclusions. They suggested, "If a nodule is detected in at least three men from a sample of 30 men aged 20 years or over, the community can be assumed to have a true prevalence of infection of 20% or more and should be included in community-based treatment."[4]

Relying on nodule palpation in a small sample of adult males became known as rapid epidemiological assessment (REA). Although REA was an improvement over skin snipping because it was quick, noninvasive, and more acceptable to communities, employing it to map the disease would require investigating nearly every village. Implementing REA widely to map the non-OCP countries would have likely meant delaying treatment of many high-risk communities that needed urgent relief from the disease. A faster, reliable method for pinpointing populations to treat was required.

TDR consultants investigated ways of accelerating REA. A 1993 study in Cameroon by Drs. Pierre Ngoumou and Frank Walsh proposed a mapping technique that required only limited basic information: "a general understanding of the ecology and behavior of the vector, the epidemiology of onchocerciasis, and knowledge of the geography of the area."[5] Their proposal led to a TDR-sponsored workshop in Ouagadougou in 1996 that refined the methodology and produced guidelines for the mapping technique, rapid epidemiological mapping of onchocerciasis (REMO). REMO got underway shortly thereafter and set the stage for launching ComDT projects focusing on "high-risk" communities.

REMO relied upon the REA concept whereby nodules in a community are a proxy for oncho prevalence as determined by levels of microfilariae in the skin, usually measured by skin snips. The technique involved nodule palpation of a sample of men 20 years or older. Age was important to ensure that the men had been exposed to fly biting for at least 10 years and for the worms to become developed in easily detectable nodules. Nodule palpation was confined to men, in part because men are on average more heavily infected than women, and to avoid having male investigators examining the bodies of women. This noninvasive, pain-free method proved to be better tolerated than skin snipping.

A premise of REMO was that nodule palpation in every village in every country was infeasible. Shortcuts were necessary. Under REMO guidelines, a sample of villages comprising 2%–5% of the total number in a wide area was sufficient to arrive at reliable results.[6] A small sample was possible by relying on the spatial-entomological characteristics of the blackfly. It was known that blackflies congregate and bite most frequently within a 10–15 km radius of a river. The first villages selected for the sample would be the highest-at-risk villages closest to river rapids where the blackfly breeds. Those villages at the front line are the most exposed to blackfly biting and the disease. A front-line community was selected every 30–50 km along a river.[7] For each front-line community, a secondary village was chosen at least 10 km farther away from the breeding sites.[8] Handheld GPS devices were used to record the coordinates of each sampled village. Results from the front-line and secondary villages were extrapolated to other villages to delineate wide-treatment areas in each country. The REMO aim was to complete mapping for an entire country within 20–25 days.[9]

In 1991, a WHO expert committee recommended treating all communities where the prevalence of onchocerciasis was ≥35%, as determined by microfilariae in the skin.[10] This threshold was the endemicity level considered necessary to treat to achieve "elimination of the disease as a public health problem"—the explicit objective of the OCP and APOC. Treating all communities with oncho prevalence ≥ 35% was equivalent to covering all "hyperendemic" and "meso-endemic" communities. Under OCP classifications, an area was hyperendemic if oncho prevalence was ≥60%, and meso-endemic if prevalence fell within the 35%–60% range. Areas where all communities had a prevalence of less than 35% were classified as "hypo-endemic." WHO experts concluded that treating hypo-endemic areas was not necessary to eliminate oncho as a public health problem.

With the advent of REA, the measure of meso-endemicity or greater became a nodule prevalence rate of ≥20%. Consequently, under REMO, the objective became to identify all communities with nodule prevalence ≥20%, by examining 30–50 adult males for nodules in each sample village. It was also determined that levels of blindness and troublesome itching were linearly related to nodule prevalence. In other words, more nodules in more people in a community meant higher levels of blindness and greater itching.

REMO turned out to be an ambitious decade-long exercise that, coupled with OCP mapping data, resulted in the first mapping of a major NTD for all of Africa.[11] The timing of REMO proved critical in planning and rapidly scaling up Mectizan-based control. REMO got underway in 1996, with the launch of APOC. Over the subsequent decade, national teams, established by each country's National Onchocerciasis Task Force (NOTF), conducted surveys in 14,473 villages and examined more than 500,000 adults for nodules.[12] The surveys were largely financed by APOC. The results were reviewed by the TCC to ensure quality standardization. Eventually, all survey teams were equipped with handheld GPS devices. Coordinates of surveyed villages coupled with pie charts of village-specific nodule prevalence levels were incorporated into a geographic information system (GIS). Data on rivers, streams, infrastructure, administrative boundaries, and population densities were added to the GIS.[13] All of the GIS information was then spatially displayed on maps for analysis in determining where to focus Mectizan treatment projects.

Areas designated as "high risk" (nodule prevalence $\geq$ 20%) were identified in 17 countries. The population in those areas was estimated to be 86 million (2011 estimate).[14] One contiguous high-risk area, exceeding 2,000,000 km^2 and covering portions of seven countries, extended from Nigeria eastward to South Sudan and southward to the DRC and Angola.[15] Half of the surface area and more than 30% of the population were found to be at high-risk for oncho in five countries— Cameroon, Central African Republic (CAR), the DRC, Liberia, and South Sudan.[16] More than 60% of the high-risk population in non-OCP Africa lived in two countries—the DRC (28 million inhabitants) and Nigeria (26 million inhabitants).[17] High-risk areas not previously known to exist were identified in Angola, Cameroon, the DRC, and Tanzania.[18] Among the 19 countries surveyed, only Kenya and Rwanda were found to have no high-risk communities.

The map below (figure 7.1) highlights the high-risk areas identified by REMO. These became staging areas for the design, preparation, and implementation of ComDT projects. For the most part, mapping proceeded quickly for the larger non-OCP countries, including Nigeria, Cameroon, Ethiopia, Uganda, and Tanzania. Consequently, projects were prepared and launched in those countries to cover most of their high-risk areas within five years of beginning REMO. However, mapping in countries experiencing political instability, including the DRC, Angola, Burundi, the CAR, and South Sudan, proceeded more slowly. Full REMO results were not available in these countries until 2005–2006, delaying treatment of their high-risk populations.[19]

Collaboration between the TDR and the CSA during the first half of the 1990s was instrumental in completing the bulk of the operational research required to launch and scale up APOC during that all-important initial 5- to 10-year timeframe. As CSA chair and Bank oncho manager, I was able to release $1.4 million from the Oncho Trust Fund to finance a CSA-endorsed program of operational research organized by the TDR's Hans Remme to lay the technical groundwork for a control effort in the non-OCP countries. That research covered four key

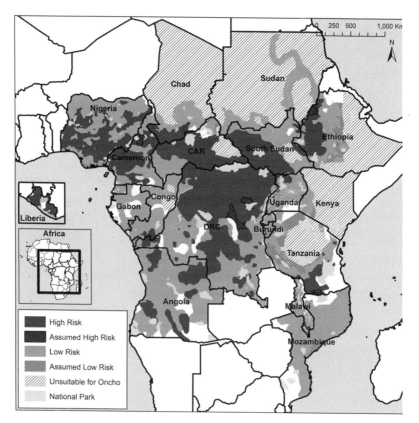

Figure 7.1. High-Risk Areas Identified through REMO. *Source*: Noma, Mounkalia, Honorat G.M. Zouré, Afework H. Tekle, Peter Al Enyong, Bertram E.B. Nwoke, and Jan H.F. Remme. "The Geographic Distribution of Onchocerciasis in the 20 Participating Countries of the African Programme for Onchocerciasis Control: (1) Priority Areas for Ivermectin Treatment." *Parasites & Vectors* 7, no. 325 (2014): 10.

areas: (1) the components of a Mectizan-based control strategy, for example ComDT; (2) preparation and implementation of a rapid-mapping scheme, such as REMO; (3) assessment of the burden of onchocerciasis in the rainforest and forest-savanna transition areas, notably onchocercal skin disease (OSD); and (4) the feasibility of vector eradication in foci in Tanzania, Uganda, and Equatorial Guinea. These studies formed the core of the CSA-TDR operational-research collaboration during 1993–1997, to prepare and commence implementation of APOC, with guidance from the programs' expert advisory committees—the OCP's EAC and the Technical Consultative Committee (TCC) of APOC.

Assessing Prospects for a New Regional Program for Sub-Saharan Africa

In 1991, John Moores, accompanied by RBF staff, came to World Bank headquarters to discuss mobilizing resources for a Mectizan delivery effort to the non-OCP African countries. The RBF was considering contributing $10 million to such an effort. We brainstormed and came up with a rough estimate of $150 million to treat the non-OCP endemic countries over a 12-year period. Based on the success in raising funds for the OCP, I felt reasonably confident that this amount could be secured from existing OCP donors. But doing so would require establishing a new program based on drug treatment rather than enlarging the OCP. That meeting set the stage for exploring prospects for a second regional effort for the rest of oncho-endemic Africa. Katherine Marshall and Jean-Louis Sarbib, the two World Bank directors for West Africa who had followed the OCP most closely over the years, encouraged me to pursue the possibility.

That year, I was elected chair of the CSA and urged the other sponsoring-agency representatives to assist in formulating the outlines of a program proposal which could be taken to the donors and the non-OCP African countries for consideration. I also initiated discussions with various partner groups during OCP meetings on the prospects and parameters for a new program. It was evident that there was support, even enthusiasm, from the sponsoring agencies, OCP management, the EAC, the MEC, and the NGDO Coordination Group for establishing a Mectizan-based program for the rest of Africa. The predominant view was that the only practical and affordable way to reach tens of millions of at-risk Africans with Mectizan would be through some form of a community-based approach.

During Bank/OCP donor visits, I sounded out donors. The successful OCP track record—evident to the donors by the early 1990s—provided impetus for a second control effort. Community-based delivery of free Mectizan was appealing to the donors due to its presumed cost-effectiveness. No other approach seemed realistic, primarily due to cost. The four largest of the non-OCP endemic countries—Nigeria, the DRC, Sudan (including South Sudan at that time), and Ethiopia—swamped the size of the 11 OCP countries in area and at-risk population. Subsequent REMO results revealed that the high-risk populations of those four countries alone exceeded 70 million. Despite the success of vector control under the OCP, the geographic size of non-OCP oncho-endemic Africa precluded such a strategy (however, Frank Walsh, former OCP entomologist, argued persuasively for vector eradication of less-common blackfly species in parts of East and Central Africa—a method that had been successful in Kenya in the 1950s). Merck representatives favored a second, Mectizan-based, program for the non-OCP countries. Dr. Samba was enthusiastic about the prospect and assigned OCP staff to assist in preparations in office space he set aside for that purpose within the OCP's Ouagadougou headquarters.

The Burden of Onchocerciasis in the Non-OCP Countries

To what extent was forest onchocerciasis a health burden? Did it impede socioeconomic development, and, if so, to what extent? Much of the research had concluded that the forest form of the disease caused considerably less blindness than savanna oncho. Some on the EAC argued that forest oncho was a nuisance, but not a serious health threat. Survey results in 1995 revealed that there were 1.3 million cases of severely-impaired vision and blindness, and 10 million cases of troublesome itching in non-OCP Africa resulting from the mix of forest and savanna oncho in the 19 endemic countries.[20]

To improve understanding of the oncho burden in the non-OCP countries, Remme proposed assessing the disease impact through a multi-country study. That assessment, which was conducted in parts of Nigeria, Cameroon, Tanzania, and Uganda, revealed a previously-underappreciated feature of forest oncho: OSD and its stigma.[21] Results showed that forest oncho caused considerable disability due to itching, inflammation, skin lesions, and disfigurement. One conclusion was that the incidence and prevalence of OSD, mainly itching, in the forest and quasi-forested areas exceeded the incidence and prevalence of blindness in the savanna areas. Troublesome itching commenced shortly after infection and worsened as victims aged up to 20 years old, when it plateaued.[22] Itching was widespread, affecting 42% of the population living where forest oncho predominated.[23] Moreover, there was significant stigma associated with OSD, frequently resulting in social ostracism.

The cumulative impact of OSD on society and local economies was found to be an economic impediment due to lost work in productive activities, health costs, and the inability to carry out basic household responsibilities. The study found that the loss of healthy life years (disability-adjusted life years, or DALYs) due to OSD was greater than the loss from visual impairment and blindness in the non-OCP countries.[24] The researchers concluded that OSD was an important public-health burden due to its "adverse psychosocial and socioeconomic effects" and should be addressed through the new program.[25]

The psychosocial impact of OSD is illustrated by the case of a 19-year-old pregnant woman, Agnes. Dr. Uche Amazigo, a senior lecturer at the University of Nigeria, Nsukka, during the 1980s, encountered Agnes while investigating disability and social isolation among oncho-infected adolescent girls and young women in the rural areas of Enugu State. Amazigo later conducted a videotaped interview with Agnes, who described her distress from OSD:

> The rashes first appeared when I was six years old. That was when the itching began. At school I couldn't concentrate because of the incessant itching. The children in class used to laugh at me, so I stopped going to school when I was nine. I married in 1989. My father arranged the marriage; my husband didn't see me before we got married. When we met and he saw my skin, he was very angry. I lived with him for a few months and became pregnant. Then my skin got worse. Despite the pregnancy, he sent me home to my parents. From the time I left until the birth of my baby, I had no support from my husband, no money for me or my baby. You can see from my skin that I am always scratching. It affects the amount of attention that I can give to my children. I can hardly sleep at night. I feel weak from the pain and nuisance that is always there. What can I do?[26]

Agnes's story represented the plight of hundreds of thousands of young women infected with forest oncho and experiencing OSD. It illustrated the anguish of unrelenting itching resulting in insomnia, weakness, and difficulty breast-feeding; the stigma undermining peer acceptance and marriage prospects; and the inability to concentrate, leading to poor academic performance and school dropout. The video portrayed Agnes's suffering—her desperation, uncontrolled scratching, and the unsightly lesions blemishing her torso, buttocks, and limbs.

We arranged to show the video at the APOC launch conference and at a WHO World Health Assembly meeting in Geneva. Agnes became the face of OSD. The video helped raise awareness of the psychosocial impact of OSD, which had been largely unknown within the international community. Following five to six years of Mectizan treatment through an APOC project, Agnes' symptoms gradually disappeared, and her husband arranged with her father to resume their relationship and restore their marriage after a separation of four years.[27] Through her experience with Mectizan, Agnes became interested in helping others receive the drug and was selected by her home community to become a volunteer community-directed distributor (CDD).

Organizing a Massive Multicountry Control Effort

By 1994, the CSA had decided the new program would rely almost exclusively on Mectizan distribution through the communities. The program would cover all of the non-OCP countries where there was an ongoing source of oncho transmission: 14 contiguous countries across Central, East and Southern Africa, plus Nigeria and Liberia in West Africa. Three additional countries, Rwanda, Mozambique, and Kenya, were impacted by infective blackflies from neighboring countries, but had no clearly identifiable local sources of transmission. These countries would be invited to participate in the program as observers.

The strategy would aim to bring the disease under control by replicating ComDT projects in hyperendemic and meso-endemic areas. The CSA concluded that it was necessary to delink the new program programmatically and organizationally from the OCP, given their differing strategies and timetables. The new program should have its separate identity. Within the CSA we referred to it as the "OCP II." World Bank Director for Western Africa, Jean-Louis Sarbib, suggested calling it "African Program for Onchocerciasis Control." It was a name that stuck, partly due to the readily accepted acronym, APOC. The name inferred that the program might eventually assume responsibility for all of oncho-endemic Africa. That implied mandate became important when several former OCP countries required support in suppressing residual transmission, and upon resuming control in Sierra Leone after its civil war. There was unanimous CSA agreement on the importance of drawing upon the extensive knowledge and control experience of the OCP over two decades. Hence, it was decided to headquarter APOC in the OCP compound in Ouagadougou, where the staffs of the two programs could interact and share information on control strategies and epidemiological and entomological surveillance.

The CSA concluded that APOC would have a duration of 12 years and a budget of $131 million. The program objective was defined as establishing within that 12-year timeframe "effective and self-sustainable community-based ivermectin treatment throughout the endemic areas" of all non-OCP African countries harboring local sources of oncho transmission. A secondary objective was to "eliminate the vector and hence the disease by using environmentally safe methods in selected foci."[28] This two-part objective was set out in the APOC Memorandum— the agreement covering the operational, institutional, and financial arrangements of the program to be signed by the participating partners.

Samba and I agreed that Azodoga Sékétéli, OCP coordinator, would assume responsibility for preparing APOC and managing it once it became operational.

Sékétéli would report to Yankum Dadzie, who was to become the new director of the OCP as well as acting director of APOC in 1995, after Samba assumed his new post as WHO regional director for Africa in Brazzaville. Sékétéli proved to be an excellent choice. He was committed, hard-working, and a strong proponent of ComDT. Sékétéli quickly began organizing APOC to help ensure its smooth takeoff in 1996. He contacted each of the African countries to urge them to participate and begin identifying ComDT projects. With guidance from the CSA and an informal working group in the World Bank, he set up the program structure and a project-review process. The latter was assigned to the TCC, a committee of independent experts and participating NGDOs. The TCC became a standing committee that met regularly over the life of APOC.

The project-preparation process involved individual NGDOs working directly with ministries of health and local communities to prepare projects based on ComDT guidelines. Once prepared, a project with accompanying budget was reviewed by the TCC and approved or returned to the country and the assisting NGDO for recommended modifications. If approved, the participating NGDO would help train district health staff and community-selected distributors, and assist in readying the project for implementation. The active involvement of the community throughout the preparation and implementation stages was fundamental to the APOC concept. A key objective was to instill grassroots ownership of the treatment process. The NGDOs played important roles in community empowerment at the design and implementation stages. They helped ensure that the project complied with ComDT guidelines and that the CDDs understood the requirements of safe and effective Mectizan treatment, including proper dosing, potential side effects, and the exclusion criteria for those ineligible to take the drug.

In parallel with preparatory operational research, CSA deliberations, and donor discussions, a small informal group was set up that met periodically at the World Bank during 1994–1995 to flesh out the APOC organizational structure. The recommendations of that group were fed back into the CSA for decision taking. Both bodies provided guidance through me to Sékétéli. The informal group consisted of: Allen Foster, Yankum Dadzie, Bernhard Liese, MDP Director Michael Heisler, and myself. The informal group brought to the task technical, organizational, and financial expertise less readily available in the CSA. The objective was to develop the outlines of a program that was accountable to the varied constituent partner groups and would foster collaboration within the partnership by ensuring that the stakeholders' roles complemented—not rivaled—one another in furtherance of the program objective.

We quickly concluded that APOC's organizational structure should be modeled on the OCP. OCP governance reflected a balance in the interests of the partner groups. Hence, APOC should retain the concept of a governing board (Joint Action Form-JAF), steering committee (CSA), expert advisory group (TCC), as well as separate fora for the donors (donors' conferences) and the Participating Countries (NOTFs). However, the APOC structure needed to reflect the far more active role of the NGDOs in control operations. We felt it was important to set up a project-preparation process that furthered collaboration between the NGDOs and the ministries of health—a relationship that, based on experience, could be a source of tension. Hence, all projects eligible for APOC support were required to be joint government/NGDO proposals. In addition, the chair of the NGDO Coordination Group would have a seat on the JAF; and a representative number of NGDOs would have membership on the TCC and be invited to the donors' conferences as observers. Given the importance of Mectizan in the control strategy, it was decided that a representative of Merck be invited to attend the JAF as an observer, and that the MDP director and the chair of the MEC become members of the TCC. In the end, it was the informal group that drafted the program document that was approved by the CSA and became the basis for the APOC Memorandum to be signed by WHO, the World Bank, the Participating Countries, and the donors during 1995–1997.

The first opportunity to test the waters with the collective OCP donor community came at a donors' conference, chaired by Sarbib, at WHO-Geneva in November 1994. A preliminary document covering the technical and organizational aspects of the new program was presented by Foster and Liese. That presentation was coupled with a document prepared by Walsh outlining the possibilities for vector eradication of select blackfly species in East and Central Africa. The message to the donors was that the knowledge base and tools existed to eliminate oncho as a public health problem throughout the rest of Africa. The donors were highly receptive to the concept of the new program, though none was yet prepared to commit to it publicly.

The Wolfensohn Presidency

Shortly after becoming World Bank president in June 1995, James D. Wolfensohn highlighted the importance of alleviating poverty, investing in people, and expanding partnership. His inaugural address to the World Bank Board of Governors emphasized these principles along with achieving results on the ground. He spoke of investments in people as the "principal engine of social and economic progress;"[29] the "power of partnerships" with the UN system, the private sector, NGOs and civil society[30]; "social and environmental benefit per capita"[31] as a measure of progress; and the "smile on a child's face" as the "real test of development."[32] The Wolfensohn presidency spanned the conclusion of the OCP and the launch and scale-up of APOC. There was greater high-level World Bank involvement in the oncho programs during his presidency than any time since McNamara's seminal role in the early 1970s. Senior Bank leadership was key at this juncture given the scale of the oncho programs that covered two-thirds of sub-Saharan Africa. High-level Bank support lent credibility to the ambitious effort to widen control of this lesser-known disease to all of endemic Africa. That support was crucial in leveraging the substantial amounts of donor funding required to implement two large control programs in parallel during the second half of the 1990s and early 2000s.

Greater high-level Bank involvement during this period was attributed to the inroads being made on the disease and to the impact of the combined effort on a larger part of the continent than any other Bank-supported initiative. Also, the results achieved aligned closely with Bank-management priorities as well as the 2000 UN Millennium Development Goals (MDGs). The oncho programs emphasized global partnership, alleviation of extreme poverty, and enhanced food security—each of which was an explicit MDG and a priority under the Wolfensohn Bank.

Once the preparation of APOC was sufficiently advanced, the CSA agreed to the launch conference taking place at the World Bank's Washington, DC, headquarters in conjunction with the December 1995 JPC. Wolfensohn readily consented to host the conference. Former minister of health of Nigeria, Dr. Olikoye Ransome-Kuti, a Bank consultant at the time, accepted to chair the working sessions, as well as the JPC plenary. I recommended that we invite former US President Jimmy Carter because of his strong interest in Africa, influence with African leaders, and his role in assisting Merck in implementing MDP. Wolfensohn knew Carter quite well and was pleased to have the former president join him in the conference wrap-up session. I also invited Robert McNamara to that session to sit at the dais with Wolfensohn, Carter, WHO Director-General Hiroshi Nakajima, and Ransome-Kuti. Nearly all of the OCP donors attended, as did all 16 of the African countries that would host APOC projects.

Wolfensohn opened the wrap-up session on December 5, 1995. He spoke of "the tremendous debt we owe President Carter for his support on the whole issue of onchocerciasis."[33] He shared his "delight" in McNamara's presence, who "represents a conscience and a sense of moral and social responsibility which is really a guiding light for our institution." Addressing McNamara, he said that "the Program is a wonderful example of the results that come from your initiative."[34] He remarked that the Bank was "particularly proud to be associated with the Program [APOC]" because "it affects the quality of people's lives . . . directly and intimately," while having "a manifest economic impact . . . in the rural communities."[35] He continued, "The . . . thing which I love about this program is that it is a true partnership," involving international organizations, the donor community, the African countries and their affected communities, NGOs, and an "exemplary" partnership with Merck.[36] Wolfensohn concluded: "So, for us, this is a prototypical, wonderful program. It deals with people, deals with poverty, deals with communities, it deals with partnership, and may I say that from the point of view of the Bank, there is nothing more significant to us than helping individual people on the ground."[37]

Nakajima referred to the OCP as "one of the largest and most successful field operations undertaken by WHO."[38] He argued that the OCP should serve as "a future model" for "our operations" and that "a similar approach has already been integrated into APOC and will help ensure its eventual success."[39] He emphasized two aspects of the OCP that were being incorporated into APOC and would bode well for its success: "harmonious and constructive partnership" and "operational research aiming at constantly improving the cost-effectiveness of field activities."[40]

President Carter recounted hearing "a lot of comments about the World Bank in my career . . . and an organization with a heart has not always been what I've heard. But I think that it's accurate to say that Bob McNamara, when the OCP was started, and now to Jim Wolfensohn, there's no doubt that the World Bank exemplifies an organization with a heart."[41] Carter described the suffering he had encountered from oncho and the relief possible by taking "one miracle tablet."[42] He concluded, "This onchocerciasis control program throughout Africa will be a major commitment of The Carter Center and a major personal commitment of me and my wife," and stressed his willingness to contact African heads of state, as needed, to emphasize the importance of implementing APOC. He closed, in saying, "I'm deeply indebted to Jim Wolfensohn for adopting this as a major commitment of the World Bank."[43]

The Carter Center became active in APOC as a participating NGDO, drawing upon its considerable expertise and hands-on experience in the Onchocerciasis Elimination Program for the Americas (OEPA). Three years prior to the APOC launch conference, The Center became a principal partner in OEPA, a regional public-private partnership similar to, though considerably smaller than, APOC. With Mectizan and RBF seed money, OEPA was launched in early 1993 under the auspices of WHO's Pan-American Health Organization to eliminate oncho morbidity and interrupt transmission in six countries (Brazil, Colombia, Ecuador, Guatemala, Mexico, and Venezuela) with an at-risk population of about 500,000.[44] The oncho parasite had been introduced into the Americas centuries earlier via the trans-Atlantic slave trade. Unlike Africa, where the disease was endemic over a vast contiguous area, oncho in the Americas was confined to 13 relatively isolated foci spread around the six countries. And, it was transmitted by blackfly species that traveled far-shorter distances than *Simulium damnosum*, the most common vector in Africa. Consequently, it was feasible to eliminate the disease in each focus through concentrated Mectizan treatment, without risk of it returning.

During the early years, the RBF served as OEPA's "parent" NGDO with administrative responsibilities for program operations.[45] In 1996, John Moores agreed to fold the RBF's programs and activities, including its OEPA administrative responsibilities, into The Carter Center. The Center also began serving as executing agency for a $4 million grant to OEPA from the Inter-American Development Bank. By 2016, after years of high coverage and bi-annual, or more frequent, Mectizan treatment, oncho was certified as eliminated in Colombia, Ecuador, Mexico and Guatemala. The major remaining challenge, as of this writing, is to wipe out oncho in the Yanomami focus in the Amazon rain forest in a border area between Venezuela and Brazil.

As of 2018–2019, there has been an active debate between those involved in OEPA and the former directors of the OCP and APOC on the extent to which methods and tools employed successfully in achieving elimination in the Americas ought to be applied extensively in Africa—despite the vastly different epidemiological situations and vectoral capacities throughout the two regions. The focus of the debate has been on the frequency of treatment with Mectizan in different epidemiological settings, and which diagnostic test and criteria to use in determining when Mectizan treatment can be stopped in pursuit of elimination.[46]

Funding and Scaling Up APOC

During 1996–1997, efforts took place to finalize the APOC Memorandum. The Memorandum legally bound the partners to the arrangements set out in the "APOC Program Document," as well as the donors to their pledges for the first six-year phase (Phase I, 1995–2001). WHO's legal counsel, Claude Vignes, who had represented WHO on the CSA since the early days of the OCP, drafted the Memorandum and secured the signatures of all 19 Participating Countries during 1996. Vignes had done a yeoman's job in providing impartial legal guidance to the CSA over the previous 15 years. He was a steady hand and an invaluable resource on the historical legal intricacies of the OCP. I felt fortunate to have his legal guidance during my years chairing the CSA.

During 1996–1997, I worked with the donors on the language defining their pledges to be incorporated in the Memorandum, and arranged for their signatures. The APOC budget in the Memorandum was $131 million over 12 years, $11 million per annum, slightly over half the average annual expenditures for the OCP.[47] APOC was later extended three years to 2010 to allow for a phasing-down period, increasing the budget to $135 million. (The Program was subsequently extended again, to 2015, to enable all ComDT projects to receive a minimum of five years in financing, the duration considered necessary to achieve treatment sustainability.) The donors pledged $20 million at the launch conference, largely sufficient to finance APOC operations through 1996–1997.

Fund mobilization efforts to scale up APOC and bring the OCP to a successful conclusion took several tracks. The first of five biennial APOC donors' conferences was convened in September 1996 at the Bank's Paris office. Donor pledges there brought in an additional $30 million for Phase I of APOC, leaving the Program $6 million short for its first six-year phase.[48] Beginning in 1997, with Wolfensohn's encouragement, I presented the first of three oral reports to the World Bank Board of Executive Directors (EDs) on progress in controlling oncho in Africa. These reports helped sustain the required funding. All of the donor countries were represented on the Board through their respective EDs, who, in most cases came from finance ministries with considerable influence over their countries' budgets.

Sékétéli and I visited donor capitals annually during 1996–2004 to keep each donor informed on progress in scaling up APOC. We undertook visits to Eastern Europe in an effort to bring in new donor countries that were starting up aid programs. Those visits resulted in agreements with Poland and Slovenia to join the donor community. Separately, I traveled to Canberra to present APOC to an Australian parliamentary committee concerned with global health. The presentation led to a follow-up meeting with Australia's minister of foreign affairs and a pledge to support APOC. Requests to Canada and AfDB, prior OCP donors, resulted in substantial funding increases. The last APOC donors' conference, hosted by Wolfensohn at Bank headquarters in June 2004, brought in sufficient funding to reduce the APOC shortfall to $13 million through its planned completion in 2010.[49] All told, fund-raising efforts secured $122 million, as against the estimated APOC budget of $135 million.

APOC operations accelerated after launch. During the decade, 1995–2004, 69 projects were established in all 16 endemic countries treating 35.6 million people in 77,000 high-risk communities—roughly equivalent to the population protected by the expanded OCP.[50] The average cost per treatment was $0.58 per person based on a 2004–2005 study in 11 geographic areas.[51] The scale-up was dramatic in Nigeria where 27 projects were underway by mid-2005 covering nearly all of the country's high-risk communities and treating 19.5 million Nigerians.[52] Nigeria's ComDT projects achieved a relatively high average coverage rate of 75%.[53]

Sékétéli later explained that the early focus on Nigeria was intended, in part, to protect the OCP area, notably neighboring Benin, by slowing reinvasion of infective blackflies westward.[54] Sékétéli remained OCP coordinator during the seven OCP/APOC overlap years (1995–2002) and was intent on protecting the gains under the OCP. He traveled to Benin in the early APOC years to meet with President Nicéphore Soglo and reassure him that the rapid scale-up in Nigeria would help minimize oncho transmission into Benin via reinvading flies from the east.[55] Sékétéli attributed the success in ramping up projects in Nigeria to the timely completion of REMO, a well-organized national team, and the leadership provided by Nigeria's National Coordinator.[56] During his travels to the APOC countries, Sékétéli encountered frequent requests from government authorities for vector control, in addition to Mectizan treatment. They were well aware of the OCP's success in largely eliminating the disease and wanted to benefit from aerial-spraying operations, as well.[57] It took repeated explanations to convince them that Mectizan treatment, by itself, with sufficiently high coverage, could bring the disease under full control.[58]

Overall, the scale-up of APOC during 1995–2004 was uneven. The stable countries with strong national teams were able to expedite REMO and achieve relatively rapid project preparation/implementation. In addition to Nigeria, these countries included Cameroon, Uganda, and Tanzania. For the most part, the high-risk (hyper/meso) areas were covered and 72% of the targeted population was receiving treatment by 2005.[59] Similarly, projects covered most of the high-risk communities in Ethiopia and Malawi by 2005, although scale-up proceeded somewhat-more slowly with treatment coverage in the 60%–68% range.[60] Angola, Burundi, the DRC, and Sudan experienced varying degrees of domestic conflict over the decade, delaying REMO and project preparation/implementation. For these countries, treatment coverage remained below 50%.[61] Liberia struggled with post-conflict during much of the decade, resulting in delays in REMO and project implementation. Less than 10% of Liberia's high-risk population was under treatment by 2005.[62] TCC-approved projects for Angola and Burundi had not yet begun treatment by the end of the decade.

Mectizan Treatment Hits a Major Snag

Post-Treatment Severe Reactions Crop Up

In 1991, an oncho-infected man in Cameroon lapsed into a coma following treatment with Mectizan. Dr. Michel Boussinesq, an ORSTOM researcher based there, learned of the incident from a colleague. The man had been living in the Pouma District, 125 km west of Yaoundé.[63] WHO's René Le Berre asked Boussinesq to investigate, but by the time Boussinesq and colleagues arrived at the hospital, the patient had died. After eliminating most possibilities, they concluded that the patient had suffered from a post-ivermectin-treatment serious adverse event (SAE) resulting from his elevated infection with loiasis, a disease affecting 35% of the population in that area of Cameroon.[64] SAEs, as defined by the US Food and Drug Administration (FDA), are side effects resulting from use of a medical product that results in a life-threatening experience, hospitalization, disability, permanent damage, or death.[65]

Loiasis is caused by the parasitic worm, *Loa loa*, which is transmitted by a deer-fly (also known as a "mango fly"). Loiasis is commonly found in the humid rainforest areas of West and Central Africa and co-endemicity with onchocerciasis occurs in up to 11 countries in that subregion. Those infected solely with loiasis are often asymptomatic or minimally symptomatic, although the disease can induce transient localized swelling on the arms and legs (referred to as "Calabar swellings"), accompanied by itching. It also results in periodic episodes of the adult *Loa loa* worm (termed "eyeworm") crawling across the white surface of the eye, which, though often alarming to the victim, usually causes no eye damage.[66]

Boussinesq and colleagues determined that the death resulted from collateral damage caused by ivermectin killing off high concentrations of *Loa loa* microfilariae (mf). Elevated levels of mf were found in the victim's cerebrospinal fluid.[67] Over the next four years, 24 similar SAEs, three of which resulted in death, were reported in the Sanaga Valley, east of Douala and slightly north of Yaoundé.[68]

TDR and MDP Sponsor Investigations

The continuing SAEs led the TDR to finance a year-long hospital-based study in Cameroon during 1993–1994. The study, led by ORSTOM researcher, Dr. Jean-Philippe Chippaux and colleagues, including Boussinesq, took place at Yaoundé Central Hospital and was published in 1995. Its principal conclusions were (1) SAEs may result in 1% of subjects with loiasis infection levels >3,000 microfilariae/milliliter of blood (mf/ml), (2) the critical level where SAEs could be expected was ≥30,000 mf/ml, and (3) SAE severity "was linked to the level of parasitemia before treatment."[69] Put simply, the greater the loiasis-infection intensity, the more likely and severe the reaction following Mectizan treatment. The study warned: the findings "should engender caution in carrying out large-scale treatment campaigns with ivermectin in *Loa loa* endemic areas."[70]

The MDP convened a meeting of experts in Paris in October 1995, to assess the problem and consider recommendations on how best to proceed. There were 18 scientific experts at the meeting, representing the MDP, the MEC, WHO, ORSTOM, the RBF, the CDC, Merck Research Laboratories, and from medical faculties of various universities. MDP Director Michael Heisler later recalled, "We wanted to keep the meeting at a scientific level and focus on the best objective information available at the time."[71] Perhaps because APOC would not be established for another two months, no one representing the new program or the CSA was in attendance. Consequently, those involved in launching APOC had only limited knowledge of the nature and scope of the potential threat to Mectizan-treatment. The meeting had at its disposal the results of the recently-completed TDR-financed hospital-based study and the two ORSTOM co-authors were attendees.

At the Paris meeting, the problem was identified as *Loa loa* encephalopathy, resulting from "abundant dead [*Loa loa*] mf blocking blood vessels in the brain."[72] Of the 24 SAEs reviewed, five were highlighted as fitting a pattern of neurological symptoms induced by the death of *Loa loa* mf, beginning with fever, headache, and myalgia within 24 hours of treatment and progressing to coma over roughly a five-day period.[73] Nevertheless, there was reluctance by some to conclude that *Loa loa* coupled with Mectizan treatment was the cause. The meeting report stated, "The consultants noted the difficulty in establishing: a) that an encephalopathic reaction was induced by the death of *L. loa* mf . . . and b) that Mectizan was the inciting cause of the reaction."[74] In addition, some participants were apparently not convinced that the problem in that area of Cameroon implied difficulties for treating oncho in the wider multicountry area endemic with loiasis. The meeting report stated: "There are no comparable reports, despite the prevalence of loiasis, from Benin, Nigeria, Gabon, Congo, Central African Republic, Chad, Uganda, Zaire, or from Cameroon west of the Sanaga Valley."[75]

The group's recommendations called for Mectizan treatment programs to: "enhance surveillance and monitoring," establish plans to transport patients experiencing SAEs to properly-equipped medical facilities, and "provide appropriate health education messages" to the local populations to prepare them for SAEs.[76] The group also recommended that the MEC/MDP pursue mapping to identify areas of heavy *Loa loa* endemicity, require information on endemicity levels in applications for Mectizan, and request NGDOs to provide guidelines for treating SAEs to the medical staff of all treatment programs.[77] Finally, the group recommended further investigations into "the potential association between *Loa* encephalopathy and Mectizan treatment in patients with very high microfilaremias."[78] Neither the implied cautions from the group nor subsequent persistent warnings from Boussinesq in MEC meetings dissuaded the Cameroonian Ministry of Health and HKI, the collaborating NGDO, from considering treatment in areas not proven to be meso- or hyperendemic for oncho, such as in hypo-endemic areas where the risk/benefit ratio of treatment was particularly high.[79]

One month before the Paris meeting, the TDR had launched a major study to better understand the cause and implications of the SAEs in Cameroon. The study, led by French scientists, Drs. Jacques Gardon and Michel Boussinesq, involved treating 17,877 inhabitants living in the Lékié area, which includes the Okola District where most of the SAEs had occurred.[80] The results, published in 1997, confirmed that the SAEs were resulting from Mectizan treatment of individuals heavily infected with loiasis. The authors stated: "This study shows that the initial *L. loa* microfilarial load was the main risk factor for the development of serious reactions, and that the risk increased with the intensity of microfilaremia."[81] The study identified a "very high risk" threshold of SAEs greater than 50,000 mf/ml. Gardon et al surmised that the lack of reported SAEs in neighboring countries may have been due to *Loa loa* mf levels below that 50,000 mf/ml threshold.[82] The authors cautioned, "In areas where loiasis coexists with onchocerciasis, ivermectin treatment should be carefully considered if the onchocerciasis found therein is not a serious public health problem."[83]

A meeting marking the launch of Cameroon's national oncho-control program under APOC took place in Yaoundé in April 1999. The meeting coincided with the launch of ComDT in central/southern Cameroon and a spate of additional SAEs in that same Lékié area. Following the meeting, APOC Director Sékétéli visited the Yaoundé Central Hospital and was struck by the number of patients undergoing treatment for SAEs.[84] Sékétéli was an entomologist, not a physician, and this first encounter with SAEs was unsettling, because, as APOC director, he was responsible for treatment in all of the APOC countries in the area where loiasis was endemic, including Cameroon. He quickly urged APOC's TCC to investigate the problem.

In October of that year, the MDP convened a meeting in Tours, France, to discuss the central nervous system (CNS) disorders in Cameroon and their implications for going forward with Mectizan treatment in areas co-endemic with oncho and loiasis. As in 1995, the meeting consisted largely of scientists, notably physicians and parasitologists, from the MDP, Merck Research Laboratories, NGDOs, ORSTOM, Cameroon's MOH, university hospitals, and WHO (AFRO and TDR), and did not include representatives from APOC or the CSA. Similar to the 1995 Paris meeting, the two-day session reviewed recent SAEs, including six fatalities occurring in Cameroon in 1999. The objective was to develop case definitions of post-Mectizan treatment SAEs in loiasis-infected patients, with the aim of improving clinical management of encephalopathic SAEs.[85] The 1995 and 1999 meetings focused on achieving greater understanding of the pathogenesis of the SAEs, with the aim of improving clinical treatment. However, little headway was made. Pursuit of that objective was handicapped by the lack of diagnostic and postmortem tissue specimens from patients and the absence of an animal model.[86]

The 1999 JAF in the Hague formally requested APOC to develop recommendations for treating oncho in loiasis-endemic areas.[87] TCC recommendations were issued in early 2000 and reissued by the MEC in a May 2000 report. The report noted that loiasis endemicity could be presumed in a wide area covering portions of 10 countries based upon environmental data related to vegetation and levels of humidity conducive to the *Loa loa* parasite and its vector. But it acknowledged that the "precise distribution of *Loa loa* in Africa is not known."[88] Consequently, the report's recommendations differed depending upon the oncho-prevalence levels of communities and their history of Mectizan treatment, rather than on the prevalence and infection levels of loiasis within those communities.

The TCC/MEC recommendations called for enhancing community awareness and providing training for CDDs and local medical personnel on ways of recognizing and responding to SAEs. In communities where there had been two rounds of Mectizan treatment covering at least 60% of the at-risk population and no reported cases of serious CNS dysfunction, the recommendation was to continue treatment.[89] For all other communities, the recommendations depended upon oncho-endemicity levels based on nodule palpation. Where a community was hypo-endemic, no treatment should be given. For meso- and hyperendemic communities, treatment should proceed, with CDDs assigned to undertake "careful observation" for a full week following treatment, supplemented by surveillance by local medical personnel "for days 3–5 after treatment." The stated objective was "early identification of CNS dysfunction and prompt referral of patients to district hospital or designated center where staff is appropriately trained and supplied for case management."[90] Authority for taking the final decision on whether to treat a specific community was left to the NOTF and the ministry of health.[91]

In October 2000, APOC financed a mission to assess compliance with the TCC/MEC recommendations in central/southern Cameroon (South West, Littoral, and Central Provinces). The mission included MDP Director Stefanie Meredith, MDP scientist Nana Twum-Danso, and CBM Medical Director Adrian Hopkins. While the mission concluded that the recommendations were being "appropriately implemented," SAE clinical management was seen as facing limitations by understaffing of health personnel, lack of transportation, and insufficient training for CDDs and nurses in early detection.[92]

Twum-Danso reported in an article in 2003 that 207 SAEs had occurred in the equatorial subregion of Central Africa between 1989 and 2001, with a disproportionate number in central/southern Cameroon.[93] Of 53 cases requiring hospitalization, eight had resulted in death.[94] During the first round of Mectizan treatment in the Bas-Congo and Tshopo provinces of the DRC in late 2003 and early 2004, 19 deaths out of 62 SAEs occurred.[95] Results from Twum-Danso's study revealed that an overwhelming proportion of SAEs occurred with the first ivermectin treatment.[96] Hence, the implication was that follow-on treatments for the same individual were unlikely to induce additional SAEs.

As awareness of SAEs spread, reticence to taking Mectizan increased. Nancy J. Haselow of HKI, the NGDO active in supporting ComDT projects in Cameroon's Central Province, presented a paper at the Scientific Working Group on SAEs in loiasis-endemic areas, in Manchester, United Kingdom, in 2002. She cited a ComDT project in the South West Province of Cameroon with a refusal rate of 27.7%—a rate she described as "closely linked to a high level of skepticism, doubt and pessimism among community members."[97] Haselow also referred to an evaluation in 2000 that found: "In the presence of SAEs, rumours and incomplete information, some community members acknowledged fear associated with even minor side effects and were understandably reticent to take ivermectin."[98] Reticence probably reduced Mectizan coverage below 65% in many communities, hindering impact on oncho transmission. The resistance to treatment in loiasis-endemic areas contrasted markedly with the enthusiastic acceptance of Mectizan elsewhere, because the drug provided relief from insufferable itching, eliminated intestinal roundworms, and contributed to overall feelings of well-being.

Shift in Emphasis toward Prevention

The focus on clinical management of SAEs shifted in the early 2000s toward prevention. A search began to find practical methods for identifying communities heavily endemic with loiasis. The TDR's Remme suggested surveying for clinical signs of loiasis, such as Calabar swellings and the presence of eyeworm. The suggestion led to a workshop in Mbalmayo, Cameroon, in December 2000 to develop a protocol for mapping loiasis based on the history of eyeworm—a technique that became known as rapid assessment (or mapping) of loiasis, or RAPLOA.[99] In 2001, Boussinesq and colleagues also concluded via a study in central Cameroon that communities with a prevalence of *Loa loa* mf ≥20% in adults had a "high probability" of SAEs.[100]

The RAPLOA technique was fully developed during 2001. Under the aegis of the TDR Task Force on OOR, Drs. Innocent Takougang, Martin Meremikwu, and Samuel Wanji, backed by TDR/APOC financing, carried out studies in two sites in Cameroon and one in Nigeria. Those studies demonstrated that loiasis prevalence could be approximated through feedback on the history of the adult *Loa loa* worm crossing the eye.[101] Community members were asked: "Have you ever experienced or noticed worms moving along the white of the lower part of your eye?"[102] Responses were confirmed using a photograph of the eyeworm in the eye. A 40% or greater affirmative response in a sample of 80 individuals, 15 years of age and above, was found to be the equivalent of ≥20% loiasis prevalence—the threshold that Boussinesq et al. flagged as exposing a community to a high probability of SAEs.[103]

Prior to RAPLOA there were only broad indications of where loiasis was endemic. The standard procedure for diagnosing loiasis infection was the thick blood smear, a method too complex and time-consuming to amass data across 10 or more countries to guide APOC in implementing Mectizan treatment projects. Consequently, RAPLOA was a breakthrough as a quick, noninvasive technique in identifying areas heavily infected with loiasis. It enabled Mectizan treatment to proceed in selected zones throughout the subregion by specifying where *Loa loa* prevalence was below 20%. The TCC reviewed RAPLOA in 2002 and recommended employing it to guide APOC operations. The method was further validated in surveys conducted in 2004 in the Republic of Congo and the DRC. Following that validation, RAPOLA was endorsed at the 2004 JAF in Kinshasa, DRC. As a result, the TCC and the MEC revised their earlier recommendations, and proposed differing levels of training for local health staff and CDDs depending upon loiasis prevalence levels determined through RAPLOA.[104]

Financed out of the APOC Trust Fund, mapping via RAPLOA got underway in 2002 and was completed by the end of the decade. Surveys were conducted in 4,798 villages randomly selected in an 11-country area covering 7,500,000 km².[105] Two sizable zones were identified as having an eyeworm history ≥ 40% and thus hyperendemic for loiasis. As shown on the RAPLOA map (figure 7.2), the

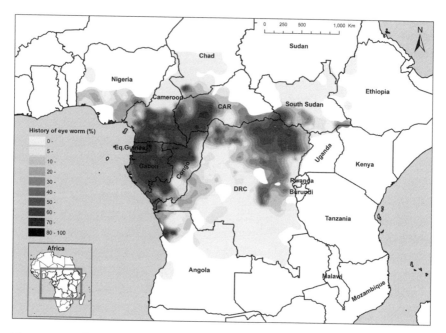

Figure 7.2. Loa loa Prevalence Based on History of Eyeworm through RAPLOA.
Source: Zouré, H. G., S. Wanji, M. Noma, U.V. Amazigo, P.J. Diggle, A.H. Tekle, and
J.H. Remme. "The Geographic Distribution of Loa loa in Africa: Results of Large-
Scale Implementation of the Rapid Assessment Procedure for Loiasis (RAPLOA)."
PLOS Neglected Tropical Diseases 5, no. 6 (June 2011): figure 4.

heavily-endemic western zone covered much of Equatorial Guinea, Gabon, cen-
tral/southern Cameroon, and parts of the Republic of the Congo, the CAR, and
Chad. The eastern zone was concentrated in northeastern DRC. All told, 10
countries had high-risk loiasis areas with a combined population of 14.4 million,
of which 80% was in DRC and Cameroon.[106] Sizable areas were found to be largely
free of loiasis: central and southern DRC, northern Cameroon, and portions of
Angola, Nigeria, Chad, and Sudan. The surveys turned up high-risk areas not
known to exist in the CAR, the Republic of Congo, and the DRC.

Information gleaned from RAPLOA was important for the DRC, where a
number of APOC-supported projects had been planned for 2003–2005. The data
enabled APOC to take precautionary steps or refrain from treatment in the DRC's
high-risk areas, containing 7.4 million people.[107] During 2004–2005, APOC ex-
perimented by integrating RAPLOA and REMO maps in four subregions of the
DRC. One subregion included the Province of Bas-Congo, identified by REMO as

hyperendemic for onchocerciasis. A number of SAEs, including deaths, as noted above, had occurred in Bas-Congo the year before, leading to a suspension of Mectizan treatment throughout the Province. Integrating mapping clarified the breadth of the problem. In two large portions of the Province, the diseases did not overlap. Oncho was severe in the eastern half, whereas loiasis was hyperendemic predominantly in the western half.[108] Consequently, ComDT projects could proceed safely in eastern Bas-Congo. A 2010 APOC assessment of this integrated mapping experiment in the DRC concluded that: "combined mapping of onchocerciasis and loiasis is an effective and essential element of sound operational planning of onchocerciasis control in the many areas in Africa where the two infections may be co-endemic."[109]

The appointment of Bjorn Thylefors as MDP director in 2001 was an important development in addressing the problem. According to Boussinesq, the MDP's view of the *Loa loa* problem "changed radically" under Thylefors.[110] Previously, the tendency had been to view the SAEs as rare occurrences and largely manageable with early detection and proper clinical treatment. After 2001, the MDP became more proactive and promoted consideration of preventive measures such as mapping via remote sensing and RAPLOA, as well as pretreatment with drugs, such as albendazole, to reduce loiasis infection levels prior to Mectizan treatment. The MDP organized the Scientific Working Group on SAEs (referenced above) and a new post of Loiasis Technical Advisor was established in Cameroon to conduct operational research and assist the MOH and the NOTF in adhering to the TCC/MEC guidelines. This strengthened institutional capacity brought greater attention to the problem and the search for solutions. During the Scientific Working Group's first meeting in Manchester in 2002, an extensive set of recommendations on preventive measures and clinical-treatment initiatives was elicited and discussed.[111] It was pointed out during those discussions, by HKI's Haselow that, given the need for greater control over Mectizan tablet inventories and the supervision of CDDs in the *Loa loa* endemic areas, the standard ComDT method of distributing Mectizan tablets was inappropriate.[112]

In addition to the history of eyeworm, another method for determining a high risk of SAEs was to measure *Loa loa* mf/ml levels in the blood. However, for the first 20+ years of the loiasis crisis, there was no quick, accurate method for doing so. In 2014–2015, a device known as a LoaScope was developed at the University of California, Berkeley, with financing from the Gates Foundation. It employed a smartphone to quantify *Loa loa* mf/ml from a drop of blood.[113] It was an important advance in measuring loiasis-infection intensity quickly in individuals at the point of care, thereby enabling implementation of a strategy known as Test and Not Treat (TaNT). In late 2015, the LoaScope was tested in a large study implementing the TaNT strategy in Cameroon. Candidates were excluded from treatment with >20,000 *Loa loa* mf/ml, the infection level determined midway through the study to be a safe cut-off level to avoid SAEs.[114]

The LoaScope enabled resumption of Mectizan treatment in oncho hypo-endemic zones in Cameroon's Okola District where treatment was suspended in 1999 due to SAEs and deaths. In implementing the TaNT strategy, 2.1% of the target population had loiasis-infection levels exceeding 20,000 mf/ml and was therefore excluded from treatment.[115] The LoaScope performed well and the TaNT strategy proved effective. No SAEs occurred in treating 92 villages with an oncho at-risk population of 22,842.[116] The LoaScope showed considerable potential in averting SAEs during treatment. However, as of this writing, the TaNT strategy with the LoaScope is not being widely deployed primarily due to cost, according to Dr. Maria Rebollo Polo, Team Leader for the Expanded Special Project for Elimination of Neglected Tropical Diseases (ESPEN), which got underway in 2017. Nevertheless, the LoaScope is being used to map loiasis-infection levels in oncho hypo-endemic areas.[117]

Looking Back

During the two decades, 1996–2015, APOC experienced 500+ cases of *Loa loa* encephalopathy and ~60 deaths in the loiasis-endemic subregion of West and Central Africa.[118] Fatal SAEs were infrequent in the context of hundreds of millions of doses of Mectizan given to more than 112 million Africans during the final years of APOC.[119] However, some SAEs might have been avoided. Warning signs that began blinking in the early 1990s were reinforced by the conclusions of the TDR-financed hospital-based study in Cameroon in 1993–1994. Nevertheless, the MDP-convened meetings of scientists in Paris in 1995 and in Tours in 1999 were cautious about both rushing to judgment on the cause of the problem and recommending suspension of Mectizan treatment in oncho-loiasis co-endemic areas, in part, no doubt, because doing so could have led to more blindness and prolonged suffering from OSD.

There may have been reluctance to highlight the problem at the Paris meeting due to the pending launch of APOC two months later. Heisler recalled, "I do remember that there was a fair amount of concern that maybe the Program was in jeopardy." APOC was an initiative of considerable international political and economic importance to the 19 non-OCP African countries, with the potential to benefit an oncho at-risk population of nearly 100 million. Given that APOC management had a major say in Mectizan treatment in the non-OCP countries, it is somewhat puzzling that officials most actively involved in APOC were not present at either the 1995 Paris meeting or the 1999 Tours meeting. Those who would have been most appropriate to include in the *Loa loa* discussions were Sékétéli, as manager-designate and later director of APOC, and Dadzie, as APOC acting director. Others who might have participated from the APOC-operations side were senior APOC staff and members of the CSA.

Not bringing into the discussion those in APOC and the CSA, with authority to determine operational policies, was inconsistent with the ethos of inclusion and collaboration that was fundamental to the oncho partnership. The vital, inextricable link between science and program operations had been demonstrated in the OCP and in the operational research fundamental to the establishment of APOC. Important perspectives leading to success are gained when consequential meetings include participants on both the science and operations side.

Participation of those involved in APOC operations in the 1995 meeting might conceivably have led to an arrangement temporarily delaying Mectizan-treatment projects in the loiasis-endemic areas, while APOC project implementation proceeded on schedule for the rest of oncho-endemic Africa. Delaying treatment would have provided additional time to investigate the problem, as recommended in Paris, without risking continued SAEs. A temporary delay might have enabled APOC management to find some way of proceeding with more limited treatment that would have reduced the risk of further SAEs. This possibility is largely conjecture, however. Those leading the APOC effort in the second half the 1990s were focused on scaling up Mectizan treatment in non-OCP Africa rapidly and generally assumed, based on the earlier large-scale Phase IV trials, that Mectizan treatment was safe in nearly all circumstances.

As it turned out, there was a price to pay in not at least temporarily delaying operations in the loiasis-endemic areas, in lives lost, neurological deficits, and reduced Mectizan-treatment compliance. That cost needed to be weighed against the benefits of continuing treatment, notably the alleviation of suffering and preventing additional blindness. David Addiss, director of the Focus Area for Compassion and Ethics (FACE) in the Task Force for Global Health, has summed up the ethical dilemma represented by the *Loa loa* issue. "How to weigh the benefits to the population versus risk to the few? It's a central problem in global health," Addiss acknowledged. "It's being played out in a very dramatic way in the *Loa loa* context."[120]

Adding Control of a Second Major Neglected Tropical Disease— Lymphatic Filariasis

At a 1996 MEC meeting at Merck's Chateau Mirabel in Riom, France, Eric Ottesen of WHO gave a presentation on recent findings on the effectiveness of two-drug regimens in treating lymphatic filariasis (LF). He noted that the efficacy of Mectizan combined with albendazole was greater than for each drug alone. Bill Foege, who was chairing the meeting, later recalled,

> The question came up, who makes albendazole? And the answer was Smith-Kline Beecham. Does anyone know anyone high enough in the company, that we could get free albendazole and actually start a program? No one did, but we kept talking about this at dinner. The next morning at 10:00, while I'm chairing the meeting, someone puts a note in front of me: 'President Carter's on the phone. Would you take the call?' So, I called for a coffee break and went in the other room, and Carter said, 'It's 5:00 in the morning in Atlanta, but I'm so excited, I had to talk to you.' He said, 'Does the name Jan Leschly mean anything to you?' And I said no, it didn't. And he said, 'Well, I had dinner with him last night in Washington, D.C., and he is the CEO of a company called SmithKline Beecham, and at dinner he told me how impressed he was with what Merck had done because he understood immediately what such an initiative means in terms of loyalty of staff.' And, Leschly asked President Carter, 'Do you have any idea of something SmithKline Beecham could do that would be similar?' And I said to President Carter, 'You're not going to believe this, but . . .' Then I told him the story. By that afternoon, he'd been back to Jan Leschly, and we had an agreement to get albendazole.[121]

It was fortunate timing. "Bill had been actively managing Merck's Mectizan Donation Program for onchocerciasis for 10 years and had been impressed with its success as a public-private partnership," David Addiss, the CDC's representative at the meeting, later remarked. "He saw it as a model of pharmaco-philanthropy and a wave of the future in addressing NTDs that impact the poorest of the poor in the developing world. Suddenly, the opportunity for replicating the model had appeared—likely by combining a donation program for albendazole with the MDP for the affected African countries—and he was determined not to let it slip away."[122] Leschly, along with his Senior Vice President of Corporate Affairs, Dr. James Hill, and several SmithKline Beecham (SB) scientists, flew to Atlanta to meet with Foege to work out the details of a donation program. Under the arrangement, albendazole tablets (donated by SB) would be distributed along with Mectizan (donated by Merck) in African countries where LF was endemic.

In 1998, Merck agreed to expand the MDP to cover LF "in African countries where onchocerciasis and lymphatic filariasis are co-endemic."[123] For the first time, two major pharmaceutical companies—normally competitors—were collaborating in a joint donation program to eliminate a major NTD in sub-Saharan Africa. And, the means of delivering the two drugs would be essentially the same as for Mectizan alone—APOC and the OCP at the regional level, and local communities via ComDT at the country and grassroots levels. A global elimination program, the Global Program to Eliminate Lymphatic Filariasis (GPELF), initially built on TDR-supported research guided by Dr. Dato C. P. Ramachandran, was developed in WHO by Drs. Eric Ottesen, Brian Duke, and Kazem Behbehani of WHO's Division for the Control of Tropical Diseases.[124] In 1996–1997, that program, coupled with the prospect of an SB commitment to donate albendazole, were instrumental in the WHO World Health Assembly issuing a declaration in May 1997, calling for the elimination of LF worldwide.

An LF partnership, known as the Global Alliance to Eliminate Lymphatic Filariasis (GAELF) was formed in 2000. The partnership consisted of the two pharmaceutical companies, international organizations (WHO, World Bank, UNICEF), donors, NGDOs, two universities (Liverpool School of Tropical Medicine, Emory University's Rollins School of Public Health), the CDC, and ministries of health in the affected countries.[125] Shortly after GAELF's first meeting in 2000, SB merged with Glaxo Welcome, to become GlaxoSmithKline (GSK). GSK upheld the SB commitment for LF and assigned Brian Bagnall as the program's first director.

WHO has ranked LF as the second-leading cause of long-term disability worldwide after mental illness.[126] LF is second only to malaria as the most widespread vector-borne parasitic disease.[127] As of 2000, 120 million people were estimated to be infected with LF, with more than 1 billion at risk of contracting the disease.[128] Roughly one-third of the total LF-infected and at-risk populations reside in Africa, with a second third in India, and the final third in three combined subregions— East Asia, the Pacific Islands, and the Americas. The LF burden on the African continent, measured by numbers of people infected, at ~40 million, slightly exceeds the 37 million calculated through REMO to be infected with onchocerciasis. Virtually all oncho-endemic countries—11 in the OCP and 19 in APOC—are also LF endemic; only Burundi has had no evidence of LF. The disease is concentrated in the rural areas, but, unlike oncho, is also found in urban areas. In Africa, the principal vector that transmits the LF parasite, *Wuchereria bancrofti*, is the *Anopheles* mosquito, found mostly in rural areas. But the parasite is also spread by the *Culex* mosquito that inhabits urban and semi-urban areas in parts of East Africa.

Similar to the oncho transmission cycle, the female mosquito picks up the LF parasite in a blood meal. While in the mosquito, LF microfilariae develop through larval stages into infective larvae that, when deposited in the skin of the next human host via mosquito bites, migrate to the lymphatic vessels, where they grow into adult worms that live for approximately five to seven years.[129] The principal manifestations of the disease result from adult worms dwelling in the lymphatic vessels and damaging the lymphatic system. Major symptoms include swelling of the limbs, known as lymphedema, resulting from fluid buildup; elephantiasis, or advanced-stage lymphedema, in which the skin and underlying tissues of the legs and feet become hard and thickened; and hydrocele of the scrotum in men, resulting from fluid buildup around the testicles. These symptoms lead to painful episodes of local inflammation including greater susceptibility to secondary infections; long-term disability; severe social stigma undermining employment and marriage prospects; and sexual dysfunction.[130]

Control and eventual elimination of LF involves pursuing two parallel strategies. The first entails blocking transmission by killing microfilariae produced by the adult worms. Research by several investigators showed that the combined treatment of Mectizan and albendazole at least once a year is close to 99% effective in eliminating LF microfilariae in the body and thereby interrupting transmission of the disease.[131] Equally effective is the combination of albendazole and DEC. The latter, however, cannot be given in most sub-Saharan African countries due to the likelihood of a Mazzotti reaction in individuals who harbor the oncho parasite. The infeasibility of treating with DEC in much of Africa was a principal reason for Merck agreeing to donate Mectizan.[132] Once LF microfilariae have been brought down to an insignificant level via Mectizan + albendazole treatment, the mosquito is unable to pick up and transmit the parasite.

The second strategy involves treating LF symptoms. Symptomatic treatment is usually individualized depending upon the symptom and its severity. Care of affected limbs involving a combination of elevation, daily washing, antibacterial and antifungal skincare, and gentle movement is commonly employed.[133] The most effective intervention for hydrocele is surgery to remove fluid buildup around the testicles.

The startup phase of the joint program encountered turbulence. "When I came to the [MDP] office in Atlanta, Merck and GSK didn't get on very well," said Bjorn Thylefors, who became MDP director in 2001.[134] He attributed the difficulties, in part, to personality clashes. However, there was a wider issue. Merck had been studying the possibility of donating Mectizan for LF for 10 years and, for various reasons, was inclined not to pursue it. GSK, on the other hand, made a quick, high-profile decision to donate albendazole for LF based on limited data. The company issued a press release in early 1998 after signing a memorandum of understanding (MOU) with WHO to donate albendazole for LF, recognizing its effectiveness when combined with either Mectizan or DEC, but needing to wait several more years for sufficient data to confirm albendazole's efficacy when given alone.[135] In taking these steps, GSK lobbied Merck to donate Mectizan for LF for all oncho- and LF-endemic countries in Africa. In the end, Merck agreed to do so, but according to Thylefors, "it was fairly long and a bit of a painful process coming to that conclusion."[136]

Despite initial tensions, the joint LF donation program for Africa eventually came to fruition and operated effectively. As GSK's Andy Wright, who helped negotiate the joint program, described the Merck-GSK relationship, there was corporate-culture complementarity. Wright gave the analogy of the only child versus the child in a large family. Merck had a long history of operating alone and in full control, whereas GSK was the product of multiple mergers and was comfortable playing backup. As Wright put it, "We were happy to be the minority partner and to slipstream Merck."[137] He thought that the negotiations over the shape of the joint program had been easier than would have otherwise been the case between two large competing pharmaceutical companies. "The negotiations probably would have been far more difficult if Merck had been negotiating with another Merck," he quipped.[138]

Following his assignment in 2000 to plan out the donation program, Wright sought out Brenda Colatrella, Manager of Product Donations for Merck, to pick her brain on organizing and carrying out a large, sustainable drug donation program. He later said, "We fully recognized we were the new kid on the block and had a lot to learn from Merck's 12-year history with the MDP. They were the first donation, had been around the longest, and were the best example of how to make a drug donation program sustainable over the long term."[139] As for GSK, "We were not so concerned about our name being on things, doing things our way, or even having control. We were happy to be a minority partner."[140] Consequently, the MDP and the MEC were retained as established by Merck, with minimal changes. The MEC was slightly modified to become the Mectizan Expert Committee/Albendazole Coordination (MEC/AC) with two LF experts (Drs. Amy Klion, NIH, and Charles Mackenzie, Michigan State University) added to the committee. GSK agreed to cofinance the MEC and several positions in the MDP.

Important similarities between oncho and LF and their treatment facilitated implementation of a joint program and enabled piggybacking the MDA of albendazole on the distribution of Mectizan via ComDT. Both diseases impact the poorest of the poor in rural areas with little or no access to health care. Both require repeated bites from their insect vectors over an extended period for an individual to become infected and for the intensity of infection to increase. Both infections take hold initially in young children and worsen into the late teens. Neither disease is fatal by itself. The MDA at least once a year for LF and oncho can interrupt transmission, provided ≥65% of the targeted population is reached over a sustained period. The timeframe required to halt transmission for each disease depends to some extent on the lifespan of the female adult worm. Combined treatment is needed for 5–7 years for LF. For oncho, the duration can vary from 8 to 20 years depending upon the percentage of the population reached with Mectizan and the infection intensity in the targeted population.[141]

Consequently, ComDT with Mectizan plus albendazole over many years has the potential to eliminate both diseases in sub-Saharan Africa. Furthermore, widespread distribution of the two drugs has the concomitant advantage of killing intestinal worms. Hence, combining albendazole with Mectizan in treating at-risk populations has the potential to eventually eliminate three of the five major NTDs as public health problems in Africa: oncho, LF, and soil-transmitted helminthiasis (STH, a.k.a. intestinal worms).

One key difference between Merck's donation of Mectizan and the GSK donation of albendazole was the involvement and control of WHO. In 1997, Dr. Kazem Behbehani, Director of WHO's Division of the Control of Tropical Diseases, drafted the first MOU between WHO and a pharmaceutical company that governed the use of a donated drug in a comprehensive disease-control program. The MOU resulted in albendazole provided through WHO rather than via an independent donation program, as was the case with the MEC and the MDP established by Merck. By 1997, WHO policy was shifting and the organization was amenable to collaborating with a large pharmaceutical company, whereas it had opposed such collaboration 12 years earlier when Merck management was exploring donating Mectizan. Senior WHO management had witnessed the dramatic impact of the Merck donation in enabling APOC to be launched and extend oncho control successfully throughout much of Africa.

By the time Gro Harlem Brundtland became WHO's fifth director-general in 1998, she and her management team were convinced of the advantages in collaborating with the pharmaceutical industry on drug donations. In her message to the first meeting of the LF Global Alliance in Santiago de Compostela, Spain in May 2000, she stated: "Some people have suggested that Industry-WHO partnerships such as these represent a conflict of interest. On the contrary, we believe such collaboration, which provides drugs for periods long enough to reach the target, are an exemplary commitment to public health in the 21st century."[142] The GSK decision to provide albendazole through WHO-Geneva put WHO in a stronger position to control the LF-elimination program than had been the case with the OCP and APOC, which were managed through the sponsoring-agency steering committee, the CSA. Given the differing institutional arrangements for accessing the two drugs and for overseeing the two programs, how could their integration best be implemented to control LF in Africa?

The LF elimination effort for Africa was discussed at the 5th JAF in the Hague, December 8–10, 1999. Dr. Maria Neira, WHO Director of the Department of Control, Prevention, and Eradication of Endemic Diseases presented the GPELF and delivered a statement on behalf of Brundtland on combining control of the two diseases. That statement read, in part: "Even if WHO is the lead agency in health . . . the broad health agenda is too big for WHO alone. That means partnerships are becoming the preferred working method—not exotic exceptions. One of the goals of the Programme [APOC] is to support primary health care development by gradually expanding community-directed treatment to the control of other endemic diseases such as lymphatic filariasis. I believe there is a potential for such integration and will follow with interest how the Programme will develop in that direction."[143]

Neira reported that WHO had investigated the safety of Mectizan plus albendazole treatment and confirmed that the combination was safe. She gave an estimated cost of $670 million to eliminate LF over a 20-year period in the 29 OCP and APOC countries endemic with the disease.[144] Anne Haddix, director of the LF Support Center at Emory University, followed with her analysis that showed that integrating LF with oncho control through the OCP/APOC would result in a savings of $62 million over the 20-year timeframe based on an assumed 50% overlap of the two diseases in the Participating Countries and would generate an ERR of 28%, due primarily to increased labor productivity.[145]

The follow-on discussions highlighted the need for mapping LF endemicity in the Participating Countries and for institutional arrangements to support combined drug treatment for LF in the context of ongoing OCP/APOC operations. It was decided, based on WHO's recommendation, that the mapping would be conducted via an antigen test, known as an immune-chromatographic test (ICT), and would be coordinated by the TDR with financing from the oncho programs.[146] An ICT was a new diagnostic tool for measuring infection levels of the

Wuchereria bancrofti parasite in minutes from a drop of blood taken from a finger-prick at any time in the field, as opposed to the late-night blood samplings required with previous tests.

There was widespread support at the Hague JAF for integrating oncho and LF control through the oncho programs, in particular APOC. The JAF final report gave a summary of key statements of support. The WHO Director General, as reported by Neira, was "convinced that APOC had the potential for such integration."[147] World Bank President Wolfensohn (in addressing the JAF via video) "underlined the opportunity . . . [for] APOC community-directed treatment to take on also the distribution of albendazole for the control of lymphatic filariasis."[148] WHO Regional Director for Africa Ebrahim Samba "saw the combined treatment as opening up opportunities for integrated mapping, integrated control, and synergistic funding."[149] As CSA chair, I summarized the sponsoring agencies' consensus that: "combining efforts to eliminate [the] two diseases . . . could yield appreciable economic benefits and prove to be highly cost-effective."[150] Finally, the delegations of the Participating Countries "expressed their wish to see the joint treatment go ahead."[151]

Three months later, I convened a special meeting of the CSA in Ouagadougou to respond to a request from the Joint JPC/JAF Session in the Hague asking the CSA to prepare an "issues paper" on integrating oncho and LF control in sub-Saharan Africa. The request specified that the paper should address "the organizational, legal, institutional, managerial, technical, funding and financial aspects of the [LF] Programme" and be submitted to the next joint session in 2000 in Yaoundé, Cameroon.[152] In Ouagadougou, WHO was represented by its regular representative, Bjorn Thylefors, director of WHO/PBL, and a special invitee, Dr. Nevio Zagaria, representing the WHO LF Elimination Program.[153] Unexpectedly, in light of the strong support voiced by Brundtland for integrating LF control into APOC, Zagaria blocked consideration of combining the two programs. Instead, he insisted that the only option for WHO was a country-by-country approach involving coordination of LF and oncho treatment at the district level within each country. It was a highly divisive meeting and a blatant exception to the consistently collegial and productive deliberations during my previous 15 years participating on the CSA. The discussion ended prematurely without any headway on the issues paper.

The deadlock presented obstacles that needed to be overcome for a viable LF program for Africa to go forward. First, WHO's position in the meeting precluded formulating an Africa-wide strategy for LF elimination in alignment with the regional approach for oncho. Second, without a regional structure for LF that could be formally linked to APOC, the World Bank could not mobilize funding for LF elimination as "fiscal agent" responsible for fundraising for APOC. Third, contributions from the 25 donor signatories to the APOC Memorandum could not be used to support an African LF elimination effort. The donor contributions in the APOC Trust Fund could not legally be drawn down to finance LF treatment without a formal link between the two programs at the central level. Fourth, in the absence of an Africa-wide structure for LF, key advantages inherent to oncho control because of its regional nature would not accrue to the LF effort. These benefits, known as "regional public goods," included intercountry collaboration, sharing of effective control methods across countries, identification of regional issues for operational research, and Africa-wide monitoring and evaluation.

The contentious CSA meeting highlighted a potential key constraint to the future integration of NTD control programs: bureaucratic territoriality. The APOC/OCP ComDT network in the 30 Participating Countries was a key asset in enabling donated drugs for NTDs to reach millions in rural areas. By the early 2000s, that network had opened up remote, desperately poor areas to access donated drugs where regular government-provided health services were scant or nonexistent. However, ComDT was a rudimentary network relying on volunteer CDDs and susceptible to overload. In the case of LF and oncho, close coordination at the central level was vital to avoid overloading that nascent network.

In order to achieve integration, WHO, as the incumbent executing agency, and its task manager(s), would need to relinquish some authority and control in order for coordination with another disease-control effort—in this case APOC—to work properly. Senior management in WHO understood the importance of partnership and the give-and-take required to make it work. However, those at the working level seemed less willing to pay the price of partnership if it meant ceding control over an ongoing disease-specific program.

The CSA meeting in Ouagadougou revealed the lengths to which a task manager might go to avoid relinquishing some control. In this case, blocking integration would mean diminished funding for LF control in Africa. The first external evaluation of APOC, led by Professor Ransome-Kuti, recognized the difficulty in pursuing integration of disease control efforts. An excerpt from the Evaluation Report presented to the Yaoundé JAF in 2000, stated, "On the subject of integration it was suggested that the concept could very well meet with resistance from the various partners in the programmes concerned and that, perhaps, priority should be given to tasks rather than to programmes as such."[154] The problem with integrating tasks rather than programs, however, was that fund-mobilization took place for entire programs, not tasks within those programs. Fundraising for specific tasks, such as mapping or drug distribution, could result in earmarking of contributions for donor-preferred tasks. Such earmarking would have made financing the oncho and LF programs excessively complicated and probably unworkable.

The aftermath of the CSA meeting involved scrambling to salvage some degree of integration between the LF and oncho-control programs to enable LF treatment to go forward. I contacted David Heymann, WHO executive director for communicable diseases, for clarification of the WHO position regarding integration. He referred to the CSA meeting stalemate as a "misunderstanding" and confirmed that the WHO position remained that LF should be "integrated into the existing onchocerciasis control framework."[155]

I also reached out to other key stakeholders in an LF-oncho program for Africa on their minimum criteria for an integrated effort. Those stakeholders included the NGDO Coordination Group, Merck, the LF Centre at the Liverpool School of Tropical Medicine, the LF Support Center at Emory University, and the MDP. There was general agreement that core LF control responsibilities should be integrated into existing oncho-control activities and managed through the OCP and APOC. Integration was seen as far preferable to two separate vertical programs in Africa, and necessary to begin addressing LF in Africa.

However, an integrated arrangement would fall short of a comprehensive approach for LF. There were nine LF-endemic countries that were not oncho endemic.[156] The group included Comoros, Eritrea, The Gambia, Madagascar, Zambia, Zimbabwe; as well as Kenya, Mozambique, and Rwanda that were part of APOC but had no local sources of oncho transmission and hence no ComDT projects.[157] Moreover, the OCP and APOC control strategies at that time confined Mectizan treatment to hyperendemic and meso-endemic areas. Drug-delivery infrastructure was largely nonexistent in the hypo-endemic areas, many of which were LF endemic. There was LF in some urban areas where oncho did not exist and where ComDT was challenging and costly to implement. Even in areas where oncho and LF control activities could be fully integrated, there was the obstacle of loiasis in some countries, limiting treatment with Mectizan. Finally, although Mectizan provided symptomatic relief for oncho-infected communities by halting itching and preventing blindness, combined drug treatment did little to ameliorate the disabling symptoms of LF. Somehow, these gaps would need to be addressed to achieve a comprehensive LF elimination effort throughout Africa.

In the end, partial integration of the LF elimination program for Africa and the oncho programs was achieved to enable LF treatment to proceed. Yankum

Dadzie, who had retired as OCP director the year before, and Johnny Gyapong, a Ghanaian epidemiologist and expert on LF, helped prepare a CSA "discussion paper" (modified name for "issues paper") for the 2000 Joint JPC/JAF Session in Yaoundé. Based on that paper, the Joint Session endorsed several key steps to integrate oncho and LF control. The oncho programs would finance LF treatment via ComDT out of their approved budgets in all co-endemic areas, except for those areas where the OCP and APOC were not operating, i.e. the oncho hypo-endemic areas.[158] This decision, by extension, meant that the World Bank would mobilize funding for LF treatment when raising financing to meet OCP/APOC budgetary obligations; and that donor contributions in the APOC Trust Fund could be drawn down to finance the MDA for LF as part of the oncho-program budgets. The Joint Session also endorsed integration at the expert advisory and national levels. The Chair of the African LF Program Review Group (PRG) would attend the sessions of the two oncho-expert committees, the EAC and the TCC; and representatives from the oncho expert committees would attend the African PRG sessions.[159] At the country level, governments were encouraged to integrate the operations of the national taskforces for the two diseases.

Dadzie continued over the next several years to pursue integration of the two control efforts with the OCP/APOC, the Global Alliance, the NGDO Coordination Group, and those responsible for each of the diseases at the national level. He served as the first chair of the Global Alliance's Technical Advisory Group (TAG) and later chair of the Global Alliance, itself. He traveled to the Participating Countries and worked to bring together the national taskforces for the two diseases in planning and implementing control activities.[160] As he later explained, he was able to convince oncho and LF national authorities that by working together they could attract greater donor funding, while economizing on resources by avoiding duplication of activities. And, in so doing, they could achieve better control results.

Mapping of LF via the ICT for all African-endemic countries proceeded more slowly than for oncho via REMO. After the first 10 years of the LF elimination program in Africa, about half of the oncho-endemic countries had been mapped for LF.[161] Nevertheless, treatments for LF scaled up rapidly, particularly in those countries that completed mapping. The Gates Foundation provided $20 million to the GPELF at the end of 2000, which enabled LF treatment to go forward in several OCP/APOC Participating Countries, including Burkina Faso, Ghana, Tanzania, and Togo.[162] Fund mobilization efforts on behalf of APOC, along with bilateral funding from USAID, helped ensure financing for the scale-up of LF treatment.

By the end of 2009, there had been 280 million cumulative treatments to 106 million Africans during the first 10 years of the effort.[163] Virtually all of these consisted of Mectizan plus albendazole treatments that took place in ex-OCP and APOC countries that were LF-oncho co-endemic. Integration of LF and on-cho treatment strategies resulted in national programs that covered entire LF at-risk populations in Burkina Faso, Ghana, Malawi, and Togo.[164] By 2017, Ma-lawi had attained sufficient progress to stop treatment for LF nationwide and Togo had become the first country in sub-Saharan Africa to be verified by WHO as having eliminated LF as a public health problem.[165]

Combining oncho and LF control strategies and activities at the regional and country levels was the first major attempt to integrate programs for two major NTDs. It paved the way for further NTD integration, much of it focused on the MDA of donated drugs from pharmaceutical companies for trachoma, STH, and schistosomiasis—in addition to LF and oncho. There was optimism within the international community that these other drugs could also be delivered cost-effectively through an integrated approach grounded in the ComDT network—the common denominator that enabled NTD programs to reach remote, rural areas in large parts of sub-Saharan Africa. International support for an NTD integrated approach received an important boost through meetings in 2003 and 2005 in Berlin, co-sponsored by the German Agency for Technical Cooperation (GTZ) and WHO. It was in the context of those meetings that the term "neglected tropical diseases" was coined.[166] The Berlin meetings also contributed to the establishment of the Department of Control of Neglected Tropical Diseases (WHO/NTD) within WHO-Geneva in 2005, with Dr. Lorenzo Savioli as its first director.[167]

Chapter 8

Deepening and Widening the Objective

The fight against river blindness is not completely won. Nor does the
challenge end there. A terrible adverse impact on development and the
quality of life can result from the diseases which maim and stigmatize
so many in Africa. . . . Through its work at the community level and its
regional approach, the river blindness program has set the stage for
results, without further extensive research, in addressing elephantiasis,
Vitamin A deficiency, trachoma, and schistosomiasis.
   —Robert S. McNamara, "Look How Successful an Aid Partnership Can
Be," *International Herald Tribune*, Thursday, December 20, 2001

New Directions, New Uncertainties

Major changes in responsibilities for the oncho-control effort took place during 2003–2006. WHO Director-General Brundtland and World Bank President
Wolfensohn left their positions in 2003 and 2005, respectively, when their terms
in office expired. Brundtland and Wolfensohn had been strong proponents of
partnership, oncho control in Africa, and NTD integration. Their replacements
lasted less than three years. WHO Director-General Lee Jong-wook died while in
office in 2006 and Bank President Paul Wolfowitz was forced to resign over ethics violations in 2007. Neither official, partly due to their limited time in office,
got actively involved in the oncho-control effort.

In addition, Dr. Sékétéli and I reached our mandatory retirement ages in mid-
2005 and late 2004, respectively. Selection committees were set up in the World
Bank and in WHO-AFRO to choose replacements for us. The AFRO selection
committee chose Dr. Uche Amazigo as the new director of APOC. Amazigo, a
biologist by training, had had a long history working on ivermectin treatment,
first as a university researcher, then as a consultant for the TDR where she developed a training program for CDDs on drug distribution and record-keeping. Previously, she had worked in APOC for a decade. Her first position was "scientist," and,
among her assignments, she participated in the TDR-sponsored ComDT study.
Subsequently, she moved up to become Chief of Sustainable Drug Distribution

under Sékétéli. Amazigo was from Nigeria, the largest and most active of the APOC countries. As the new APOC director, she became the first woman to have a senior management role in either the OCP or APOC.

The World Bank panel chose Dr. Ousmane Bangoura, a medical doctor from Guinea, for the position of Oncho Coordinator (the title reverted to Coordinator from Manager). Prior to joining the World Bank, Bangoura had held the position of Guinea's secretary-general in the ministry of health, second to the minister. He had been hired into the World Bank in 1994, as a health-sector task manager, by Ok Pannenborg, Bank division chief for health and education for the Sahelian countries, who was also responsible for the oncho programs. The selection of Bangoura appeared logical for someone working on a major disease-control effort covering much of sub-Saharan Africa.

Bangoura had a solid understanding of NTDs and health-care projects at the country level. He had worked in Bank country offices in Mauritania and Cameroon in implementing country strategies to improve health care.[1] However, he had little background in donor coordination and fundraising. It does not appear that the World Bank panel gave much, if any, weight to the Bank's statutory responsibilities in relation to APOC in selecting the new Coordinator. The foremost responsibilities of the Bank under the program agreements, as oncho fiscal agent, were fund mobilization, financial management of the Trust Fund, and donor coordination. Instead, the panel's emphasis was on health-related skills associated with disease control—an area that overlapped with the responsibilities of APOC management. To my frustration, the division chief responsible for oncho did not permit me to assist in preparing the terms of reference for the position to guide the panel in making its selection.

The upshot was that Bangoura focused on program activities in the APOC countries and gave far less attention to donor support. Bernhard Liese, consultant in the Oncho Unit working with Bangoura, later commented, "Ousemane had no interest in donor fundraising."[2] The resulting inattention to APOC financing led to declining donor support during the second half of the 2000s. And, the increased involvement of the Bank in program-implementation issues precipitated infighting and disagreements between Bangoura and first, Sékétéli, and then Amazigo.[3] The resulting tensions dampened interest among the APOC directors in participating in joint Bank/APOC donor visits.[4]

Prior to beginning retirement, I sent an email to Bangoura, with copies to the Bank oncho team, recommending that the Oncho Unit undertake several fund-mobilization activities for 2006. The most important of these was to organize an

APOC donors' conference at World Bank headquarters in June 2006.[5] Since Bank-chaired donors' conferences had been convened biennially during the previous 20 years, and the last one had occurred in June 2004, the next conference was due to take place in 2006. I saw convening and organizing an APOC donors' conference as the Bank's most important oncho task that year. The funding would be necessary for the Program to continue to scale-up. Equally important, the conference would provide an opportunity to introduce the new senior oncho team, Amazigo and Bangoura, to the donors.

At the 2005 JAF in Paris, participants "expressed concern on the repeated absence of some donors at APOC meetings and requested that the World Bank as the fiscal agent . . . rekindle the interest of all existing donors in APOC meetings, Donor Conferences, and Programme operations, and aim to attract new donors."[6] At that meeting, the new chair of the CSA, Dr. James Mwanzia from WHO/AFRO, "announced that a Donors' Conference was being planned for June 2006 . . . to mobilize resources for the financial shortfall to complete APOC."[7] In the end, no donors' conference took place in 2006. Moreover, no donors' conference was convened by the Bank during the last decade of APOC. Additionally, less than 10 Bank/APOC missions were undertaken to meet with different donor delegations in capitals during 2006–2015. By contrast, 12–16 missions had been carried out every year in donor capitals by the Bank with oncho program directors during the previous two decades.

The absence of donors' conferences and donor visits had a detrimental impact on donor support. Funding for APOC began declining and donor interest waned. During 2006–2011, 12 donors dropped out. Reaching agreement on policy proposals within the partnership became more problematic because there was no donors' forum to discuss them and arrive at a consensus position. The final evaluation of APOC, led by Gilbert Burnham of Johns Hopkins University's Bloomberg School of Public Health, stated, "There were perceptions that beyond 2004, the cessation of donors' conferences hampered relationships with the donors and failed to sustain their interest in the programme. In the final years of APOC, some donors and countries indicated that they were feeling sometimes excluded from the decision-making process."[8]

Bangoura's replacement in 2009, Dr. Donald Bundy, later argued that donor financing and participation suffered primarily because of the global financial crisis during 2008–2009.[9] The crisis was unquestionably an important factor. Nevertheless, donors began leaving prior to 2008, and some remained throughout the crisis but left afterward. In any case, the Bank's efforts to mobilize funding for

APOC declined beginning in 2005 through the end of the Program, even though the World Bank was obligated under the APOC agreement (Memorandum) to secure the funding required to implement APOC. The agreement specified the Bank's role as: "[reaching] an understanding" annually, or biennially, with "each Contributing Party on the amount" "to be contributed by it" to obtain the funding "required to be paid in annually or biennially . . . for implementation of the Programme."[10]

The absence of a donor forum eventually led to alternative ways to communicate with the donors. The concept of "expanded CSA meetings" was developed, whereby the largest donors and some participating countries were invited to attend select CSA sessions. Employing the CSA for donor communication modified the functions and membership of the CSA from those specified in the APOC agreement.[11] It was no longer exclusively a steering committee led by the sponsoring agencies focusing on policies, strategic plans, program budgets, and interim decision-making on behalf of the JAF. The CSA's executive function was weakened, as it became a vehicle for communicating with select donors and Participating Countries. Moreover, some donors did not regard expanded CSA sessions as an adequate substitute for previous donors' conferences, which had included all donors and covered all financing issues. The final APOC evaluation team wrote: "Some donors were increasingly unhappy with their perceived peripheralization in financial matters at APOC. The donors felt they had difficulty getting a true financial picture of the project, and how the funds were being used."[12]

Two important developments during 2007–2010 helped rescue APOC financially. One involved a Merck decision to contribute to the APOC Trust Fund. As Merck's Director of Global Health Partnerships, Kenneth Gustavsen, described it: "In 2007, two things came together nicely. There was a $50 million gap in the Trust Fund that coincided with the 20th anniversary of the MDP. We saw this as an opportunity to do something that would be partly commemorative of the 20th anniversary and would be catalytic in helping the Bank in closing the financing gap. So, we took the initiative to contribute 50% of the financing gap and let the rest figure itself out."[13] Merck's contribution of $25 million was pledged at the 2007 JAF in Brussels and paid into the APOC Trust Fund over 2008–2015. The Merck pledge was coupled with a statement by World Bank President Robert Zoellick, in a press release at the Brussels JAF, that "the World Bank, as fiscal agent and one of the largest donors of APOC, remains committed to mobilize additional contributions from the other contributing parties in order to effectively achieve the funding goals necessary to complete this worthy effort."[14]

The other development was Amazigo's personal involvement in fundraising. After initially trying to convince Bangoura to organize a donors' conference without success, she began working with select donor representatives with whom she had a personal rapport to secure additional financing for the Trust Fund.[15] She succeeded in getting increased commitments from the Netherlands; CIDA; the Champalimaud Foundation in Portugal; General Theophilus Danjuma, a wealthy Nigerian, through the local NGDO, MITOSATH; and AfDB.[16] The AfDB contribution was substantial, totaling $22.9 million during 2009–2015.[17] Based on these additional commitments and a projected budget of $114 million during 2008–2015, Bangoura was able to report to the 2008 JAF in Kampala, Uganda, that a financing gap of "about $20 million" remained for the last seven years of APOC.[18]

APOC Makes Major Inroads on Onchocerciasis

SCALING UP TREATMENT

Amazigo's experience in working with the TDR and APOC was well suited to the needs of the Program during 2006–2011. She had developed skills and knowledge related to strengthening the capacity and sustainability of ComDT; enhancing gender awareness; and empowering local communities. Each of those skills came into play during her five-year tenure. The principal objective over those years was to strengthen ComDT sustainability to eventually transfer Mectizan-treatment responsibilities to the Participating Countries. Enhanced ComDT capacities were needed to deliver health-care interventions in addition to Mectizan and albendazole in the rural areas. The Program also became more attentive to the needs of at-risk adolescent girls and young women; and efforts were stepped up to recruit women as CDDs.

Despite financial strains, APOC continued to scale up rapidly during Amazigo's tenure. APOC-supported projects increased distribution of Mectizan from 35.6 million people through 77,000 communities during 2004–2005 (the year before she assumed the directorship) to 80.2 million people in 142,000 communities in 2011 (the year she retired).[19] And, the average coverage rate was 76.7%.[20] Only one country, Angola, had coverage below 60%. The number of people treated reached 90% of the "high-risk" population identified by REMO. By the end of 2011, the Program was approaching coverage of all of the heavily endemic populations in the 17 Participating Countries (South Sudan gained independence and joined the Program in 2011).

ELIMINATING THE VECTOR

During the preparation of APOC, consultant entomologist Frank Walsh had identified four foci where oncho vectors could potentially be eliminated. They were in Uganda, Equatorial Guinea, and Tanzania. Walsh had recommended a strategy for elimination based, in part, on the successful elimination of the blackfly species, *Simulium neavei*, from Kenya during the 1950s. Elimination of vectors turned out to be an expeditious and sustainable method of interrupting oncho transmission, but the strategy was only feasible where blackfly species were isolated and traveled shorter distances.

In 1995, APOC initiated large-scale ground larviciding with temephos in the Itwara focus in western Uganda near the DRC border, an area of 600 km² with a population of ~80,000 inhabitants[21] The target was *Simulium neavei*, an efficient vector that lays larvae on freshwater crabs in rivers. Oncho transmission levels were high in the Itwara area.[22] Efforts had been made to reduce transmission through Mectizan treatment prior to APOC, with little success.[23] Larviciding was completed in 2003. Assessments since have not found any blackflies or vector-invested crabs in the Itwara focus.[24] The parasite reservoir in the population was on schedule to die out by 2016.[25]

Adjacent to Itwara, in Uganda was the Mpamba-Nkusi focus, with the same *Simulium neavei* vector. Mpamba-Nkusi was about half the size of Itwara, with a smaller population. Despite annual Mectizan treatment in 330 communities in the area for more than a decade, "infection remained relatively high."[26] Ground larviciding with temephos was launched in 2002, supplemented with Mectizan treatment. Since 2008, crabs in the area have been negative for *Simulium naevei* larva, and no biting blackflies have been caught there since 2010.[27] Recent surveillance has shown that the vector, and hence, transmission, have been eliminated in the Mpamba-Nkusi focus.[28]

The vector elimination project in the Tukuyu focus, an area of 3,000 km², in southern Tanzania near the border with Malawi, appears to have been less definitive in wiping out the local vector, *Simulium thyolense*, in large part due to nearby sources of potential vector re-invasion. Large-scale ground larviciding was undertaken in 2003 and 2005. The result was "drastically reduced" blackfly biting rates in the area.[29] Larviciding was complemented by Mectizan treatment through a Sightsavers-supported ComDT project. The result has been near-elimination of the disease, though the threat of the vector returning remains.

The most ambitious of the vector-elimination efforts was on the Island of Bioko, part of Equatorial Guinea. Bioko, with an area of 2,017 km² and 334,463 inhabitants (2015 census), lies 32 km off the closest mainland in Cameroon. Bioko was the only island in the world to be oncho endemic. Mectizan treatment began in 1990 and reduced OSD morbidity, but did not interrupt transmission. With the launch of APOC in 1995, preparatory studies confirmed that the vector, a local form of *Simulium yahense*, was sufficiently isolated to enable an attempt at elimination. Ground-based larviciding with temephos commenced in early 2001, but had to be supplemented by helicopter spraying in 2003 and 2005 due to the inaccessibility of large parts of the island. The last local blackfly was caught in 2005 and none has since been found.[30] A study carried out during 2016–2017, found no evidence of active infection or recent transmission. The study's authors concluded that WHO criteria for stopping Mectizan treatment had been met and recommended that WHO commence three years of post-treatment surveillance to confirm elimination of the disease.[31]

Broadening and Extending the APOC Mandate

At CSA initiative, a summit of APOC partners was organized in Yaoundé, Cameroon, in September 2006. The summit arose out of the 2005 APOC external evaluation, which recommended that the JAF and the CSA consult with APOC partners, such as governments, international organizations, donor agencies, and NGDOs, on how to ensure continuing ComDT project support after APOC's conclusion—at the time, planned for 2010.[32] The evaluation team was concerned about implementation delays in conflict and post-conflict countries and in loiasis-endemic areas, and with the resulting inability to provide project support for the minimum five years considered necessary to achieve self-sustaining Mectizan treatment. Self-sustainable community-directed treatment was a key APOC objective referenced in the Memorandum. The other concern was perceived donor reluctance to extend the Program beyond 2010.[33] The donors were seeking a larger Participating Countries budgetary commitment to support treatment sustainability, before agreeing to extend APOC.[34]

In preparation for the Yaoundé Summit, the CSA set up the Working Group on the Future of Onchocerciasis Control in Africa. The task of the group, chaired by Catherine Hodgkin of the Netherlands' Royal Tropical Institute, was to respond to recommendations from the 2005 Evaluation to take stock of the future of APOC, including the focus of its activities, its geographic mandate, and its sources of financing. The group's recommendations in each of these areas were endorsed by the MOH ministers at the Yaoundé Summit in a "Declaration on Onchocercia-sis." Those recommendations included (1) extending APOC from 2010 to 2015; (2) establishing sustainable ComDT projects in all oncho-endemic countries, notably widening inclusion to the former OCP countries; (3) developing "an evidence base" for determining when and where to stop Mectizan treatment; and (4) encouraging APOC to "promote . . . co-implementation" of interventions through ComDT projects "to provide multiple health benefits to large populations."[35]

The group also recommended exploring new funding opportunities, including Participating Countries commitments, which resulted in a statement in the Yaoundé Declaration, that "urge[d] endemic countries to make annual budgetary commitments for onchocerciasis control activities."[36] This statement helped satisfy the donors' concern for greater budgetary support from the Participating Countries going forward. And, it enabled the Yaoundé Declaration to endorse the Working Group's recommendation to extend APOC through 2015 to fulfill the objective of establishing sustainable ComDT projects in all oncho-endemic African countries.

The Working Group refocused attention on the former OCP countries. Five of the ex-OCP countries (Benin, Ghana, Guinea, Sierra Leone, and Togo) had received Mectizan treatment support in the Special Intervention Zones (SIZ) since the closure of OCP in 2002. The SIZ were areas experiencing ongoing transmission after the OCP closed. Treatment in the SIZ was financed out of the $6.4 million reserve remaining in the OCP Trust Fund. After five years of treatment, surveillance showed that transmission indicators and prevalence levels in the SIZ in Benin, Guinea, and Togo had been brought down to acceptable levels.[37] Elsewhere, however, the situation required attention.

It was known by the OCP's closure, that Sierra Leone would require at least 10 years of Mectizan treatment to halt transmission, which had resumed throughout the country during its lengthy civil war.[38] The Working Group's report referred to the situation in Sierra Leone as "very alarming."[39] Treatment coverage rates were also unacceptably low in the SIZ in Ghana. Entomological surveillance during 2005 showed blackfly-infectivity in the Pru River basin to exceed acceptable levels.[40] In the non-SIZ countries of Guinea-Bissau and Côte d'Ivoire, civil conflicts during the late 1990s and early 2000s had led to a resurgence of transmission and there was concern that it could spread beyond Ivoirian borders into Mali and Burkina Faso.

The Working Group recommended that the APOC mandate be expanded to cover the ex-OCP countries and provide them with surveillance and technical support to protect the gains achieved under the OCP. The 2006 JAF in Dar es Salaam,

Tanzania, approved the Working Group's recommendations to address an "epidemiological situation [that] requires urgent attention."[41] The 2007 JAF in Brussels, Belgium, approved an amended APOC Memorandum to provide the legal authority to include the ex-OCP countries, and to extend APOC, including the Trust Fund, through 2015.[42] By 2009, three million people were still being treated annually in former OCP areas with APOC financial and technical support.

It can be argued, given the need for continuing control in the former OCP countries, that the OCP was concluded prematurely. After 2000, there was general agreement within the CSA and OCP management that closing the OCP in 2002 was important to demonstrate to the donors that the Program was time-bound, as they had been told, and would conclude once the long-promised results of eliminating the parasite reservoir in the OCP area had been achieved (with the exception of Sierra Leone due to the civil war). The OCP had been underway for nearly 29 years—well beyond its initial 20-year timeframe. After 1995, the donors were asked to double up their support by financing the OCP and APOC in parallel. It was my view that the level of contributions being asked of the donors could not be sustained beyond the seven-year overlap of the two programs (1996–2002). There was also concern that extending the OCP beyond 2002 could jeopardize the rapid scale-up of APOC. It was generally thought in the early 2000s by those of us involved in the management of both programs that any residual transmission in the former OCP countries could be suppressed through Mectizan treatment, coupled with ongoing surveillance via the Multi-Disease Surveillance Center (MDSC).

However, unanticipated issues complicated the control effort in the ex-OCP countries.[43] First, there was a tendency within the governments of the former OCP countries to conclude that the oncho problem had been solved, based on the decision to close the Program. That mindset made it difficult to commit scarce government resources to address residual transmission. Second, with the closure of the OCP, there was the absence of a forum for discussing oncho-related problems and for advocating for action to address them. Third, given the emphasis on vector control, NGDO involvement in the former OCP countries was patchy, limiting the availability of resources for community-directed treatment. Fourth, unexpected conflicts, particularly in Côte d'Ivoire, resulted in oncho resurgence in non-SIZ areas. Finally, financial resources for the MDSC were unexpectedly constrained during the post-OCP years. The plan was to have the MDSC provide surveillance for oncho and cerebral spinal meningitis in the ex-OCP countries, utilizing the offices and laboratories in the former OCP compound in Ouagadougou. The MDSC was established and survived for a number

of years but did not receive adequate funding from WHO/AFRO, potential donors, or the APOC Trust Fund to carry out the multicountry surveillance anticipated. By the end of 2010, the Center lacked the financing to cover staff salaries
for the team responsible for oncho surveillance.[44]

Major Studies Provide Justification for Widening and Deepening Control Efforts

DISEASE CONTROL INTEGRATION

Based on ComDT's success in achieving high coverage with Mectizan for oncho
and with Mectizan plus albendazole for LF and STH in countries where the three
NTDs were co-endemic, there was increasing interest within the TDR and APOC
in investigating the potential to deliver other health-care interventions. There was
a rapidly-growing need for cost-effective ways of delivering health care to the rural
poor, who, historically, had lacked access to it. Effective drugs were coming on
stream in the early 2000s through pharmaceutical donation programs, but the infrastructure was inadequate to get them to the populations in need. Consequently,
the TDR's Hans Remme proposed a follow-on study to the 1994–1996 community-
based study that established ComDT to deliver Mectizan. This new study would
assess the capacity of ComDT to deliver additional "community-directed interventions" (CDI) to address "major public health problems in Africa."[45] The stated objective was "to determine the extent to which the CDI process currently being used
for ivermectin treatment of onchocerciasis in Africa can be used for the delivery of
other health interventions with differing degrees of complexity."[46]

The three-year CDI study got underway in 2005. It included 2.4 million people
in Cameroon, Nigeria, and Uganda at seven sites covering 35 health districts.[47]
ComDT had been delivering Mectizan treatment at each of the sites for several
years. The capacity of ComDT was tested by adding one new intervention to ongoing Mectizan distribution during year one and year two of the study. Four interventions with varying degrees of complexity were tested. The interventions were:
malaria treatment, insecticide-treated bed nets, vitamin A capsules (to prevent
childhood blindness and mortality), and directly observed treatment of tuberculosis (DOTS). In the third year, the study assessed the capability of ComDT to deliver
all four interventions, in addition to Mectizan. Each research site encompassed
five health districts, enabling comparisons across districts. Four districts were
used to try out differing interventions and to compare the effectiveness of delivering them with the one district where conventional means of delivery were de-

ployed.[48] Interventions were graded based on generally-accepted quantitative indicators, levels of coverage, and standard qualitative indicators.

The findings demonstrated the superiority of ComDT over conventional methods regardless of the type and complexity of the intervention. ComDT was more cost-effective and achieved higher coverage in delivering all interventions, except DOTS for tuberculosis. With DOTS, coverage via ComDT was equivalent to the traditional approach. Overall, the study demonstrated that communities are fully capable of delivering complex interventions and sustaining them, if the communities receive proper training and support.

Surprisingly, when the four interventions were combined with Mectizan delivery in the final year, Mectizan-treatment coverage increased by 10%.[49] The JAF had expressed concern that adding interventions could over-load ComDT, and weaken Mectizan treatment. But the opposite occurred—apparently due to greater community engagement engendered with a CDI package that addressed multiple health concerns.[50] The study also revealed that CDDs were more motivated by "intrinsic incentives," such as recognition and status, than by material incentives.[51] The constraints encountered usually resulted from shortages of drugs or other intervention-related materials.[52] The study's summary recommendation read, "In areas with experience in community-directed treatment for onchocerciasis control, the CDI approach should be used for integrated community-level delivery of a broader range of appropriate health interventions."[53]

In 2010, an evaluation of APOC was conducted by an independent team of experts led by Dr. Sam Adjei, former deputy director-general of the Ghana Health Service. The evaluation concluded that APOC was well-managed, successfully achieving oncho control through its commitment to the sustainability of Mectizan treatment, and working toward multi-disease control integration.[54] The evaluation highlighted ComDT's effectiveness as a platform for community-directed interventions. It cited co-implementation of interventions for malaria, LF, Vitamin A supplementation, and STH; and noted that in 2008, 37.5 million Africans benefited from non-oncho health interventions in conjunction with Mectizan treatment.[55] The evaluation concluded that one of APOC's important achievements had been the contribution of ComDT to "Primary Health Care systems strengthening for integrated service delivery."[56] It cited APOC's development of a curriculum and training module on ComDT to be introduced into the curricula of 34 faculties of medicine and nursing schools in 20 African countries as an important step in spreading knowledge about the CDI.

ELIMINATION OF ONCHOCERCIASIS

The first empirical evidence on the feasibility of oncho elimination with ivermectin in Africa was published in 2009.[57] Those results were part of a longitudi-
nal study on elimination, organized by the TDR Task Force on OOR and financed
by the Gates Foundation. The study was carried out by a research team from the
MOHs of Mali and Senegal, with support from Remme who coordinated the research. The follow-on report of final results was published in 2012 and became
known as the "Proof-of-Principle Study on Onchocerciasis Elimination."[58]

The two reports provided evidence that Mectizan alone could interrupt transmission over a sufficiently-long period to eliminate oncho in a circumscribed area
without risk of it returning. The research took place over 2006–2011 and covered
131 villages and 29,753 people in three hyperendemic foci in eastern Senegal and
western Mali, that were among the first areas to receive large-scale Mectizan treatment in Africa.[59] By 2006, the three foci had received 15–17 years of continuous
treatment. Interim evaluations showed the prevalence of oncho infection falling to
"very low levels."[60] The objective of the study was to determine whether oncho infection and transmission after lengthy treatment had fallen so low "that transmission would be unlikely to sustain itself." That hypothesis was tested by stopping
treatment and conducting surveys for three years to confirm that there had been
no recrudescence of infection and transmission. The 2012 published results
showed that infection levels in all three foci had fallen to zero and transmission
had not resumed more than three years after stopping treatment.

Importantly, treatment was stopped in all three foci before the prevalence of
microfilariae had declined to zero. This led to the finding that there is an infection "breakpoint" below which transmission is no longer self-sustaining and oncho infection will die out of its own accord.[61] Studies during the OCP had indicated that it was safe to stop vector control when the prevalence of microfilariae
reached ≤1.4%.[62] The three study foci were located in the northern half of the
OCP western-extension area that had never benefited from vector control.
Hence, the impact on transmission and infection levels was determined to have
resulted solely from long-term treatment with Mectizan.

The Proof of Principle Study led to a fundamental change in the perception of
Mectizan as a tool to eliminate oncho. ONCHOSIM simulations had indicated that
elimination with the drug was theoretically possible. But there were doubts within
the expert community about whether it was feasible in hyperendemic areas where
the vector was highly efficient, as was the case in the study foci.[63] The findings

were the first empirical evidence that the ONCHOSIM predictions regarding ivermectin and elimination had been accurate. They also highlighted the importance
of epidemiological and entomological evaluations in determining when to stop
treatment, and, after stopping, whether treatment cessation could be permanent.

The study ushered in a fundamental shift in APOC strategy. During the study
years, interim results were reported by Remme to the TCC and the JAF. The
2007 JAF in Brussels recommended applying the study's guidelines on evaluations of stopping treatment in other countries.[64] The APOC Memorandum was
amended by the JAF by adding a clause to the program objective, namely: "[to]
develop the evidence base and assist countries to determine when and where
ivermectin treatment can be stopped."[65] Amazigo reported to the 2008 JAF in
Kampala, Uganda, that for the first time scientific evidence existed that oncho
transmission could be eliminated, "using ivermectin treatment alone delivered
by African communities themselves."[66] It had the makings of an important leap
forward, similar to the breakthrough with ComDT. Like ComDT, the challenge
would be finding concrete ways to put it into action.

That same JAF requested APOC management develop a working definition of
"elimination" and begin undertaking epidemiological evaluations to assess progress toward elimination in ComDT projects and assist in determining where
and when Mectizan treatment could be stopped.[67] Although elimination had
been achieved in the three foci after 15–17 years of Mectizan treatment, the final
study report emphasized that the duration required in other areas would depend
on pre-control endemicity levels. In areas of low endemicity, elimination might
be achieved in less than a decade, whereas areas of very high endemicity might
require annual treatment for 20–25 years.[68]

In February 2009, an Informal Consultation on Elimination of Onchocerciasis
Transmission with Current Tools in Africa was organized by APOC. The session
was financed by APOC, with support from the Gates Foundation and the MDP. The
participants arrived at a definition of elimination: "Reduction of *O. vovulus* infection
and transmission to the extent that interventions can be stopped, but post intervention surveillance is still necessary."[69] The consultation group concluded it would be
difficult to achieve elimination in all of endemic Africa and that APOC "should
proceed gradually, targeting elimination where it is considered feasible."[70] The 2009
JAF in Tunis, Tunisia, at the recommendation of the TCC, endorsed pursuing elimination via a project-by-project strategy.[71] Consequently, epidemiological and entomological surveillance became key in determining which project areas were candidates for eliminating transmission and stopping treatment.

In response to the 2008 JAF request for APOC to begin identifying where Mectizan treatment could be stopped, the Program, with the assistance of Remme, assembled an operational guide to prepare for cessation of treatment. That document, entitled "Conceptual and Operational Framework of Onchocerciasis Elimination with Ivermectin Treatment," set forth procedures for decision-makers in the elimination process. A series of epidemiological and entomological evaluations was recommended over three phases.[72] The first (Phase 1.a.) involved assessing declines in infection levels to predict when the "breakpoint" might be reached. The second (Phase 1.b.) entailed evaluations to determine that the breakpoint had been reached and that treatment could be stopped safely. The third (Phase 2) involved surveillance over at least three years after stopping treatment to confirm that recrudescence had not occurred. And, the last (Phase 3) entailed routine epidemiological surveillance to detect possible recurrence of infection and transmission.

Research supported by modeling in the OCP had indicated that the entomological breakpoint was one infective fly per 2,000 and the epidemiological breakpoint was an average prevalence of microfilariae of 1.4%.[73] Below these thresholds, vector control could be stopped without recurrence of transmission. The thresholds for stopping treatment in the Mali/Senegal elimination studies were similar, though somewhat lower, at 0.92 infective flies per 2,000 and average microfilariae prevalence in the 0.1%–0.8% range.[74]

In light of the new elimination objective, JAF deliberations focused on strategies for accelerating it. At the 2008 Kampala JAF, participants recommended the APOC and former OCP countries "work toward achieving" treatment coverage of "at least 80% instead of the current threshold of 65%."[75] The 2011 Kuwait JAF urged APOC management to scale-up alternative-treatment approaches, including twice-annual Mectizan distribution, which appeared to accelerate oncho elimination in the Americas.[76] The Kuwait JAF encouraged management to "speed up" treatment in "problematic areas," and to focus on cross-border areas, which were important because of the large number of rivers with breeding sites that defined borders, yet were difficult to treat due to the intercountry collaboration required.[77] "Problematic areas" referred to conflict and post-conflict countries and loiasis-endemic areas in West and Central Africa.

Even with these recommended improvements, there remained the hypoendemic areas, which took on new importance with the shift to elimination. In a number of the Participating Countries, these areas would need to be investigated for active sources of transmission for possible treatment. However, nodule palpation, used for REMO, lacked the precision to detect local sources of transmission in hypo-endemic areas. Hence, other mapping methods would need to be employed, which would be time-consuming and expensive. While the JAF had taken the decision to pursue elimination, the cost implications had not been fully assessed. Mapping the hypo-endemic areas had not been accounted for in APOC budgets, and financial strains in the later years of the Program made it difficult to add such new expenditure items.

Nevertheless, it was reported at the 2012 JAF in Bujumbura, Burundi, that entomological surveillance suggested that six ex-OCP countries (Benin, Guinea, Guinea-Bissau, Mali, Niger, and Sierra Leone) might have already halted transmission countrywide and reached the infection breakpoints to enable them to stop treatment and begin post-treatment surveillance.[78] At that same JAF, Remme reported on progress toward elimination in the APOC countries. Out of 34 ComDT projects evaluated during 2008–2012, 12 projects, covering an at-risk population of 17.6 million, had "probably" achieved elimination.[79] Furthermore, preliminary results from epidemiological surveys in Malawi and Chad had confirmed elimination, indicating they could undergo entomological evaluations to determine whether treatment could be stopped.[80]

The International Community Embraces Integrated NTD Control

In addition to elimination, there was a growing interest within the APOC partnership in widening the effort to deliver other health-care interventions, and, in the process, strengthen primary health care. The Kuwait JAF in 2011 framed the combined objective for APOC's remaining five years: "JAF reaffirmed its endorsement for the Programme to pursue the elimination of onchocerciasis in Africa as well as co-implementation of preventive chemotherapy interventions for other selected NTDs in the context of increased support to community level health system strengthening." The 2008 CDI study demonstrated the potency and cost-effectiveness of ComDT in delivering multiple health-care interventions. There was near-unanimous agreement that ComDT should play a central role in co-implementing interventions and thereby facilitate integration of NTD control and elimination. However, there was less agreement on the role that APOC should play in managing NTD integration.

Partly as a result of efforts to integrate oncho and LF control in Africa via APOC during the early 2000s, WHO and the international community began focusing on integrated approaches for controlling and eliminating NTDs. In 2012, the WHO/NTD office, under the direction of Savioli, produced "Accelerating

Work to Overcome the Global Impact of Neglected Tropical Diseases: A Road-map for Implementation" (the Roadmap). The targets for the major NTDs were based on World Health Assembly resolutions during 1997–2011 covering 11 NTDs, including the five largest—LF, oncho, STH, schistosomiasis, and trachoma. According to the Roadmap, the total number of Africans estimated to require "preventive chemotherapy" (periodic drug treatment) for four of the largest NTDs (LF, oncho, STH, and schistosomiasis) exceeded 1 billion, counting more than once individuals infected with two or more of the diseases.[81]

The Roadmap targets became the objectives of a major high-level gathering in London at the Royal College of Physicians in January 2012, cosponsored by WHO Director-General Margaret Chan and Bill Gates. The assembly included pharmaceutical companies, donors, endemic countries, and NGDOs, along with officials from WHO and the World Bank. The meeting produced the London Declaration that committed most of the partners in attendance to controlling, eliminating, or eradicating 10 NTDs through drug access programs, collaboration among the partners, and increases in funding and technical support for integrated NTD control.[82]

The two largest bilateral aid programs at the London meeting, USAID and Britain's DFID, were also the principal remaining country donors in APOC. Both had launched major initiatives to finance national NTD programs. The USAID program began in 2006 and initially focused on LF, trachoma, and oncho in five "fast-track" countries: Burkina Faso, Ghana, Mali, Niger, and Uganda. Over time, the program scaled up to cover five major NTDs in 10 of the former OCP countries, seven of the largest APOC countries, and 14 countries in Asia and the Americas, with an annual budget of $100 million during 2014–2018. The DFID program committed £50 million for bilateral NTD control during 2009–2014.[83] Both programs gave primary focus to the five largest NTDs for which there were drug donations, and to sub-Saharan Africa; and their goals, in line with the Roadmap, called for elimination of LF and trachoma by 2020, and onchocerciasis by 2025. USAID initially set up an arrangement to work through an implementing organization, Research Triangle Institute (RTI International); and, as the program expanded with two additional projects in Africa and Asia, worked with a second NGDO, FHI 360, to assist in project implementation.[84]

With the momentum created by the London Declaration, the 2012 JAF in Bujumbura, Burundi, discussed at length NTD integration and coordinated actions with other NTD programs. The focus was on the big five NTDs with drug donations that had the potential to achieve elimination—referred to as "preventive chemotherapy and transmission control (PCT)" NTDs. Those diseases, the drugs to treat them, and the donating pharmaceutical companies were (1) onchocercia-sis (ivermectin donated by Merck); (2) lymphatic filariasis (albendazole + iver-mectin donated by GSK and Merck; or albendazole plus DEC donated by GSK and Eisai, a pharmaceutical company in Japan); (3) trachoma (azithromycin do-nated by Pfizer); (4) schistosomiasis (praziquantel donated by Merck KGaA, a pharmaceutical company in Darmstadt, Germany); and STH (mebendazole or albendazole, donated by Johnson & Johnson and GSK, respectively). The chal-lenge was to find the most cost-effective arrangement acceptable to the partner-ship to manage a multi-disease control/elimination effort, relying on the ComDT platform to sustain progress toward oncho elimination. The WHO/NTD office had taken the position at the 2010 Abuja JAF that, while it favored APOC con-solidating achievements in oncho control, it did not support APOC becoming "the lead institution to manage multiple diseases."[85]

Extension of the Regional Effort?

With the shift in the objective to elimination, government representatives be-gan arguing for extending APOC by 10 years. At the 2010 JAF in Abuja, Nigeria, the Cameroon delegation stressed the need for a 10-year extension and a con-certed focus on cross-border areas, to achieve elimination.[86] The statement of the president of Nigeria, Dr. Goodluck Jonathan, at the opening of the JAF, sup-ported extending APOC beyond 2015.[87] The report of the External Mid-Term Evaluation of APOC, which was presented and discussed in Abuja, reinforced the case for an extension. One of the report's conclusions read, "It is contradic-tory to expect APOC to exit the scene by 2015 and yet to expect to protect invest-ments and attain the anticipated results. There will be a continuing need for re-gional and technical oversight and coordination. This evaluation supports the need for a 'transformed APOC' for the future beyond 2015."[88]

At the Kuwait JAF in 2011, CSA advisory groups presented the results of anal-yses requested by the JAF the year before. Professor Mamoun Homeida, TCC chair, summarized the conclusions of the Advisory Group on Onchocerciasis Elimination in stating that, while some ComDT projects were on schedule to stop treatment by 2015, no APOC country would achieve elimination by then. Nevertheless, 12 APOC countries and all 11 former OCP countries were on track to eliminate oncho by 2020, protecting a population of 60 million.[89]

Dr. Sam Adjei, who led the 2010 midterm evaluation, presented four sce-narios on behalf of the advisory group on the future of APOC. They included

(1) extending APOC in its existing form to 2025 to achieve oncho elimination; (2) transforming APOC into a "technical agency" for 2015–2025; (3) extending the APOC mandate to 2025 and transforming the Program into "an NTD hub," focusing on health systems strengthening; and (4) have APOC continue on its ongoing track and conclude in 2015.[90] Following discussion of the four scenarios, the JAF reported a "clear consensus" among the African governments in favor of option 3, described as "continuing a dynamic APOC to 2025 for onchocerciasis elimination with co-implementation for NTDs and health system strengthening."[91] The Kuwait JAF requested that APOC management with CSA guidance prepare for the next JAF in Bujumbura, a "concept note" delineating the role of APOC and actions it could take to pursue elimination while collaborating with other NTD programs in Africa; and a Strategic Plan of Action and Budget to achieve elimination during 2016–2025.

The concept note and strategic plan were prepared under the new APOC director, Dr. Paul Samson Lusamba-Dikassa, who was selected by the AFRO to replace Amazigo upon her retirement in 2011. Guidance during preparation was provided through the Expanded CSA, chaired by AFRO's Chris Mwikisa, which included both African country and donor representation. The concept note laid out the rationale and framework for a new regional entity to replace APOC, which "should focus primarily" on the elimination of oncho and LF, while supporting interventions for other preventive chemotherapy (PC) NTDs in Africa, "within the context of national PC programs."[92] The activities of the new regional entity would take place within the framework of the London Declaration and the WHO Roadmap.

The final version of the strategic plan turned into a program proposal for the new entity, including implementation phases, governance structure, and an indicative budget over a 10-year timeframe. The entity was given the name, "Programme for the Elimination of Neglected Diseases in Africa" (PENDA). PENDA was put together by a small group of consultants with input from many, but not all, of the APOC partners through a series of meetings, including two Expanded CSA sessions. Contributors included the three sponsoring agencies at the time (World Bank, WHO, AfDB), two donors (USAID, DFID), two pharmaceutical companies (Merck, GSK), and the most active NGDOs in APOC.[93]

The objective of PENDA was threefold: (1) eliminate LF in Africa by 2020, (2) eliminate onchocerciasis by 2025, and (3) strengthen national programs to combat NTDs.[94] The targets would be achieved principally through full treatment coverage for both diseases, and by enhancing the capacity of national NTD programs to sustain progress toward elimination.[95] The geographic scope would be widened to include all African countries endemic with oncho or LF—potentially 10 additional countries. The key guiding principles were country leadership based on national strategies, partnership, and community empowerment including gender equity.[96] The PENDA document argued for a regional approach to ensure the weakest national programs and post-conflict countries received focused support, cross-border issues were given special attention, up-to-date information and knowledge were shared across countries, and the necessary resources were mobilized.[97]

The most controversial feature of the proposal was the indicative budget. It purported to cover the investment required to eliminate oncho and LF over the 10-year period, most of which would finance PENDA activities. The total budget came to $813,960,000, an average of $81.4 million per annum.[98] Costs were front-loaded beginning at $143 million in 2016 and declining to $30 million in 2025. Accounting for the costs likely to be financed by the African governments and NGDOs, PENDA expenditures averaged $75 million per annum during the first five years—more than double the peak-budget years for the OCP or APOC.[99] Given that the oncho donor community was vastly smaller in the closing years of APOC, it was highly improbable that the few remaining donors could finance PENDA. Hence, going forward with PENDA, as proposed, would have almost certainly required convening a major donors' pledging conference and the prospects for securing the amount proposed would have been highly uncertain, at best.

The 2013 JAF in Brazzaville approved the PENDA document as well as the budget "as presented."[100] The JAF received a statement from GAELF endorsing PENDA, and calling for "full and equal partnership" between the LF and oncho communities during implementation. The JAF donors' group requested that APOC management and the World Bank prepare a plan for resource mobilization and suggested organizing "a donor replenishment forum" in 2015.[101] The donors also called for the CSA to organize an independent management review of the existing APOC structure to determine the best organizational arrangement given the objectives and responsibilities proposed for PENDA.[102]

The management review was carried out by consultants and completed in July 2014. It analyzed the existing APOC structure in light of the PENDA proposal. The review determined that APOC's organizational structure needed to be extensively transformed into a model that supported country ownership and leadership. It called for a shift from project management to supporting country-led NTD programs. According to the review, the new program necessitated "a fresh approach to communication and openness to function, including greater transparency."[103] The authors concluded that "because of the extensive transformation required for the formation of PENDA, its management system should not be evolved from APOC by adding-on, cutting-back, or re-organizing."

In October 2014, three months after submission of the management review, USAID and DFID issued a "Joint Statement on Support for Onchocerciasis Elimination in Africa" to the CSA. The statement criticized APOC management and the PENDA proposal for failing to define "a regional role for PENDA that reflects current realities, has a clear implementation strategy, or structure capable of achieving this new mandate [elimination of oncho and LF]."[104] The Statement referred to "APOC's history of a closed approach to results management and data disclosure . . . non-transparency, and an apparent reluctance to advance the elimination agenda."[105] The two agencies expressed "reservations" about going forward with the PENDA proposal "that is merely a relabeling of the current structure."[106] The statement called for the adoption of recommendations as a condition for the two agencies deciding whether to support PENDA. Those recommendations included "a new level of transparency," a "decentralized entity capable of using the institutional memories of both APOC and GPELF," "a re-direction from operational management to one of enabling countries to make their own decisions based on evidence available," and "the sharing of all data in real time."[107]

I met with the USAID officials responsible for NTDs, who drafted the Statement, a year after it was issued. They were Emily Wainwright, senior operations advisor for NTDs, and Darin Evans, technical advisor for onchocerciasis and schistosomiasis. It was clear that some of the issues highlighted in the joint statement had been festering for several years—notably nontransparency and lack of urgency in pressing forward on elimination for both oncho and LF. Wainwright spoke to the reason behind issuing a statement separate from the wider donor group: "We felt like we had to, at a certain point, step alone because the messages we were trying to convey to the JAF and leadership at APOC through the donors' working group were being softened. And we were saying, look, systematically, year after year, we in USAID are starting to give less money. We've been telling the APOC leadership we're not happy with where it's going. We're raising the issue in the donors' group, and somehow, nobody's getting this."[108] The donors' group referred to a meeting of donors that took place at JAF sessions on the side of the plenary, whereby donors would state their views on issues and their levels of support for APOC. The problem, alluded to by Wainwright, was that in the process of amalgamating various donor positions, those of individual donors were watered down, and, in the case of USAID, the agency's concerns were not being conveyed clearly to APOC management and the CSA.

The inability of donors to get their messages across and the issue of non-transparency highlight the post-2005 problem of the lack of a robust donors' forum, along the lines of the donors' conferences during the first decade of APOC and throughout most of the OCP. Neither the expanded CSA meetings nor the JAF donors' group were suitable substitutes for the donors' conferences. The CSA was a committee under the APOC and OCP agreements, intended to have an executive function, with the sponsoring agencies, as the sole permanent members, having a management role. Inviting select donors to periodic CSA meetings fell far short of the forum required by the donors. The JAF donors' group only provided an opportunity for donors to state positions and levels of support. It did not allow for give-and-take with program management to better understand operational and financing issues or for extensive discussion of such issues with the other donors.

The donors' conferences, on the other hand, provided for comprehensive data disclosure related to program policies and progress; a full day-and-a-half to ask questions to program management and staff and exchange views with other donors; and the opportunity to reflect upon, clarify, and state positions. The conferences were chaired by the World Bank at a high level, which helped ensure that donor views and positions were followed up, and adhered to, by APOC (and previously, the OCP) management. A key component of donors' conferences was pledging. Pledging was vital for the World Bank to assess total commitment levels in order to plan fund mobilization efforts. An important audience was APOC (and the OCP) management and staff. A donor's pledge of support, often with explanations, was a way of communicating about program aspects that the donor approved of, or wanted changed.

One of the concerns expressed by the USAID officials was that APOC did not evolve after 2009. The Program went from being at the forefront on disease control to becoming outdated.[109] An argument can be made that if there had been a robust donors' forum during those years enabling donor views to be conveyed to APOC management, with follow-up by the World Bank through the CSA, APOC might have evolved and remained more relevant to changes in the foreign-assistance landscape.

The other major USAID concern, which helped trigger the Joint Statement, was the proposed PENDA budget of $75 million per annum. It was regarded as excessive and lacking transparency. Evans stated, "It did not take into account what others in the partnership were doing. We're already spending tens of millions of dollars on NTDs in country, and DFID is doing the same."[110] After the joint statement was issued, the CSA set up a subcommittee for interested partners to look at various scenarios and their costs, taking into account other work on NTDs financed elsewhere. As Evans described it, "We spent several months creating different scenarios. We worked with an economist in trying to figure out where the costs were, what is actually getting paid for by APOC now, what's getting paid for by others. And, we said to APOC, okay, here's the three scenarios. What budget do you think you need for these? And they came back with $70 million, $72 million, and $74 million," as annual budgets. Evans was under the impression that the APOC director, Dr. Jean-Baptiste Roungou, remained "pretty adamant" about holding to the original PENDA proposal.

In the final analysis, the budget appears to have been the final straw that doomed PENDA and forced closure of APOC at the end of 2015. There was one major player that might have provided the leadership to resolve the budget issue and arrive at an agreement on an alternative PENDA scenario: The World Bank. But, as Remme remarked, "In the later years of APOC, the World Bank did not play the leadership role it had throughout the OCP years and during the first half of APOC. As a result, the Program was undermined by criticisms from various corners of the partnership, some of which were unfair, and was unable to stay on course."[111] Remme's comment reflected a general feeling in the NTD community that the Bank, as the sponsoring agency go-between with the donors, could have led the way in ensuring that APOC and any follow-on regional entity were more responsive to donor interests and concerns, both with regard to the budget and the need to provide support to national integrated NTD programs. Patrick Lammie, director of the NTD Support Center at the Task Force for Global Health, remarked, "with a little bit of vision and leadership," APOC could have established itself as an integrated NTD platform, particularly when LF scale-up was stagnating in some oncho countries. He commented, "I feel like the more recent history of APOC was one of missed opportunities and a leadership failure."[112]

There were also decisions taken at the senior level in the World Bank during the later APOC years that had the effect of undermining support for the elimination effort. In April 2010, the council of the World Bank's Development Grant Facility (DGF) under Bank President Robert Zoellick decided to phase out all long-term, DGF-financed programs to "free up funding for new and innovative proposals," with funding to APOC to cease by 2014 (FY15).[113] The DGF was the sole source of Bank funding to the APOC Trust Fund and for the Bank's Oncho Unit. Ok Pannenborg, former division chief responsible for oncho, who was advising the Oncho Unit at the time, remarked that termination of DGF support "affected the Bank's involvement and contribution to APOC significantly by critically reducing staff interest and engagement. Without the Oncho Unit budget to fund travel, the staff lost interest in working on the Program."[114]

The loss of DGF support was compounded by a protracted reorganization under Bank president, Jim Yong Kim. During that reorganization no one at a senior level in the Bank was focusing on arrangements for a new oncho program, or even whether the Bank would be willing to continue to serve as the fiscal agent for a new entity. MDP Director Adrian Hopkins, who was participating in the working group on scenarios for PENDA, said in April 2015 in reference to the Bank reorganization: "I think it's a mess in trying to find an acceptable arrangement [for PENDA] because this was really a time when we needed a lot of guidance from the World Bank as to what they could put into this and how they could help this whole process."[115]

By the late spring of 2015, with APOC scheduled to close at the end of the year, the international community was working frantically on a successor organization to take up the mantle of NTD elimination in Africa. That new program would become the Expanded Special Project for Elimination of Neglected Tropical Diseases (ESPEN), based in Brazzaville under AFRO and its regional director, Dr. Matshidiso Rebecca Moeti. After a transition year in 2016, ESPEN got fully underway in 2017, with the objective of eliminating the five major PCT NTDs in Africa.

There were several reasons why the decision was finally taken to close APOC at the end of 2015 and not to proceed with PENDA. Around 2009, a major shift began to occur within the foreign-assistance community toward supporting national integrated NTD programs. The TDR-sponsored multicountry study on CDI had just been completed and the results demonstrated that integrated NTD programs based on the ComDT platform were eminently feasible and cost-effective. USAID and DFID launched major programs to support national integrated NTD programs in the second half of the 2000s. And, with the global financial crisis, donors were seeking more cost-effective approaches to NTD control. Moreover, for some donors, priorities were changing toward mortality reduction instead of endemic-disease control. France was emphasizing control of HIV-AIDS rather than endemic diseases in its assistance program.[116] USAID was giving high priority to reducing maternal and child mortality.[117] Supporting national NTD programs was seen as less expensive, in part because integrated control was thought to be more cost-effective and because national programs relied more heavily on recipient government resources and capacities. Regional programs such as APOC were effective and had many advantages, but maintaining the regional infrastructure was costly. Transparency was also an important consideration. During the later years of APOC, it was unclear to some donors exactly what their financing was being used for. USAID's Wainwright commented: "The majority of our funding goes to the national level because we know we can see the results for it. For APOC, we just can't get the results out of it. Whereas, at the country level we can tell you by disease, at the district level, exactly what diseases we supported."[118]

This time frame, 2009–2015, coincided with the shift of the APOC objective from sustained control to elimination. The studies showed elimination was feasible with Mectizan alone, but the donors were not seeing a concrete plan being implemented. In our 2015 interview, Wainwright commented, "APOC came close to achieving its objective of eliminating blindness as a public health problem. But the transition from supporting a public health elimination agenda to a true elimination agenda (i.e., elimination of the disease) never really happened. It was talked about a lot over five years, but a plan really was never presented for how we move from elimination as a public health problem to elimination of the disease, and how you do that in the context of other elimination programs going on in the region."[119] The Johns Hopkins University-led team that conducted the final evaluation of APOC came to a similar conclusion: "An opportunity was missed with the shift from control to elimination to thoroughly assess what this paradigm shift entailed, both operationally and from the costs aspects, and to address these upfront."[120]

The fewer donors that remained with APOC after 2010 were not seeing a plan backed by data for achieving elimination, and no appropriate donors' forum existed for APOC management to convince them otherwise. Hence, when they were presented with the far more costly PENDA proposal, which they saw as a relabeled, expanded APOC, they balked. A lighter and far-less costly regional program that complemented the national NTD programs they were supporting might have been acceptable. But PENDA did not fit that bill.

The ESPEN program which emerged in 2016 was more to their liking. It is a coordinating entity that provides support to national integrated NTD programs to accelerate elimination of the five PC NTDs. Unlike the OCP and APOC, which were quasi-independent programs cosponsored by three or four international organizations, ESPEN is part of WHO AFRO, under the authority of the AFRO Regional Director. Its operations are overseen by a steering committee consisting of representatives from the endemic countries, NGDOs, pharmaceutical companies, donors, and WHO. The steering committee makes recommendations to the Regional Director regarding ESPEN's priorities, work plans, and budget allocations to recipient countries. It also has responsibility for assisting the program in resource-mobilization efforts based on disease-elimination targets and the estimated cost of ESPEN operations.[121]

ESPEN's expenditures over the first two years, 2016–2017, totaled $7.8 million.[122] It operated during that period with a full-time professional staff of five, led by ESPEN Team Leader, Dr. Maria Rebollo Polo.[123] The ESPEN trust fund is managed by WHO Geneva. The World Bank plays no active role. Former APOC donors, USAID, the Kuwait Fund, DFID, Merck, and Sightsavers have become ESPEN donors, along with the Gates Foundation, the END Fund, and the Arab Bank for Economic Development in Africa.[124]

APOC Achievements

By 2017, two years after APOC closed, the total population treated in the APOC countries reached 116.8 million (substituting treatment data for 2016 for the CAR and Chad, which lacked data for 2017), with a coverage rate of 69.6%.[125] The population treated in the APOC countries surpassed the goal of 90 million established at the Abuja JAF in 2010. Populations receiving treatment in the former OCP countries numbered an additional 29.5 million.[126] The population treated in all 31 oncho-endemic African countries totaled 146.3 million in 2017— 72% of the estimated 204 million people living in at-risk areas, i.e., areas subject to potential transmission of the parasite.[127]

It is worth noting that the population treated in 2017 was approximately 23% greater than the population treated in 2014, the year before APOC closed. This increase suggests that APOC has been relatively successful in establishing self-sustaining ComDT projects, since much of that increase occurred during 2016– 2017 when APOC was no longer providing project support and ESPEN was just getting underway. Moreover, data presented by WHO at the final JAF in Kampala in 2015, showed that sustained treatment was occurring at a relatively high coverage rate. Since 2010, 12 of the original APOC countries had maintained a coverage via ComDT above 71% of the targeted population.[128] The scale-up of Mectizan treatment coverage over the life of APOC was rather remarkable, based on its achievement in a relatively short period of time. That scale-up went far toward eliminating widespread oncho blindness, impaired vision, troublesome itching, and skin disfigurement in sub-Saharan Africa in only one generation.

A thorough analysis of APOC progress in achieving elimination was carried out during 2008–2015 by a group of researchers led by APOC epidemiologist Dr. Afework Tekele. The team performed epidemiological evaluation surveys during 2008–2015 in 58 areas with ComDT projects that provided at least six years of annual Mectizan treatment in 12 Participating Countries.[129] The team gathered data on declining infection and prevalence levels and compared progress toward elimination with results predicted by ONCHOSIM. The question was whether treatment, given pre-control levels of infection, was leading to declines in transmission and infection levels that were approaching, or had already achieved, the infection breakpoint, so that transmission could no longer sustain itself.

The overall results that were published in 2016 were better than expected in terms of progress toward elimination. For 13 areas, containing 7 million people, the infection breakpoint had been reached and the epidemiological criteria had been met for stopping treatment.[130] The evaluations showed that another 20 areas with a population of 21 million were "close to elimination," and that some of those areas might have already achieved elimination.[131] Another 18 areas with more than 17 million people were "on track" to reaching the infection breakpoint, but required more years of Mectizan treatment to achieve elimination.[132] Seven areas with a population of 10 million were found to have made "unsatisfactory progress" toward elimination, primarily due to low-treatment coverage.[133]

The conclusion was that all areas in the 12 APOC countries that had received "adequate annual treatment coverage" were making "satisfactory progress" toward elimination. Many of those areas, with a population of 28 million, were either close to, or had already achieved, elimination. The evaluation team stated, "Hence, onchocerciasis elimination now appears feasible in most, if not all, endemic areas in Africa."[134] Data presented by WHO at the 2015 JAF in Kampala showed that, based on entomological and epidemiological evaluations, Guinea-Bissau, Malawi, Mali, Niger, and Senegal had probably achieved elimination.[135]

The evaluation team also concluded that the original APOC objective of eliminating onchocerciasis as a public health problem had been achieved. They drew this conclusion based on a 1991 study by Dadzie et al. that cited a CMFL of 10 microfilariae per skin snip (mf/s) as the cutoff level above which blindness begins to become a public health problem. The evaluations in all areas with more than three-years treatment showed CMFL levels to be below 10 mf/s.[136] In fact, two thirds of the villages surveyed had CMFL levels below 0.5 mf/s—a level at which no oncho blindness has been known to occur.[137] As for OSD, notably troublesome itching, no quantitative indicators are available for determining the level that constitutes a public health problem. However, given the more than 132 million at-risk and oncho-infected people regularly receiving Mectizan treatment at the end of APOC and the known near-immediate and salutary effect of the drug on itching, it is probable that OSD has also been largely eliminated as a public health problem throughout much of sub-Saharan Africa.[138]

Chapter 9

Learning from the Past, Looking to the Future

This once commonplace image of blind adults being led from place to place by children is progressively becoming a scene from the past.
—Inscription at the base of the *Riverblindness Statue* in the World Bank's James D. Wolfensohn Atrium, Washington, DC

Fortunately, we live in a time when science is validating what humans have known throughout the ages: that compassion is not a luxury; it is a necessity for our well-being, resilience, and survival.
—Joan Halifax, Upaya Institute and Zen Center, Santa Fe, New Mexico, "The Precious Necessity of Compassion," *Journal of Pain and Symptom Management*

Prospects for Eliminating Oncho throughout Africa

The oncho prevalence maps for 1975, 2002, and 2015 (figures 9.1, 9.2, and 9.3), based on epidemiological surveys, show the prevalence rates for all oncho-endemic countries in Africa during the first and last years of the OCP (1975, 2002) and the final year of APOC (2015). The 1975 map shows pre-control endemicity levels. The maps for subsequent years present a snapshot of a rapidly changing situation in which both the prevalence and intensity of onchocerciasis infection are declining in most areas in nearly all countries as Mectizan treatment is sustained at the relatively high levels reached during the later years of APOC. It should be noted that the prevalence levels on the maps tend to overstate oncho severity during the year in question because they lag the declining trend in infection intensity as measured by the CMFLs. The CMFLs, which reflect the risk of severe disease manifestations, are falling faster than the prevalence levels over time, and even faster with ComDT than with vector control as shown in figure 3.2.[1]

Every OCP country had areas that were hyperendemic (prevalence rate ≥60%) in 1975 when OCP operations began. Large parts of the 11-country OCP area were among the most heavily endemic in the world. By completion of the

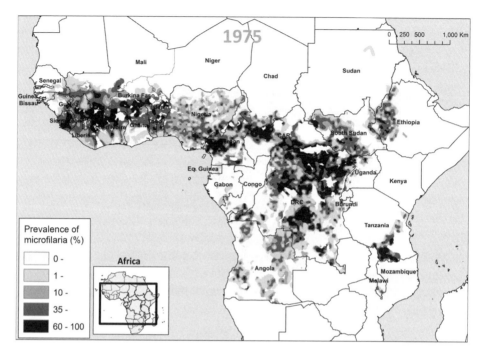

Figure 9.1. Oncho Prevalence, 1975. *Source*: World Health Organization African Programme for Onchocerciasis Control. "Progress Report." PowerPoint presentation, JAF doc. 21, Kampala, Uganda, December 15–16, 2015.

OCP in 2002, all of the high-prevalence areas (prevalence ≥35%, constituting a public health problem) had disappeared, with the exception of Sierra Leone, where control operations were suspended in the mid-1990s due to the country's civil war, and two other hyperendemic foci. One focus was on the Côte d'Ivoirian border with Liberia, in the Cavelly Region, in a forest zone slightly outside the OCP operational area and beyond the reach of vector control. That focus eventually received concentrated treatment with Mectizan, and recent results indicate satisfactory progress toward elimination.[2] The other focus was on the northern Togo-Benin border. This was a SIZ that experienced residual transmission after the OCP closed and received Mectizan treatment well beyond 2002; by 2015, prevalence had declined to zero. (figure 9.3, Prevalence Map, 2015). One focus in the southwest corner of Burkina Faso (Comoé Province) cropped up after the OCP closed, as shown on the 2015 map, and has been receiving Mectizan treatment. It is unclear whether its reappearance was due to recrudescence or reinvasion from Côte d'Ivoire or, conceivably, elsewhere.

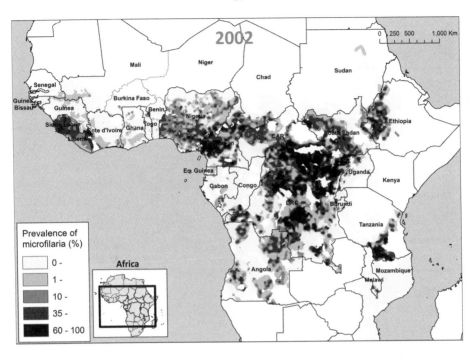

Figure 9.2. Oncho Prevalence, 2002. *Source*: World Health Organization African Programme for Onchocerciasis Control. "Progress Report." PowerPoint presentation, JAF doc. 21, Kampala, Uganda, December 15–16, 2015.

Regarding the APOC countries, by December 2015, when the 2015 map was produced based on current survey data, Mectizan treatment had eliminated large foci with prevalence ≥35% (meso-endemic or hyperendemic). By then, there had been a major decline in prevalence nearly everywhere, but further progress was needed in the DRC, South Sudan bordering the Central Africa Republic (CAR), Angola, northern Uganda, and the Republic of the Congo. In the 12 other APOC countries, high-prevalence areas leading to blindness and severe OSD had disappeared: oncho had been largely eliminated as a public health problem in Cameroon, Chad, CAR, Sudan, Nigeria, Ethiopia, Tanzania, Burundi, Malawi, Equatorial Guinea, Gabon, and Liberia. (figure 9.3, prevalence map, 2015). Predictions for these countries will have to be adjusted when and where more recent empirical data become available, since the December 2015 survey data have been the latest accessible for this analysis.

In 2009, the original APOC objective of eliminating onchocerciasis as a public health problem was stepped up to the more ambitious goal of eliminating the

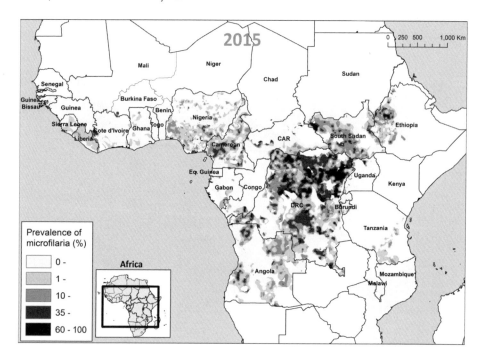

Figure 9.3. Oncho Prevalence, 2015. *Source*: World Health Organization African Programme for Onchocerciasis Control. "Progress Report." PowerPoint presentation, JAF doc. 21, Kampala, Uganda, December 15–16, 2015.

disease entirely, where feasible. Under this new objective, "disease elimination" meant elimination of infection and transmission. This goal was deemed attainable with Mectizan alone, based on studies in Mali, Senegal, and Kaduna, Nigeria. During the final five years of APOC, significant progress was made toward this objective, although no African country had achieved elimination by the end of 2015—however, many countries were close.

The report of the CSA Advisory Group on Onchocerciasis Elimination (see chapter 8) submitted to the 2011 JAF in Kuwait summarized the progress toward elimination and estimated which countries would achieve it, and when, based on ONCHOSIM predictions. The conclusion was that 12 APOC countries plus all 11 former OCP countries were on track to achieve elimination by 2020.[3] Collectively these countries had an estimated at-risk population exceeding 100 million. To reach the goal by 2020, the advisory group report concluded that these countries needed support beyond continued Mectizan treatment. They required assistance in conducting evaluations to determine where and when treatment could be stopped.[4]

For a number of countries, Mectizan treatment needed to be extended into areas where oncho prevalence was below 35% in all communities (the hypo-endemic areas). The APOC mandate for the first 14 years called for treating exclusively the hyper- and meso-endemic areas that constituted a public health problem—areas with prevalence ≥35%. The advisory group's report concluded that extending into the hypo-endemic areas would involve treating an additional 5%–20% of the targeted population and that transmission could be interrupted relatively quickly, given the low pre-control endemicity levels.[5]

These areas had been identified as hypo-endemic by REMO in the late-1990s to mid-2000s timeframe. When APOC staff investigated some of these areas after 2010, they discovered that some pockets of infection had dissipated. This was the case in parts of Burundi, Malawi, Chad, and mainland Equatorial Guinea. The disappearance fit the theory that transmission stemming from low-infection areas will eventually die out unless fed by transmission from high-infection areas nearby.[6]

To achieve elimination in a hypo-endemic area, only those foci with active locally-sustained transmission need treatment.[7] Four former directors of the OCP and APOC (Dadzie, Amazigo, Boatin, Sékétéli) recommended in 2018 that the onchocerciasis operational research (OOR) "further quantify thresholds for sustained local transmission in low endemic areas" to better identify these foci for treatment.[8] Work has been underway recently to develop an "elimination-mapping" strategy with the goal of identifying all possible transmission foci in the hypo-endemic areas.[9] It would employ a new, more sensitive diagnostic tool known as OV16, a serological test that detects antibody reactions to the oncho parasite. OV16 is capable of identifying low infection levels and possible sources of transmission that nodule palpation and skin snipping are insufficiently sensitive to locate. Because it picks up historical exposure to the oncho parasite, OV16 may result in false positives by showing antibody responses in individuals no longer harboring active infection. This is less likely to occur if the diagnostic test is confined to children, the best population cohort to reveal signs of recent transmission.

There were areas in four APOC countries with high pre-control endemicity, where elimination was predicted to lag unless control efforts were intensified. They were in southern/central Cameroon (Central Province), eastern Nigeria (Benue State), southern Tanzania (Ruvuma Region), and northern Uganda (Kitgum and Pader Districts). The 2011 Advisory Group Report recommended increasing treatment frequency to twice a year, exploring ways of enhancing treatment compliance, and focusing greater attention on cross-border foci. Cross-border areas are the Achilles's heel of a comprehensive elimination effort, because they require close collaboration between countries sharing borders in conducting treatment and surveillance to assess progress and determine when to stop treatment. The emphasis on cross-border areas highlights the importance of retaining a strong regional focus in post-APOC elimination efforts.

Countries considered unlikely by the advisory group's report to achieve elimination by 2020 were the CAR, the DRC, Liberia, Gabon, and South Sudan. Angola needs to be added to this list given the lack of treatment progress to-date and a reported national-coverage of under 5% as of 2017.[10] The population at-risk in these countries (including Angola) was approximately 36 million according to earlier REMO data.

Several factors were expected to contribute to delay. The DRC, the CAR, Liberia, and South Sudan are post-conflict countries and have experienced lags in project preparation and implementation, as well as low treatment coverage. Except for Liberia and the CAR, these countries have loiasis-endemic areas inhibiting Mectizan treatment. The Angolan Government has consistently demonstrated a lack of commitment in pursuing control. Gabon and mainland Equatorial Guinea, with relatively small at-risk populations, are both loiasis hyperendemic and oncho hypo-endemic, a combination precluded from Mectizan treatment under TCC/MEC guidelines. Ground-based larviciding might present an effective alternative in suppressing transmission in some foci. For the loiasis-endemic countries, an option might be to employ the LoaScope in mapping where Mectizan treatment could proceed safely, which might accelerate control operations, but by itself would probably not lead to elimination.

The advisory group's report concluded that there were areas in the DRC, South Sudan, and the CAR that may not achieve elimination by 2025. These were areas of high pre-control endemicity and subject to civil unrest. Accelerating elimination will require increased resources, higher treatment coverage, and possibly alternative treatment strategies, such as biannual treatment, complementary vector control, and treatment with newer drugs, such as doxycycline and moxidectin. Doxycycline is an antibiotic effective against *wolbachia*, a parasitic microbe required for the survival of the adult worm. Doxycycline appears safe in loiasis-endemic areas because the *Loa loa* parasite does not contain *wolbachia*. Though effective in clinical trials, use of doxycycline remains restricted based on the impracticality of required daily treatment for at least four weeks, and on contraindications for young children and women of childbearing age.[11] Moxidectin is an alternative microfilaricide that delays repopulation of microfilariae in the skin, with somewhat longer-lasting effects than ivermectin. Moxidectin was approved by the FDA for treatment of onchocerciasis in 2018 for patients of 12 years of age or older, though cost and availability remain issues for the foreseeable future. The LoaScope might be employed in loiasis-endemic areas in the DRC and South Sudan under a TaNT strategy to accelerate Mectizan treatment.

As the former OCP/APOC directors argued in their 2018 article, extensive knowledge has been gained over the past 45 years regarding effective control and elimination of oncho. That knowledge includes: vector control and ivermectin treatment as control/elimination tools, the reproductive lifespan of the female worm, the flight range of vectors, the effectiveness of ComDT, and entomological/epidemiological evaluation procedures for assessing progress and taking decisions on elimination. To this list should be added ONCHOSIM, an invaluable predictive tool in a range of epidemiological and entomological situations, and OV16 to strengthen mapping of hypo-endemic areas. Consequently, the technical parameters are in place and the tools and knowledge exist to complete oncho elimination in Africa. Achievement of that objective requires the application of the many tools developed and lessons learned during the past 45 years of the OCP/APOC experience, backed by international leadership, resource mobilization efforts, and political will, which have been central to past oncho-control/elimination progress in Africa.

On the 2015 prevalence map (figure 9.3), the darker areas showing prevalence of 10% or greater are where the follow-on effort will need to focus to advance elimination. Assuming Mectizan treatment is sustained at least at the same level as during the last five years of APOC, ONCHOSIM predicts that oncho prevalence will decline significantly nearly everywhere over the coming years. This progress is shown on the map for 2025 (figure 9.4). Virtually all of the areas of high prevalence (≥ 35%) in 2015 will be wiped out by 2025. Hence, based on the trajectory of Mectizan treatment since 2010, ONCHOSIM simulations predict that elimination of onchocerciasis will be substantially achieved throughout Africa by 2025.

A Monument to the Oncho Partnership

After launching the River Blindness Foundation (RBF) in the early 1990s, John Moores searched for a meaningful gift to thank RBF donors. RBF's CEO Bill Baldwin had sketched out a stick-figure drawing of a child leading a blind adult to serve as the RBF logo.[12] Moores contacted sculptor R.T. "Skip" Wallen, whose larger-than-life size sculpture of an Alaskan brown bear Moores had admired, and asked if Wallen could produce 15 two-foot (61 cm) tall bronze statues (maquettes) based

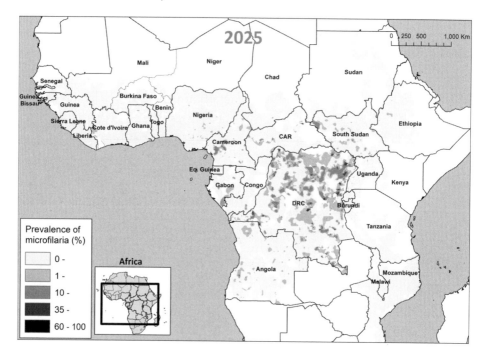

Figure 9.4. Oncho Prevalence, 2025. *Source*: World Health Organization African Programme for Onchocerciasis Control. "Progress Report." PowerPoint presentation, JAF doc. 21, Kampala, Uganda, December 15–16, 2015.

on the logo. Wallen volunteered his time and Moores underwrote the foundry costs to produce the maquettes. RBF named the sculpture "Sightless among Miracles," partly in reference to the "miracle drug" ivermectin.

In anticipation of Vagelos's retirement in 1995, Merck's public affairs division contacted Moores about acquiring one of the maquettes for the Merck board to give to Vagelos as a retirement gift. Moores suggested Merck contact Wallen about sculpting a bigger version of the maquette for the gift.[13] The end result was an 8-foot (2.44 m) high bronze sculpture, which was placed in the entrance to Merck's world headquarters in Whitehouse Station, New Jersey. The sculpture was a powerful symbol of compassion and partnership in the face of a highly threatening, disabling disease. Anyone coming to Merck headquarters would see the statue and either remember or learn of the company's instrumental role in helping to defeat oncho in Africa.

I first saw the "Riverblindness Statue" in the garden of The Carter Center, where a duplicate of the Merck statue was dedicated in 1996. I had seen photos of the statue, but seeing it in person was awe-inspiring. The imposing sculpture depicts a child leading a blind adult by a stick. The man holding onto the stick has opaque eyes, the unmistakable trait of a blind oncho victim. His eyes resemble "Mara"—the "lion's stare" in Bambara, Mali's widely spoken local language. The man is tentatively lifting his left foot, unsure of where to step, and he is starting to raise his left hand, fingers slightly spread, to catch himself should he fall. Based on his physique, he looks to be in his prime. The boy appears healthy but may already be infected without any overt signs of infection.

During the dedication ceremony, I met Wallen, who told me that the sculpture mold could produce up to five statues. Hence, three more were feasible. I realized then that if I could secure the financing to purchase those three, it would be possible to donate them to three additional partners in the oncho programs and have that iconic sculpture placed in an agency representing nearly all of the partner-groups in the partnership—private sector (Merck), NGDOs (The Carter Center), Executing Agency (WHO), Sponsoring Agencies (World Bank), and donors (Netherlands). Doing so would raise awareness of a still relatively unknown disease along with the achievements of the partnership. The statues might also help lock in the highly effective oncho partnership for the duration of APOC, and possibly beyond to address other challenges. I pursued that objective over the next nine years, and by 2005, statues had been placed and dedicated in all of the key partner groups represented in the OCP and APOC, with the exception of the Participating Countries. In parallel with the placement of the Wallen sculptures, the government of Burkina Faso commissioned a similar larger-than-life size bronze statue sculpted by Burkinabé artist, Guiré Tasséré, which stands in a prominent square in Ouagadougou.

With financial support from Moores, the World Bank Art Society, and NGDOs participating in APOC, oncho statues were unveiled during 1997–2005 in ceremonies variously attended by President Carter, World Bank President Wolfensohn, and WHO Director-General Brundtland, in the atrium of the World Bank headquarters in Washington, DC; at the entrance to WHO headquarters in Geneva; and at the Royal Tropical Institute (Koninklijk Instituut voor de Tropen—KIT) in Amsterdam. The Netherlands was chosen because it was the largest donor in Europe, the largest donor country on a per capita basis, and one of the most active donors in the oncho programs. Unexpectedly, the Wallen mold was able to produce a sixth statue, which was placed in another APOC NGDO, the Lions Club International, at their world headquarters in Oak Brook, Illinois, in 2007.

These statues are monuments to partnership. The boy and the blind man are trusted partners, just as many individuals, organizations, and governments have been trusted partners in battling the disease. The sculptures are appropriately larger than life, as the oncho endeavor has been bigger than any one person or organization; in fact, its success—even its survival over several decades—depended on close collaboration among more than 100 partners and thousands of individuals.

Looking Back

How do the benefits from the oncho-control/elimination effort stack up against the costs of implementing it? The returns have been multifold: economic and health improvements; lessons for large-scale programs and partnerships; and global-health externalities in promoting pharmaco-philanthropy and addressing other NTDs. What, then, were the key actions and inflection points that enabled the effort to expand from a sub-regional program confined to the Sahel countries to all of endemic Africa? Answers to these questions begin with an assessment that takes into account the economic investment and return; motives behind the most significant decisions; and the core characteristics of the partnership involved in this endeavor.

Economic Costs and Benefits

The total cost of the oncho-control/elimination effort (1974–2015) attributed to donor support, was $824 million, or slightly more than $19 million per annum. The total broke down into $556 million for the OCP over 29 years (1974–2002), and $268 million for APOC over 21 years (1996–2015).[14] That donor support provided virtually all of the financing to cover program expenditures over the 43-year timeframe. There were other costs associated with the effort, notably NGDO expenditures, Participating Countries budgetary support, and Merck's donation of Mectizan.

The value of the drug donation has been substantial, but difficult to quantify because the cost of producing the drug is unknown, and is proprietary information. Data exist for a rough approximation of that value based on certain assumptions. By the end of 2018, Merck had donated 3.6 billion treatments of Mectizan for oncho and LF since the MDP began in 1988.[15] Assuming a cost of production of $0.10 per tablet (a price that Merck considered charging for the 6 mg tablet prior to the donation), and an average of 2.8 tablets per treatment,[16] a ballpark estimate of the value of the Mectizan donation for 1988–2018, comes to $1 billion.

From the standpoint of official foreign assistance, support for the oncho programs has been cost-effective and the impact substantial. The OCP was protecting an estimated at-risk population of 35 million in 10 countries by the time it closed in 2002 (excluding Sierra Leone due to the civil war) and continued to do so after closure because transmission had been interrupted throughout most of the Program area. The annual cost per-person protected averaged out to $0.57 over the life of the Program. In establishing a sustainable drug-delivery network via ComDT, APOC financing had enabled ongoing treatment for an estimated at-risk population of 132.5 million in 31 countries by 2016, the year following its closure.[17] The average cost per treatment under APOC through the ComDT network was $0.58 per person.[18]

By protecting and treating large populations, the two programs have contributed importantly to rural development. In West Africa, OCP operations opened up better quality land to settlement and cultivation. Additional productive land combined with a larger and healthier labor force resulted in increased agricultural production, yielding an economic return that more than justified the sizable investment in the OCP. Both the OCP and APOC led to increases in the amount and quality of labor through reductions in blindness, visual impairment, premature death, and OSD.[19] The largest disease burden in the APOC countries was pervasive itching. APOC has succeeded in largely eliminating that burden, resulting in productivity increases in a population exceeding 100 million.[20] Analysis by researchers at Erasmus University in 2013, projected that APOC would have prevented productivity losses equivalent to $1.7 billion from troublesome itching by its conclusion—three times the losses averted from blindness.[21]

KEY DECISIONS, CRITICAL JUNCTURES

Three key decisions during the 40+ year control/elimination effort altered its course and propelled it toward its ultimate objective. The first was World Bank President Robert McNamara's decision in 1972 to launch a regional effort to control oncho throughout a multicountry West African subregion, in collaboration with WHO, the UNDP, and the FAO, and with the backing of bilateral donors. It entailed a new and unprecedented mandate for the World Bank to spearhead a multi-decade regional program focusing on health and based on grant financing rather than lending. It was the Bank's first foray into health. Nothing of that scope and duration had been attempted before and there were doubts that it would succeed. Because of the OCP's eventual success, the international community was prepared to underwrite an expanded effort for all of oncho-endemic Africa.

The second was Roy Vagelos's decision in 1987 for Merck to donate Mectizan to treat onchocerciasis. This unprecedented pharmaceutical donation enabled the OCP to be brought to a successful conclusion on schedule and APOC to eliminate the disease as a public-health problem in the rest of Africa, including the continent's largest countries. The Merck donation launched an era of pharmaco-philanthropy that changed the character of foreign assistance in global health. Other pharmaceutical companies eventually followed suit with donations for the most widespread NTDs. Even as foreign assistance later shifted away from endemic-disease control, NTDs remained a priority for key donors, given the availability of indispensable, high-value drug donations. As a USAID official remarked, "We have to put so little money in to leverage a large expense, it would be crazy not to be supporting NTDs."[22] USAID reports that every $1 invested in its NTD program leverages $26 in donated drugs.[23]

The third game-changing decision was taken by Ebrahim Samba, director of the OCP, in 1992 to adopt "community self-treatment," as it was termed at the time, as the principal method for delivering Mectizan in the OCP countries. He pushed for this approach despite doubts from many quarters that assigning full responsibility for Mectizan treatment to the communities would be safe and effective. As OCP director, Samba requested the TDR's Hans Remme to investigate the best way forward to achieve a viable community-led approach that would have broad applicability across sub-Saharan Africa. The resulting TDR-sponsored research led to ComDT becoming the principal method for delivering Mectizan through nearly 200,000 rural communities to an at-risk population exceeding 100 million. ComDT also enabled combined Mectizan/albendazole treatment to reach tens of millions of Africans at risk for LF; and was shown in a TDR-led follow-on study to be a cost-effective, operationally feasible approach to deliver other vital interventions and strengthen basic health care in rural communities in Africa.

SALIENT FEATURES OF HIGHLY EFFECTIVE, LARGE-SCALE PROGRAMS

What aspects of the oncho programs contributed to their success? One notable feature was partnership. Both the OCP and APOC encompassed a diverse, cohesive partnership that had the backing of a committed, broad-based donor community. What started out as a limited partnership in the early 1970s—with the four co-sponsoring agencies, nine donors, and seven beneficiary countries—expanded in successive stages and thrived for nearly 40 years. By 2002, the oncho programs had scaled up into one of the largest partnerships of any development program in history. It was a complex and potentially unwieldy partnership. However, it functioned relatively smoothly for several decades, and in the process produced important synergies by bundling the comparative advantages of the various partners.

There were three basic reasons why the partnership remained cohesive and productive. First, the program objective and the strategic goals for achieving it were kept clear, simple, and relatively consistent over time. From the beginning, the stated program objective was to eliminate onchocerciasis, first as a public health problem, and then as a disease. The principal strategic goal was to halt transmission. The exception occurred during the first half of APOC when, due to the perceived lack of a tool to stop transmission, the strategic goal was dialed back to morbidity control. The means for halting transmission evolved as new tools became available, from vector control to Mectizan treatment.

Relative consistency in program objectives and the strategic goals for achieving them prevailed over time even though fundamental changes had to occur in program structure to evolve from a high-tech, top-down vector-control operation to the bottom-up, community-based operation necessary to deliver Mectizan in remote areas throughout the continent. Clarity, simplicity, and consistency in objectives and strategic goals were important in ensuring that the diverse, disparate group of 100+ partners remained in alignment over decades. As a consequence, the partners tended to pursue activities that were both complementary and consistent with the broader program objectives and strategic goals.

Second, each partner was given a "seat at the table," in some fashion. For most, this meant a seat on the governing board (JPC, JAF). For others, it meant participation on committees which were integral to the larger operation. Moreover, until the second half of APOC, every partner group had its own forum, in which positions were consolidated and fed into the final governing-board decision-making phase. Guaranteeing a seat at the table for each partner helped ensure buy-in, ownership, and long-term commitment to the program effort.

Third, collaboration among key players was strong and transcended institutional allegiance. In the book *Real Collaboration*,[24] Mark Rosenberg and his team analyze a range of global health partnerships, which they classify across a spectrum of cohesiveness and teamwork. The oncho programs are cited as falling in the category of "close collaboration," in which individuals identify more strongly with the partnership and its objectives than with the institutions they represent.[25] In their research, Rosenberg et al. use APOC to help frame the "close collaboration" prototype.[26]

Over my years working on the OCP and APOC, identification with, and allegiance to, the program mission were powerful motivators for those on the core team that met regularly in the CSA. Others with similarly-strong allegiance to the partnership and its mission were actively involved through the TDR, the MDP, the NGDO Coordination Group, the EAC and the TCC. One core team member stands out for his commitment to oncho control/elimination. After retiring from WHO in the early 1980s, Dr. Ole Christensen worked for free as a consultant to the OCP and APOC for more than two decades. Throughout, he remained an Afro-optimist and a strong believer in Africa and its people. He headed up the OCP/APOC Liaison Office in WHO-Geneva for many years and served as secretary for CSA, JPC, and JAF meetings throughout my tenure. The partnership was extremely fortunate to have Christensen's tireless dedication to the oncho mission during 1984–2004.

Another salient feature of effective large-scale programs is a strong regional (or global) focus, which is important in addressing problems comprehensively that are regional (or global) in nature and transcend national boundaries and interests. A regional approach was imperative for effective control of onchocerciasis via vector control in the West African subregion during the 1970s-1990s. The predominant vector, *Simulium damnosum*, could travel up to 500 km. It would have been excessively complicated and costly to have addressed the disease on a country-by-country basis.

The regional approach required relying on grant financing from a range of donors rather than on loans/credits—the traditional source of World Bank financing. Borrowing was infeasible because there was no official entity at the regional level to guarantee repayment of the loan/credit, and official guarantees are required under Bank procedures. Theoretically, there could have been 11 separate loans/ credits to the OCP countries, but that arrangement would have been excessively complicated, perhaps unworkable. Lending to the 17 APOC countries in pursuit of oncho elimination regionwide would have been even more complex.

Grant financing from a range of donors was more time-consuming and staff-intensive to secure than lending, but it presented distinct advantages that became increasingly apparent over time. One was the oncho-trust-fund arrangement, involving donor contributions pooled in Bank-held trust funds. It was a cardinal Bank rule that no contributions could be earmarked, such as for a designated country or activity. The prohibition against earmarking was to ensure that program management retained maximum flexibility in directing financing where most needed to achieve region-wide elimination. Pooling non-earmarked donations also allowed for maximum resource-allocation efficiencies, not possible if donors restrict usage of their contributions. It was only at the tail end of APOC that the Bank's oncho coordinator, perhaps in an effort to secure greater funding, permitted earmarking, or "ring-fencing," donor contributions for specific countries.

Similar to the financing flexibility achieved through the trust-fund arrangement, the OCP agreement, and to a lesser extent the APOC agreement, provided for operational flexibility by allowing for the passage of resources, including Program staff, equipment, and drug supplies, across the Program area. Particularly with the OCP, operations were unencumbered by border restrictions between countries in the Program. The regional approach also fostered equity in the burden sharing of the costs and benefits of protecting the regionwide population.

One of the most striking and unique advantages of predominantly regional programs is the output of regional public goods (RPGs) that have wide-ranging benefits. Public goods are commodities, services, or resources which when consumed by one user do not become less available to other users. Clean-air and police protection are often cited as illustrations. Shielding populations across countries from transmission via vector control is a prime example. Sharing information, knowledge, and best practices in regional meetings; and the standardization of methods, processes, and indicators across the oncho-endemic countries are other important instances. These advantages do not exist or are far more limited in strictly national programs.

One of the potentially problematic issues with public goods is the "free rider problem"—meaning that an individual, group, or country can benefit from a public good without paying for it. This can lead to under-financing. To overcome under-financing, governments levy taxes to fund public goods, such as police protection or streetlighting. In the case of oncho, broad-based grant financing promoted equity across the donor community in paying for the RPGs. That is a reason why the World Bank's role in mobilizing financing was important. The Bank, through its convening authority and finance ministry contacts, could secure the required funding to produce the RPGs, while ensuring that the costs were widely distributed by soliciting support from a wide range of donors. Also important were broad-based budgetary commitments across the Participating Countries to limit free-riding, as in the Yaoundé Declaration. Because no single donor or African country was dominant, the programs could only function highly effectively if each donor and Participating Country pulled its own weight in support of the program objectives.

The OOR was an RPG, largely inherent to the regional nature of the programs, and it also became a best practice. It was conducted both within the programs and by the TDR in a way that was highly responsive to program-implementation needs. It enabled the OCP to discover and implement alternative larvicides to overcome a crisis of insecticide resistance in the mid-1980s, and to employ state-of-the-art computer modeling to guide control operations and predict outcomes to inform program management, governments, the CSA, and the donors.

The TDR-sponsored OOR was instrumental in enabling Mectizan treatment to be operationalized throughout sub-Saharan Africa; and it provided many of the findings essential to launching APOC, refining its architecture, and enhancing its operations over time. During 1987–2008, the TDR designed and led nine studies: ivermectin community trials (1987), the importance of OSD (1993), the viability of ComDT (1994), vector-elimination feasibility (1994), rapid mapping of oncho via REMO (1994), the impact of ivermectin on OSD (1996), rapid mapping of loiasis via RAPLOA (2002), ComDT capability to deliver multiple health-care interventions (2004), and the feasibility of elimination via ivermectin (2008). The funding built up in the OCP Trust Fund during the 1980s-1990s played an important role in the execution of this OOR program. In 1994, when the TDR Task Force for the OOR had exhausted its budget of $250,000, I was able to transfer $1.4 million out of the sizable OCP contingency reserve to enable many of these studies to be completed.[27]

A symbiotic relationship developed between the TDR-led OOR and operational needs. This occurred, in part, because Remme, who managed the TDR's Task Force for the OOR, had worked in the OCP and understood oncho-control strategies and modeling through ONCHOSIM. The task force chair was Professor Oladele Olusiji Kale of the University of Ibadan, who knew well the challenges of oncho control beyond the OCP. The task force's research agenda was closely coordinated with the expert advisory committees, the EAC and the TCC which Kale also chaired. Remme gave reports on ongoing OOR to every meeting of those committees during 1994–2008.[28] The advisory committees, in turn, ensured that operational priorities were factored into research protocols, while providing rigorous peer review of studies underway. The TDR's OOR program was developed and executed to maximize control results across Africa. Without that program, it is probable that APOC would not have had the beneficial impact it did on tens of millions of Africans.

Another advantage of the regional approach was the introduction of competition through peer review. Project proposals were vetted in the TCC by independent experts and NGDO representatives. NGDOs involved in project design and preparation worked to produce quality proposals to be reviewed and approved for financing by their peers. Countries also reported on progress in preparing and implementing projects at JAF sessions. That reporting process in a high-profile regional forum exerted peer pressure on health ministries and their staffs to deliver higher quality project results.

Countries also reported on capacity-building training programs in JAF sessions. The final evaluation of APOC, led by Burnham of Johns Hopkins University, concluded that "capacity building was a major achievement of APOC."[29] It was according to the evaluation, "a central part of APOC's programme design."[30] As reported in the evaluation, the training had a cascading effect: "The central level programme managers then trained regional level implementers, who then trained district and frontline health workers. The community distributors were trained by frontline health workers, under the supervision of district health workers, assisted by NGDOs."[31] According to the evaluation, 537,000 district and frontline health workers and 4,711,000 CDDs were trained over the life of APOC.[32] In addition, OCP and APOC financed the training of hundreds of epidemiologists and entomologists to prepare health ministries to assume responsibility for control and elimination.

Combining regional collaboration with health system strengthening through capacity building at the national, district, and community levels turned out to be a highly effective model. In a paper on RPGs in official development assistance, commissioned by the Inter-American Development Bank in 2001, Dr. Marco Ferroni argued that the OCP, including its extension under APOC, is "perhaps the best example of what a judicious combination of national and regional approaches can achieve."[33] He had high praises for the programs: "The river blindness coalition has been held together by a strong sense of purpose shared by the participants, the right combination of leadership and submission on the part of individual contributors in accordance with their comparative advantages, a step-by-step approach following precisely defined and phased objectives, and the right amount of flexibility and compromise in execution."[34]

Reinforced by CDD training and retraining, ComDT, as an RPG resulting from regional collaboration, became critical in progressing toward Africa-wide elimination. Following Merck's commitment, the TDR undertook research via ONCHOSIM to determine the Mectizan coverage level required to interrupt transmission. The TDR-led OOR concluded that ComDT could achieve and sustain that level. Consequently, ComDT became APOC's principal vehicle for delivering Mectizan. By 2015, APOC had established delivery networks in 190,000 communities treating 119 million people per annum, and the Program was on track to eliminate oncho in nearly all of Africa in another decade.[35]

My interview with USAID officials indicated that an important reason for the donor shift to bilateral support for NTDs, was the lack of transparency experienced with APOC during the last few years. Reduced transparency was, in part, a consequence of erosion in APOC autonomy. WHO-AFRO became the permanent chair of the CSA in the APOC later years. Previously, the CSA had followed the practice, based on a WHO legal counsel decision, that WHO could not chair the CSA because it was also the executing agency. Having the director, a WHO employee, report to a committee chaired by WHO, was deemed a conflict of interest. The problem did not arise when other sponsoring agencies chaired the CSA. World Bank chairing of the CSA did not present a similar conflict of interest even though the Bank was also the programs' fiscal agent, because the programs' budgets were prepared by the OCP/APOC staff, not the Bank. And, the Bank's fund-mobilization responsibilities did not fall within the purview of the CSA: they were financed separately out of the World Bank's administrative budget rather than through the Trust Fund. During the last several years, WHO-AFRO was selecting the APOC directors from AFRO senior staff which also infringed on program autonomy, whereas most previous directors had come up through the ranks in the OCP or APOC or were appointed from the outside.

With AFRO chairing the CSA and appointing the program directors, APOC became more accountable to AFRO and less accountable to the donors and, to some extent, the Participating Countries. The combination of diminished accountability and discontinued donors' conferences, resulted in a growing donor disconnect with program operations. Prior to these changes, OCP and APOC directors had been diligent in ensuring that the donors were kept well informed and up-to-date, particularly with regard to program expenditures and budget forecasts that had implications for donor financing.

The donor shift away from the multilateral approach toward bilateral support presents risks for oncho elimination. By relying principally on bilateral support, there is a risk of gaps in an Africa-wide effort that could undermine the comprehensiveness required for elimination. Even the largest of the bilateral donors, USAID, supported NTD programs in only 17 out of the 31 oncho-endemic African countries at the end of APOC.[36] Consequently, there is the likelihood that one or more oncho-endemic countries will receive little or no bilateral donor support on an ongoing basis. Gaps in comprehensive control will make it more difficult to achieve continent-wide elimination, and to prevent recrudescence in countries lacking support, that could spread to neighboring countries given the capability of the oncho vector to travel long distances.

With the conclusion of APOC, the Participating Countries have expressed dismay over the loss of advantages that accrued through the regional effort. In October 2015, three months prior to APOC closure, I interviewed Burkina Faso's Minister of Health, Amédée Prosper Djiguimde, who voiced concern that the regional oncho structure, in place for more than four decades, might be abandoned and the long-term gains lost, particularly in Burkina's cross-border areas. An evaluation of USAID's NTD Program by Johns Hopkins University's Bloomberg School during 2016–2017, reported, "A common theme of in-depth interviews and country visits [to Burkina Faso, Cameroon, Ghana, Uganda, Tanzania] was that, since the demise of APOC, there is a lack of regional mechanisms to bring countries together for joint epidemiological review and planning."[37] The evaluation continued, "Country NTD leadership in the countries visited expressed a desire for more regional and sub-regional consultation and collaboration on NTD issues."[38]

Contributing to the dissolution of regional capacity was the phaseout of financing long-standing programs from the World Bank's DGF. Bank grants via the DGF have long been a key source of funding for regional programs, such as the OCP, APOC, and the TDR; and for regional/global public goods in general. Other programs negatively impacted by the phaseout included Roll Back Malaria and Research and Development in Human Reproduction.[39] Closure of the DGF funding window is a major loss. It was uniquely effective in strengthening development at regional levels and enhancing the mix of regional/global public goods, notably through research. Traditional Bank lending instruments are not designed to address the special requirements and complexities of regional efforts. Since establishing the oncho programs, some progress has been made in designing arrangements for regional programs that mix Bank lending with bilateral grant financing. Reducing the complexity of these endeavors remains a challenge. A concern for the World Bank with the phaseout of the DGF is the loss of policy leverage in ongoing and future long-term regional programs and associated fora.

Principles, Structure, and Processes

The advantages of a large, diverse partnership are major. If managed well, they yield synergies by combining the comparative strengths of various, expert-partner groups. They enable widespread burden-sharing. And, they enhance international visibility of the problem and the effort to address it.

For partnerships to endure and remain directed toward the end objective, they should adhere to certain principles, structures, and processes. These include

1. Clearly specified, realistic, shared goals.
2. Transparency, to instill trust essential for holding a large coalition together.
3. Delineated partner roles and responsibilities, based on comparative advantages that promote complementarity and minimize overlap and rivalry.

4. A legal framework defining the program structure and its institutional components, for example, committees, and the roles and responsibilities of those components.

5. Continual service by management to the partners. This includes providing information proactively and responding to questions to keep the participating countries and donors informed and engaged over time.

6. Credit spread liberally and frequently among the partners to maintain broad-based commitment. This was important in mobilizing funding from the donor community and keeping the donors on board and committed. Advertising each donor's support as contributing significantly to the success of the effort allowed them to maintain support from their constituencies "at home" and remain with the program over the long term.

7. Recognition that distinct benefits for all parties are important; altruism is not adequate for sustained commitment. Every partner seeks some gain from their participation. By recognizing the motivation of each partner, those interests can be catered to, to sustain commitment.

8. Program independence and autonomy that help ensure that staff and resources remained directed toward program objectives.

9. Strengthened institutional memory for programs that span decades, to ensure that collective knowledge and best practices are retained and inform ongoing and future operations, recognizing that institutional memory erodes with time and personnel turnover, diminishing the overall effectiveness of a long-term effort.

10. Inclusion of fund-mobilization capacities and expertise to weather crises and to incorporate new technologies and control tools over time to maximize effectiveness.

11. Program implementation according to detailed medium-term plans that are monitored regularly and evaluated at key junctures by independent experts.

Former World Bank director for human development for Africa Birger Fredriksen recognized in his work on education in OECD, the UN Educational, Scientific and Cultural Organization, and the World Bank, similar ingredients for success in long-term partnerships. He cited "staff continuity and strong personal commitment" as critical to partnership cohesion and effectiveness.[40] He emphasized the importance of keeping all partners "well informed about program challenges, outcomes, and successes," via World Bank convening authority. He stated doing so was "essential in maintaining the partners' ownership and long-term commitment."[41]

Consequential Compassion

During the many interviews for this book, I was struck by a powerful common thread: compassion. Speaking with John Moores, I asked why he established and funded the RBF. He responded, "There's something enormously compelling about people who are utterly helpless. I could not see any downside in trying to help people at the end of the road who have miserable lives by scratching themselves to death or becoming blind. Getting ivermectin to these people would alleviate suffering and possibly enable them to work. You could only make lives immeasurably better by supporting delivery of the drug. I feel better about starting the River Blindness Foundation than anything else I've ever done."[42]

In a follow-up interview, Moores spoke of having been deeply affected as a child when his father abandoned him, his mother, and his two siblings. "After that, I just felt helpless because I couldn't help my mother or my siblings. That experience has been the driving force of my life. Ever since, I've had empathy for those suffering from helplessness. I want to help alleviate that suffering to enable others to gain control over their lives."[43] Difficult experiences in childhood, it seems, can be powerful in inducing empathy in individuals who later can act on that empathy to reduce suffering in others—a notion referred to as "consequential compassion" by Bill Foege."[44]

I had a similar childhood experience that became a potent force in motivating me to pursue the alleviation of suffering in others I saw as disadvantaged through no fault of their own. After returning from World War II in early 1946, my father became executive secretary of the community fund association to benefit the poor and disadvantaged in the Greater Lynn area of northeast Massachusetts. One afternoon in September 1948, he came down with a severe sore throat at the office. He saw a doctor on his way home and was given a shot of penicillin. Once home, he went to bed. While my mother and I were eating dinner at the kitchen table, he emerged from the bedroom unable to breathe. My last images of him were of him on his knees on the kitchen floor gasping for air. My mother pulled me out the door as we ran to a neighbor to call an ambulance. Mother told me the next day that my father had died. I was five years old.

Although the cause of his death was initially thought to be "acute respiratory infection," it later became apparent that my father died from an allergic reaction to penicillin—still an experimental antibiotic in 1948. His sudden loss at 33 years old shocked everyone, including the Greater Lynn community that had benefited from a surge in social services during his two-year stint as head of the association.

He looked to have an extremely promising career as a social work executive, and had been named director of the Washington, DC, United Communities Service the day he died—a major promotion in his field. I did not learn about the specifics of that job offer until researching for this book, although I dwelled on what might have been for years after his death.

Similar to Moores, I felt helpless—in particular to comfort my mother—and agonized over the loss into my teens. I was fortunate to have had the abiding, unconditional love of my mother and two sets of grandparents throughout those years. Their care and concern helped mollify bitterness over my plight compared to relatives, schoolmates, and friends with fathers.

In an unexpected way, that experience became an important credential for me later. I empathized with others I perceived as disadvantaged and found ways to sublimate that earlier loss into compassion. The oncho position in the World Bank became a vehicle for acting on that compassion. It provided an opportunity to help improve the well-being of millions disadvantaged and suffering from a devastating disease.

There are many other examples of consequential compassion in the oncho story. Sékétéli first encountered blind oncho victims along the Red Volta River while receiving WHO training in 1975. He later remarked that he was "deeply troubled" by the anguish he encountered and sought to work in the OCP to address it.[45] While lecturing at the University of Nigeria in Enugu State in the 1980s, Amazigo met Agnes, a 19-year-old, oncho-infected, pregnant woman suffering from unrelenting itching and the stigma of oncho dermatitis (see chapter 7).[46] Amazigo became a passionate, tireless advocate for oncho-infected women, whom she regarded as having no voice.[47] After assuming leadership roles in the oncho-control effort, Amazigo recruited women, including Agnes, as CDDs to deliver Mectizan in their communities. The compassion and commitment of Drs. Sékétéli and Amazigo became apparent to me while working closely with them during the late 1990s and early 2000s. But they were far from unique in the oncho community. There were many in management and on the staffs of the OCP and APOC, and among the NGDOs, who were driven by compassion to alleviate suffering from the disease.

It appears that Robert McNamara was endeared to the oncho program, in part, because it fulfilled his sense of compassion for the extreme poor in Africa. His son, Craig McNamara, recently described that connection: "My father spoke frequently about the riverblindness program at home. It was dear to his heart. He had an abiding concern for the poor. He and my mother established a family foundation in

1954—15 years before he became World Bank president—to address poverty and hunger. My father saw the riverblindness program as achieving those objectives as well as alleviating tremendous suffering. I remember that years later he kept a small statue of an adult blinded by the disease led by a child by a stick prominently on our coffee table at home to remind him and visitors of the Program he was so proud of establishing."[48] Shortly after encountering the oncho-infected rural poor in Upper Volta in 1972, Robert McNamara established as a priority for the World Bank eradication of "absolute poverty" in the developing world by focusing assistance on the rural areas. That strategy was introduced in his speech to the Board of Governors at the Bank's annual meeting in Nairobi, Kenya in September 1973.

As noted earlier, compassion is also relevant to the Merck decision to donate Mectizan. In 2015, I interviewed Merck CEO Kenneth Frazier. Frazier reflected on the reasons behind the donation: "MDP is a manifestation of core values that Merck people subscribe to, best exemplified by the George W. Merck quote that 'medicine is for the people, not for the profits.' Our core reason for existing is to relieve human suffering." In commenting on Vagelos's compassion for the patient having influenced his decision, Frazier responded: "I would like people to think of Merck as a compassionate company. That resonates very strongly with what I believe is true of the company."[49]

The positive experience with the MDP marked the beginning of a series of Merck humanitarian programs. Most have been in Africa, because, as Frazier remarked, "That is where so much of the human suffering is."[50] In 2000, Merck took on the challenge of HIV/AIDS in Botswana where HIV prevalence rate was one of the highest in the world. Partnering with the Gates Foundation, Merck donated anti-retroviral drugs, and, with Gates, provided $166.5 million to support the effort. As of April 2019, Merck had completed the testing of an Ebola vaccine (V920 Ebola Zaire Vaccine) and had donated 145,000 doses in response to an outbreak of Ebola in the DRC in 2019.[51] Regarding the vaccine, Frazier remarked, "This is very much because of the precedent of MDP. Each generation at Merck wants its own humanitarian initiative to be proud of."[52]

On the benefits to Merck, Frazier stated, "These kinds of programs pay for themselves many times over because of the people who have chosen Merck because they think of it as a compassionate, caring company. In pursuing these humanitarian programs, you get a greater level of discretionary effort from the employees. They become imbued with a sense of purpose that allows the company to weather unpleasant times, such as a restructuring or downsizing. The

MDP and the Botswana program helped Merck weather the Vioxx storm" (when Merck was sued over Vioxx, a drug that CEO Raymond Gilmartin eventually pulled from the market).[53]

Will Merck hold to the Mectizan commitment until oncho has been eliminated? "Absolutely and unambiguously, yes," Frazier replied. "We intend to live up to the initial commitment that we will donate Mectizan wherever needed for as long as needed, and that commitment is not wavering in any way. Actually, it's stronger now because we are closer to that goal of elimination."[54]

Recognition

In August 2000, while on vacation with my family, I received an email message from Wolfensohn requesting a background briefing on the OCP and APOC. I had never received a message directly from a World Bank president, but clearly, I could not delay responding, so we put our vacation on hold while I prepared and sent the briefing. Six weeks later, I received a copy of a Wolfensohn memo sent to all Bank staff announcing that he would be making a Special Presidential Award to me for my long-term commitment to the elimination of riverblindness in Africa. I was stunned—though elated. The oncho programs were not regarded as mainstream Bank operations; for that reason, I did not think that senior Bank management would consider them worthy of such recognition. The presidential award would be the first ever to an individual in the World Bank and the first involving a special program.

At the November 2000 award ceremony, Wolfensohn cited my long-term efforts to build and sustain the oncho partnership "as managers, ministers, and presidents come and go."[55] In my remarks, I emphasized that the program achievements were the result of that extraordinary partnership, and central to its effectiveness had been exceptionally competent, collegial program directors of high integrity. The directors of the OCP and APOC at the time, Drs. Boatin and Sékétéli, honored me by traveling to Washington, DC, to participate in the ceremony.

The award highlighted the value and power of partnership. By cosponsoring a health program with WHO, the World Bank brought rural development, food production, and poverty alleviation into the equation, which, in turn, enhanced the overall development impact of the disease-control effort. Those extra dimensions enabled the programs to attract higher levels of donor support than possible for a strictly health-focused program. In addition, the Bank brought to the partnership powerful convening authority as well as connections with finance ministries with control over purse strings in donor countries. These advantages made it possible to mobilize the substantial funding required to carry out a control effort covering most of Africa.

The oncho success provided strong evidence that dedicated staff continuity—in my case, two decades—can produce results far greater than when Bank task managers rotate in and out of projects. Effective large-scale programs entail long learning curves, require nurturing years-long relationships, and involve the development and retention of long-term institutional memory that can be tapped into to maximize results. These requirements demand staff continuity. It was ironic that the first World Bank Special Presidential Award was given to a staff member who bucked the system by not rotating, and staying in the same position for two decades. In fact, the award was given largely because of that sustained commitment.

The award was also deeply satisfying on a personal level. I had struggled for several years to secure a long-term position in the World Bank. At one point, I was rejected by a World Bank Economist Panel for a tenured position. But one of the economists on the panel spotted the paperwork describing my background and thought I would be a good fit for the oncho job. Moreover, from time to time, the OCP and APOC were neglected by senior Bank managers because they were "special programs"—not traditional country-focused initiatives. At last, these programs were receiving recognition. The award was acknowledgment at the highest level within the World Bank that regional, grant-based programs can have an important development and humanitarian impact.

People Interviewed, October 2014–August 2019

Merck

Roy Vagelos (former CEO and Chairman of the Board)

Kenneth Frazier (CEO and Chairman of the Board)

William Campbell (former Senior Scientist, Animal Health Division, MRL)

Charles Fettig (former Director of Marketing for Cardiovascular Medications)

Alfred Saah (Director, Merck Investigator Studies Program & Scientific Engagements and Education)

Philippe Gaxotte (former Medical Director, Mectizan Program, Paris Office)

Brenda Colatrella (Associate Vice-President, Corporate Responsibility)

Kenneth Gustavsen (former Manager, Global Health Partnerships)

Kenneth Brown (former Executive Director, Anti-infectives and Vaccines, MRL)

GlaxoSmithKline

Andy Wright (former Vice President of Global Health Programmes)

Task Force for Global Health, Mectizan Donation Program (MDP), Mectizan Expert Committee (MEC)

William Foege (former Director of the Centers for Disease Control and Prevention, founder of the Task Force for Child Survival, and Chair of the Mectizan Expert Committee)

Mark Rosenberg (former President and CEO, Task Force for Global Health)

David Ross (President and CEO, Task Force for Global Health)

Adrian Hopkins (former MDP Director and Medical Director of CBM)

Bjorn Thylefors (former MDP Director, former Director of WHO Office for the Prevention of Blindness, and former ophthalmologist in OCP)

Stefanie E.O. Meredith (former MDP Director)

Michael Heisler (former MDP Director)

Yao Sodahlon (MDP Director)

Eric Ottesen (Program Director, Envision, RTI International and senior advisor of the Neglected Tropical Diseases Support Center, Task Force for Global Health)

David Addiss (Director, Focal Area for Compassion and Ethics, Task Force for Global Health)

Patrick Lammie (Director for the Neglected Tropical Diseases Support Center, Task Force for Global Health)

Joni Lawrence (Sr. Associate Director, Programs, MDP)

Onchocerciasis Control Program (OCP), African Program for Onchocerciasis Control (APOC)

Yankum Dadzie (former OCP Director)
Azodoga Sékétéli (former APOC Director)
Boakye Boatin (former OCP Director)
Uche Amazigo (former APOC Director)
Laurent Yaméogo (former APOC Coordinator)
David Baldry (former Entomologist, OCP)
John Davies (former Entomologist and Acting Chief, VCU, OCP)
Grace Fobi (former Community Ownership and Partnership Officer, APOC)
Afework Tekle (former Epidemiologist, APOC)

Nongovernmental Development Organizations

Allen Foster (former Chairman of the Coordination Group, former Medical
    Director of CBM)
John Moores (Philanthropist and founder of the River Blindness Foundation)
Michel Pacqué (Director of Sightsavers for Africa)
Caroline Harper (Chief Executive, Sightsavers)
Catherine Cross (former Manager of International Programs, Sightsavers)
Simon Bush (Director, Neglected Tropical Diseases, Sightsavers)
Elizabeth Elhassan (Epidemiologist, Sightsavers, Accra, Ghana office)
Victoria Sheffield (President and CEO, International Eye Foundation)
John Barrows (Vice President, Programs, International Eye Foundation)
Julie Jacobson (former Senior Program Officer, Infectious Diseases, Global Health
    Program, Bill & Melinda Gates Foundation)
Ellen Agler (Chief Executive Officer of the END Fund)
Bernard Philippon (Secrétaire General, Organisation de la Prevention de la Cécité,
    and former Chief, VCU, Onchocerciasis Control Program)
Frank Richards (Director, Malaria, River Blindness, Lymphatic Filariasis and
    Schistosomiasis Programs, The Carter Center)
Paul Derstine (former President, Interchurch Medical Assistance)

Experts at Universities and Research Entities

Danny Haddad (Director of Global Ophthalmology with the Emory Eye Center at
    Emory University, Director of the International Trachoma Initiative, and Helen
    Keller International Advisor)
Jesse Bump (Executive Director of the Takemi Program in International Health and
    Lecturer on Global Health Policy at the Harvard T. H. Chan School of Public Health)
Gilbert Burnham (Professor, Bloomberg School of Public Health, Johns Hopkins
    University and Chair of the Mectizan Expert Committee)
Della McMillan (associate research scientist in the Department of Anthropology,
    Center for African Studies, University of Florida)
Michel Boussinesq (Director of Research, Institut de Recherche pour le Développe-
    ment, Montpellier, France)

Deborah McFarland (Professor, Department of International Health, Rollins School of Public Health, Emory University)
Philip Coyne (former Associate Professor of Tropical Public Health, Uniformed Services University)
Paul Cantey (US Centers for Disease Control and Prevention)
Janelle Winters (Wellcome Trust Fellow and Researcher on the OCP, University of Edinburgh)
Amy Klion (Laboratory of Parasitic Diseases, National Institutes of Health)
Andy Crump (Kitasato University, former TDR Communications Officer)

World Health Organization (WHO)
Jacques Hamon (former Assistant Director-General and PAG Mission Leader)
Ralph "Rafe" Henderson (former Assistant Director-General)
Dirk Engels (former Director, Department of Control of Neglected Tropical Diseases)
Tony Ukety (former NGDO Coordinator for Onchocerciasis Control)
Xavier Daney (Senior Legal Officer, Office of the Legal Counsel)
Chris Ngenda Mwikisa (former Acting Director, APOC, WHO AFRO)
Jan "Hans" F. Remme (former Manager, TDR Task Force for Onchocerciasis Operational Research; former Chief, Biostatistics, OCP)
Marc Karam (WHO representative, Committee of Sponsoring Agencies; former epidemiologist, OCP)
Annette Kuesel (Scientist, Intervention and Implementation Research, TDR)
Jamie Guth (former Communications Manager, TDR)
Rosemary Villars (former WHO PAG Mission Programme Officer)
Addulai Daribi (APOC/AFRO Liaison Office)
Pamela Drameh (former NGDO Coordinator for Onchocerciasis Control, Prevention of Blindness Department)
Maria Rebollo Polo (Team Leader, Expanded Special Project for Elimination of Neglected Tropical Diseases, AFRO)

World Bank
James D. Wolfensohn (former President)
Jean-Louis Sarbib (former Senior Vice-President, Human Development and Vice-President, Africa Region)
Katherine Marshall (former Director, Sahel Country Department, Africa Region)
Birger Fredriksen (former Director, Human Development Department, Africa Region)
Merza Hasan (Dean of World Bank Board of Executive Directors)
Bernhard Liese (former Principal Tropical Disease Specialist)
Steven Denning (former Chief, Sahel Country Division)
Larry Hinkle (former Chief, Sahel Country Division)
Jean-Paul Dailly (former Onchocerciasis Coordinator, Sahel Country Division)
Dirk Mattheisen (former Research Assistant, Oncho Unit, Sahel Country Division)

Thomas Blinkhorn (former Division Chief, Public Affairs Division, Information and Public Affairs Department)

Eva Jarawan (former Sector Manager, Africa Health, Nutrition and Population)

Timothy Evans (former Senior Director of Health, Nutrition and Population)

Donald Bundy (former APOC Coordinator, African Region, Human Development Department)

Andy Tembon (Oncho Team Member, African Region, Human Development Department)

Ok Pannenborg (former Chief Health Advisor, Africa Region)

Alireza Azimipour (former Co-financing Analyst, Oncho Unit, African Region, Human Development Department)

Bilkiss Dhomun (former APOC Financial Analyst, Oncho Unit, African Region Human Development Department)

Donor Representatives

Abdlatif Y. Al-Hamad (Director-General of the Arab Fund for Economic and Social Development)

Emily Wainwright (Senior Operations Advisor for NTDs, USAID)

Darin Evans (Technical Advisor for Onchocerciasis and Schistosomiasis, USAID)

Christian Bailly (former Chef du Bureau Santé, Ministère des Affaires Etrangères, France)

John Gibb (former Programme Analyst and Manager, DFID)

Philip Steven Mason (DFID representative)

Camilla Ducker (former Health Advisor, DFID)

David Molyneux (former Director of the Liverpool School of Tropical Medicine, DFID Delegation, and Chair, Expert Advisory Committee of OCP)

Scott Hardie (DFID)

Catherine Hodgkin (Royal Tropical Institute, the Netherlands)

Abdulwahab A. Al-Bader (Director General, the Kuwait Fund)

Marwan A. Th. Al-Ghanem (Deputy Director-General, the Kuwait Fund)

Thamer Al-Failakawi (Regional Manager for West African Countries, the Kuwait Fund)

A.M. Bahman (Agricultural Advisor, the Kuwait Fund)

Mohammed Sadeqi (Engineering Advisor, the Kuwait Fund)

Reem Al-Mutwawa (Media Officer, the Kuwait Fund)

Shareefa Jaber Al-Sabah (Media Officer, the Kuwait Fund)

Participating Country Officials

Amédée Prosper Djiguimde (Minister of Health, Burkina Faso)

Soungalo Traoré (Coordonnateur National du Programme de Lutte contre l'Onchocercose, Burkina Faso)

Daniel Boakye (Medical Entomologist, Noguchi Memorial Institute for Medical Research, Accra, Ghana)

Michael Wilson (Department of Parasitology, Noguchi Memorial Institute for Medical Research, Accra, Ghana)

Other

Diana Masieri McNamara (Wife of Robert McNamara, 2004–2009)
Craig McNamara (Robert McNamara's son)
Curt Strand (Robert McNamara's close friend in Snowmass, Colorado)
RT "Skip" Wallen (Sculptor of Riverblindness statues)
Lynn Wallen (Business Associate and Wife of RT Wallen)

Acronyms and Abbreviations

ABR	annual biting rate
AfDB	African Development Bank
AFRO	WHO Regional Office for Africa
APOC	African Program for Onchocerciasis Control
ATP	annual transmission potential (of biting blackflies)
AVV	Autorité des Aménamagements des Vallées des Volta (Volta Valley Authority of Upper Volta)
B.t. H-14	*Bacillus thuringiensis*
CAR	Central African Republic
C/B	cost-benefit analysis
CBM	Christoffel-Blindenmission
CDD	community-directed distributor
CDI	community-directed intervention
CDTI	community-directed treatment with ivermectin
CFA (franc)	Communauté financière d'Afrique (currencies used in parts of West and Central Africa)
CICRED	Committee for International Cooperation in National Research in Demography
CIDA	Canadian International Development Agency
CMFL	community microfilarial load (measure of community infection levels)
CNS	central nervous system
ComDT	community-directed treatment
CSA	Committee of Sponsoring Agencies (steering committee of the OCP and APOC)
DALYs	disability adjusted life years
DDT	dichlorodiphenyltrichloroethane
DEC	diethylcarbamazine
DFID	Department for International Development (UK)
DGF	Development Grant Facility (of the World Bank)
DOTS	directly observed treatment, short course for tuberculosis
DPD	Directorate of Pharmacy and Drugs (France)
DRC	Democratic Republic of Congo

EAC	Expert Advisory Committee (of the Onchocerciasis Control Program)
ECOWAS	Economic Community of West African States
EDs	executive directors of the World Bank
EDF	European Development Fund (foreign assistance agency of the European Community / Union)
EG	Ecological Group (of the Onchocerciasis Control Program)
EPI	Epidemiological Unit (of the Onchocerciasis Control Program)
ERR	economic rate of return
ESPEN	Expanded Special Project for Elimination of Neglected Tropical Diseases
FAC	Fonds d'Aide et de Coopération (Fund for Aid and Cooperation, foreign assistance agency of France)
FACE	Focal Area for Compassion and Ethics at the Task Force for Global Health
FAO	Food and Agriculture Organization
FDA	United States Food and Drug Administration
FIDES	Fonds d'Investissement pour le Développement Economique et Social des Territoires d'Outre-mer (Fund for Investment in Social and Economic Development for the overseas territories of France)
GAELF	Global Alliance to Eliminate Lymphatic Filariasis
GIS	geographic information system
GPELF	Global Program for the Elimination of Lymphatic Filariasis
GSK	GlaxoSmithKline
HKI	Helen Keller International
IAPB	International Agency for the Prevention of Blindness
ICOPA	International Congress of Parasitology
ICT	rapid immunochromatographic test
IDA	International Development Association (of the World Bank Group)
IDB	Inter-American Development Bank
IEF	International Eye Foundation
IFPRI	International Food Policy Research Institute
JAF	Joint Action Forum (of APOC)
JCC	Joint Coordinating Committee (governing board of the Onchocerciasis Control Program during the early years)
JPC	Joint Program Committee (governing board of Onchocerciasis Control Program)
LF	lymphatic filariasis
LSR	Land Settlement Review
LTS	long-term strategy (for the Onchocerciasis Control Program)
MDA	mass drug administration
MDGs	United Nations Millennium Development Goals

MDP	Mectizan Donation Program
MDSC	Multi-Disease Surveillance Center
MEC	Mectizan Expert Committee
mf	microfilariae
mf/ml	microfilariae per milliliter of blood
mf/s	microfilariae per skin snip
MEC/AC	Mectizan Expert Committee/Albendazole Coordination
MOH	ministry of health
MOU	memorandum of understanding
MPH	Master's in Public Health
MRC	Medical Research Council (UK)
MRL	Merck Research Laboratories
NGDO	nongovernmental development organization
NGO	nongovernmental organization
NIH	National Institutes of Health (US)
NOC(s)	National Onchocerciasis Committees (of the Onchocerciasis Control Program)
NOTF(s)	National Onchocerciasis Task Forces (of the African Program for Onchocerciasis Control)
NTD(s)	neglected tropical disease(s)
OCCGE	Organisation de Coordination et de Coopération pour la lutte Contre les Grandes Endémies (Organization for Coordination and Operation to Combat Major Endemics)
OCP	Onchocerciasis Control Program
OCRC	Onchocerciasis Chemotherapy Research Center
OCT	Onchocerciasis Chemotherapy Project
OED	Operations Evaluation Department (of the World Bank)
OEPA	Onchocerciasis Elimination Program for the Americas
ONAT	Office d'Aménagement des Territoires of Burkina Faso (Office of Land Management for Burkina Faso)
OOR	onchocerciasis operational research
OPEC	The Organization of the Petroleum Exporting Countries
ORZs	onchocerciasis reference zones (of the FAO Demographic Study)
OSD	onchocerciasis skin disease
ORSTOM	Office de la Recherche Scientifique et Technique Outre-Mer (Office of Scientific and Technical Research Overseas for France)
PC	preventive chemotherapy
PCT NTDs	preventive chemotherapy and transmission control NTDs
PENDA	Program for the Elimination of Neglected Diseases in Africa
PLANOPS	Plan of Operations of Phase III of the Onchocerciasis Control Program
RAPLOA	Rapid Assessment Procedure for Loiasis
RBF	River Blindness Foundation

REA	Rapid Epidemiological Assessment
REMO	Rapid Epidemiological Mapping of Onchocerciasis
RMC	Research Management Council
RPGs	regional public goods
PAG	Preparatory Assistance to Governments mission
PHN	Population, Health, and Nutrition (World Bank sector office)
PLANOPS	plan of operations (of the Onchocerciasis Control Program)
SAEs	severe adverse events
SB	SmithKline Beecham
SED	socioeconomic development
SGHMP	Service Général d'Hygiène Mobile et de Prophylaxie (General Service of Mobile Hygiene and Prophylaxis of France)
SIZ	special intervention zone (of the Onchocerciasis Control Program)
SSZ	Sudano-Savanna climactic zone
SSPH	severe symptomatic postural hypotension
STH	soil-transmitted helminthiasis
TaNT	test and not treat
TCC	Technical Consultative Committee (of African Program for Onchocerciasis Control)
TDR	Special Program for Research and Training in Tropical Diseases (sponsored by UNICEF, UNDP, World Bank, and WHO)
TOR	terms of reference
UNDP	United Nations Development Programme
USAID	United States Agency for International Development
VCU	Vector Control Unit (of the Onchocerciasis Control Program)
VHW	village health worker
WHO	World Health Organization
WHO/PBL	WHO Office of the Prevention of Blindness

Notes

CHAPTER 1: **The Challenge**

Epigraph. John Wilson, "Blind Eyes and Seeing Hands," *West African Review* 1392, no. 3 (1950), quoted in Jesse Boardman Bump, "The Lion's Gaze: African River Blindness from Tropical Curiosity to International Development" (PhD diss., John Hopkins University, 2004), 202.

1. Jerome Goddard, "Black Flies and Onchocerciasis," *Infectious Medicine* 18, no. 6 (2001).

2. I am indebted to Jesse Bump for his research during 2001–2004 on his PhD dissertation for Johns Hopkins University, entitled "The Lion's Gaze: African River Blindness from Tropical Curiosity to International Development." He conducted that research while separately working as a research assistant in the World Bank's Onchocerciasis Unit that I was managing at the time. His research spanned the earliest work on onchocerciasis through the launch of the Onchocerciasis Control Program in 1974. I have relied on Bump's research as presented in "The Lion's Gaze" for parts of chapter 1 and have cited his work accordingly. Bump, "The Lion's Gaze," ii.

3. Bump, "Lion's Gaze," ii.

4. Bump, "Lion's Gaze," 64.

5. Bump, "Lion's Gaze," 69.

6. Andy Crump, Carlos M. Morel, and Satoshi Ōmura, "The Onchocerciasis Chronicle: From the Beginning to the End," *Trends in Parasitology* 28, no. 7 (2012): 283.

7. Bump, "Lion's Gaze," 113.

8. Bump, "Lion's Gaze," 103.

9. Crump, Morel, and Ōmura, "Onchocerciasis Chronicle," 282.

10. Crump, Morel, and Ōmura, "Onchocerciasis Chronicle," 282.

11. Bump, "Lion's Gaze," 107.

12. John Coles, *Blindness and the Visionary: The Life and Work of John Wilson* (London: Giles de la Mare, 2006), 44.

13. Lady Jean Wilson (wife of the blind activist Sir John Wilson), discussion with the author, April 2, 2015.

14. Coles, *Blindness and Visionary*, 44.

15. Lady Jean Wilson, discussion, April 2, 2015.

16. John Foster Wilson, *Travelling Blind* (London: Hutchinson, 1963), 43.

17. Bump, "Lion's Gaze," 174.

18. Bump, "Lion's Gaze," 185.

19. Bump, "Lion's Gaze," 190–191.

20. Bump, "Lion's Gaze," 192.

21. Bump, "Lion's Gaze," 199.

22. Bump, "Lion's Gaze," 190.

23. Coles, *Blindness and Visionary*, 49.

24. Wilson, *Travelling Blind*, 44.

25. Lady Jean Wilson, discussion, April 2, 2015.

26. Coles, *Blindness and Visionary*, 50.

27. Lady Jean Wilson, discussion, April 2, 2015.

28. Lady Jean Wilson, discussion, April 2, 2015.

29. Bump, "Lion's Gaze," 203.

30. Bump, "Lion's Gaze," 208–209.

31. Bump, "Lion's Gaze," 209.

32. Bump, "Lion's Gaze," 210.

33. Bump, "Lion's Gaze," 210.

34. Bump, "Lion's Gaze," 211.

35. Bump, "Lion's Gaze," 211.

36. Bump, "Lion's Gaze," 212.

37. Crump, Morel, and Ōmura, "Onchocerciasis Chronicle," 283.

38. Crump, Morel, and Ōmura, "Onchocerciasis Chronicle," 284.

39. Bump, "Lion's Gaze," 246.

40. Crump, Morel, and Ōmura, "Onchocerciasis Chronicle," 284.

41. Crump, Morel, and Ōmura, "Onchocerciasis Chronicle," 284.

42. Bump, "Lion's Gaze," 296.

43. Crump, Morel, and Ōmura, "Onchocerciasis Chronicle," 284.

44. Bump, "Lion's Gaze," 218.

45. Jacques Hamon, email message to author, February 21, 2018.

46. Helen Bynum, *Success in Africa: The Onchocerciasis Control Programme in West Africa, 1974–2002* (Geneva: World Health Organization, 2002), 18.

47. Bump, "Lion's Gaze," 305.

48. Bump, "Lion's Gaze," 306.

49. Bump, "Lion's Gaze," 307.

50. Bump, "Lion's Gaze," 318.

51. Bump, "Lion's Gaze," 320–321.

52. Bump, "Lion's Gaze," 326.

53. Bump, "Lion's Gaze," 353.

54. Bump, "Lion's Gaze," 338.

55. Ebrahim M. Samba, *The Onchocerciasis Control Programme in West Africa: An Example of Effective Public Health Management* (Geneva: World Health Organization, 1994), 11.

56. Samba, *Onchocerciasis Control Programme*, 11.

57. Samba, *Onchocerciasis Control Programme*, 11.

58. Bump, "Lion's Gaze," 339–342.

59. Bump, "Lion's Gaze," 340.

60. Bump, "Lion's Gaze," 342.

61. Bump, "Lion's Gaze," 342.

62. Jacques Hamon and Rosemary Villars, email message to author, February 21, 2018.

63. Bump, "Lion's Gaze," 354.

64. Samba, *Onchocerciasis Control Programme*, 12.

65. Bump, "Lion's Gaze," 358.

66. Diana Masieri Byfield McNamara, discussion with the author, August 27, 2016.

67. Robert S. McNamara, "To the Board of Governors, Washington, D.C. September 30, 1968," in *The McNamara Years at the World Bank: Major Policy Addresses of Robert S. McNamara, 1968–1981* (Washington, DC: World Bank, 1981), 12.

68. Roger Chaufournier, "The World Bank/IFC Archives Oral History Program," interview by Robert W. Oliver, The World Bank, July 22, 1986, 67.

69. Chaufournier, interview by Robert W. Oliver, 1986, 68.

70. Chaufournier, interview by Robert W. Oliver, 1986, 68.

71. Bernard Philippon (former ORSTOM/OCCGE Entomologist and Chief of VCU), discussion with the author, March 25, 2015.

72. Robert McNamara, "The World Bank's Venture into the Onchocerciasis Program," in *Roger Chaufournier and the Onchocerciasis Program: A Tribute to One of its Founding Fathers*, working paper, 1994.

73. Donald Easom, "River Blindness Foundation Newsletter," 1992.

74. René Le Berre, "Contribution a L'Étude Biologique et Écologique de *Simulium Damnosum*," dissertation, Docteur ès Science Naturelles: Maître de Recherches à L'ORSTOM, 1996, 182.

75. Samba, *Onchocerciasis Control Programme*, 12.

76. McNamara, "The World Bank's Venture."

77. Bump, "Lion's Gaze," 362.

78. Bjorn Thylefors (former director of WHO's Office for the Prevention of Blindness and former ophthalmologist in the OCP EPI Unit, 1974), discussion with the author, March 25, 2015.

CHAPTER 2: **Launching and Scaling Up the Onchocerciasis Control Program**

1. James W. Wright (former Chief of Vector Biology and Control Unit) and Lucien Bernard (former Assistant Director-General of WHO) as communicated to Jacques Hamon, email to author, February 21, 2018.

2. Rosemary Villars (former PAG Mission Administrative Officer), email to author, February 21, 2018.

3. Jacques Hamon (former PAG Mission Leader and Assistant Director-General of WHO), discussion with the author, March 25, 2015.

4. "Onchocerciasis Control in the Volta River Basin Area," UNDP, the FAO, the IBRD, WHO doc. 73.1, 1973, 1.

5. "Onchocerciasis Control," 2.

6. Hamon, discussion, March 25, 2015.

7. "Onchocerciasis Control," 2.

8. Hamon, discussion, March 25, 2015.

9. Hamon, discussion, March 25, 2015.

10. "Onchocerciasis Control," 2.

11. "Onchocerciasis Control," 2.

12. Hamon, discussion, March 25, 2015.

13. Hamon, discussion, March 25, 2015.

14. Ebrahim M. Samba, *The Onchocerciasis Control Programme in West Africa: An Example of Effective Public Health Management* (Geneva: World Health Organization, 1994), 16.

15. Bjorn Thylefors (former director of WHO's Office for the Prevention of Blindness and former ophthalmologist in the OCP EPI Unit, 1974), discussion with the author, March 25, 2015; Azodoga Sékétéli (former APOC director), discussion with the author, October 3, 2015; Rosemary Villars (former program officer in the OCP director's office), discussion with the author, March 21, 2015.

16. Jesse Bump, email to author, November 22, 2017.

17. Agreement Governing the Operations of the Onchocerciasis Control Programme in the Volta Basin Area, at 201, November 1, 1973. 1126 U.N.T.S. 17537.

18. World Bank, "Transcript of Meeting of the Executive Directors of the Bank and IDA Held on Tuesday, May 1, 1973: Onchocerciasis in Western Africa" (Board Transcript, Washington D.C.: World Bank Group, May 1, 1973), English, 30. http://documents.worldbank.org /curated/en/513621496833276816/Transcript-of-meeting-of-the-Executive-Directors-of-the -Bank-and-IDA-held-on-Tuesday-May-1-1973-Onchocerciasis-in-Western-Africa.

19. Bump, "Lion's Gaze," 366.

20. Bump, "Lion's Gaze," 364.

21. Bump, "Lion's Gaze," 367.

22. Hamon, discussion, March 25, 2015.

23. Bump, "Lion's Gaze," 367.

24. Merza Hasan (dean of the World Bank Board and executive director), discussion with the author, February 24, 2016.

25. Marwan A. Th. Al-Ghanem (director of operations for the Kuwait Fund for Arab Economic Development), discussion with the author, January 25, 2016.

26. Abdlatif Y. Al-Hamad (director-general of the Arab Fund for Economic and Social Development), discussion with the author, January 26, 2016.

27. Thomas Blinkhorn and Jamie Martin, producers, *A Plague Upon the Land* (1973, Burkina Faso: World Bank/ International Finance Corporation, 1984), VHS.

28. Al-Hamad, discussion, January 26, 2016.

29. Thomas A. Blinkhorn, "The Making of a World Bank Movie: Troubles Plague 'A Plague Upon the Land' Amateur Filmmakers but Everything Turns Out All Right in the End," bank notes, October 6, 1973.

30. Thomas A. Blinkhorn (former World Bank staff member), discussion with the author, September 17, 2017.

31. Thomas A. Blinkhorn, "The World Bank Group Archives: Oral History Program," interview by Robert P. Grathwol, The World Bank, June 16–18, 2008, 22.

32. Al-Hamad, discussion, January 26, 2016.

33. Al-Hamad, discussion, January 26, 2016.

34. A. M. Bahman, "Investment Costs of Developing Irrigated Land," *International Journal of Development Research* 5, no. 11 (2015): 6084.

35. Thamer Al-Failakawi (regional manager for West African Countries), discussion with the author, January 25, 2016.

36. Onchocerciasis Control Program, "25 Years of OCP" (Government document, Ouagadougou, Burkina Faso, 1999), 20.

37. Jesse Bump, "The Crosskey-Davies Experiement and Onchocerciasis in West Africa," *PLoS Neglected Tropical Diseases* 8, no.10 (2014).

38. Bump, "Crosskey-Davies Experiment," 2.

39. World Health Organization (WHO), *Onchocerciasis Control Programme in the Volta River Basin Area*, pt. 1, evaluation report, O.C.P. doc. 78.2 (1979), 22.

40. WHO *Onchocerciasis Control Programme*, supra note 43, 22.

41. John B. Davies, email to author, October 28, 2019.

42. Davies, email, October 28, 2019.

43. Bernard Philippon (former ORSTOM/OCCGE entomologist and chief of VCU), discussion with the author, March 25, 2015.

44. Davies, email to author, October 28, 2019.

45. Philippon, discussion, March 25, 2015.

46. WHO, *Onchocerciasis Control Programme*, supra note 43, 23.

47. WHO, *Onchocerciasis Control Programme*, supra note 43, iii.

48. WHO, *Onchocerciasis Control Programme*, supra note 43, 23.

49. WHO, *Onchocerciasis Control Programme*, supra note 43, iii.

50. WHO, *Onchocerciasis Control Programme*, supra note 43, iii.

51. David Baldry, email to author, February 15, 2015.

52. Garms et al., "Studies of the Reinvasion of the OCP in the Volta River Basin by *Simulium damnosum* s.l. with Emphasis on the South-Western Areas," *Tropenmed Parasitol.* 30 (1979): 360; WHO, *Onchocerciasis Control Programme*, supra note 43, iii.

53. WHO, *Onchocerciasis Control Programme*, supra note 43, iii.

54. Bump, "Crosskey-Davies Experiment," 2.

55. Bump, "Crosskey-Davies Experiment," 2.

56. Bump, "Crosskey-Davies Experiment," 2.

57. Bump, "Crosskey-Davies Experiment," 2.

58. René Le Berre, "Contribution a L'Étude Biologique et Écologique de *Simulium Damnosum*" (dissertation, Docteur ès Science Naturelles; Maître de Recherches à l'ORSTOM, 1966), 182.

59. Samba, *Effective Public Health Management*, 12.

60. Bjorn Thylefors (former director of WHO's Office for the Prevention of Blindness and former ophthalmologist in the OCP EPI Unit, 1974), discussion with the author, March 25, 2015.

61. Thylefors, discussion, March 25, 2015.

62. Thylefors, discussion, March 25, 2015.

63. Thylefors, discussion, March 25, 2015.

64. Philippon, discussion, March 25, 2015.

65. Rosemary Villars, email to author, February 21, 2018.

66. Thylefors, discussion, March 25, 2015.

67. Villars, email, February 21, 2018.

68. Bernhard Liese (former World Bank Principal Tropical Disease Specialist), discussion with the author, September 9, 2014.

69. Sékétéli, discussion, October 3, 2015.

70. Sékétéli, discussion, October 3, 2015.

71. Sékétéli, discussion, October 3, 2015.

CHAPTER 3: **Expansion and Rescue**

1. World Health Organization (WHO), "Independent Commission on the Long-Term Prospects of the Onchocerciasis Control Programme," (August 1981), iii.

2. WHO, "Independent Commission," iii.

3. WHO, "Independent Commission," iii.

4. WHO, "Independent Commission," iii.

5. WHO, "Independent Commission," iii.

6. WHO, "Independent Commission," 22.

7. WHO, "Independent Commission," 22.

8. WHO, "Independent Commission," 22.

9. WHO, "Independent Commission," annex B.

10. WHO, "Independent Commission," 32.

11. World Health Organization (WHO), "TDR's Contribution to the Development of Ivermectin for Onchocerciasis: Third External Review," prepared by Tomoko Fujisaki and Michael Reich in Takemi Program in International Health, Harvard School of Public Health, Reference Document: 3 (n.p.: World Health Organization, 1998), 5.

12. WHO, "Independent Commission," annex E.

13. WHO, "Independent Commission," 64.

14. Webb et al., "External Review of the Onchocerciasis Control Program" (unpublished external review, October 1990), 17.

15. Webb et al., "External Review of the Onchocerciasis Control Program," unpublished external review, October 1990, 17

16. Onchocerciasis Control Program, "25 Years of OCP" (government document, Ouagadougou, Burkina Faso, 1999), 20.

17. Jean-Paul Dailly (former Onchocerciasis Coordinator in the Sahel Division of the Western Africa Department), discussion with the author, September 11, 2017.

18. World Health Organization (WHO), "Onchocerciasis Control Programme in the Volta River Basin Area," evaluation report, pt. II, doc. 78.2 (1978), iii.

19. WHO, "Onchocerciasis Control Programme," iii.

20. WHO, "Onchocerciasis Control Programme," v-vi.

21. WHO, "Onchocerciasis Control Programme," vi.

22. WHO, "Onchocerciasis Control Programme," iii.

23. WHO, "Onchocerciasis Control Programme," vii.

24. OECD Sahel and West Africa Club, "The Socio-Economic and Regional Context of West African Migrations" (2006), 25.

25. OECD, "West African Migrations," 17.

26. Economic Community of West African States (ECOWAS), "Agricultural Potential in West Africa" (2008), 22.

27. ECOWAS, "Agricultural Potential," 22.

28. Della E. McMillan et al., "Settlement and Development in the River Blindness Control Zone," In *Series on River Blindness Control in West Africa*, World Bank Technical Paper 200 (June 1993), 8.

29. McMillan, "Settlement and Development," 8.

30. McMillan, "Settlement and Development," 9.

31. Joint Coordinating Committee of the Onchocerciasis Control Program (JCC), "Onchocerciasis Control Program: Economic Review Mission," fifth sess., pt. 2, in *Evaluation Report: Economic Aspects*, appendix III, 3 (1978).

32. JCC, "Onchocerciasis Control Program: Economic Review Mission," appendix III, 3.

33. J. H. F. Remme, and J. B. Zongo, "Demographic Aspects of the Epidemiology and Control of Onchocerciasis in West Africa," in *Demography and Vector-Borne Diseases*, ed. Michael W. Service (Boca Raton, FL: CRC Press, 1989), 367–386.

34. JCC, "Onchocerciasis Control Program: Economic Review Mission," Provisional Agenda Item 11, 7.

35. Steve Denning (World Bank Division Chief of the Sahel Countries and the OCP), discussion with the author, September 4, 2017.

36. Rosemary Villars, email with author, March 3, 2018.

37. Azodoga Sékétéli (former APOC director), discussion with the author, October 3, 2015; Yankum Dadzie (former OCP director), discussion with the author, October 5, 2015.

38. Ebrahim M. Samba, personal conversation with author, 1987.

39. Ebrahim M. Samba, "Ebrahim M. Samba: Curriculum Vitae," 1988.

40. Bernhard Liese (former World Bank Principal Tropical Disease Specialist), discussion with the author, February 8, 2018.

41. Azodoga Sékétéli (former APOC director), discussion with the author, October 3, 2015.

42. Jean-Paul Dailly (former Onchocerciasis Coordinator in the Sahel Division of the Western Africa Department), discussion with the author, January 22, 2018.

43. Dailly, discussion, January 22, 2018.

44. David Knox, "Opening Statement: Meeting of Contributors to the Onchocerciasis Fund," speech, Paris, October 11–12, 1982; World Bank Archives, Washington, DC, 1300674, 1.

45. Dailly, discussion, January 22, 2018.

46. Knox, "Opening Statement," 5.

47. Liese, discussion, February 8, 2018.

48. Dailly, discussion, January 24, 2018.

49. Dailly, discussion, January 24, 2018.

50. Samba, personal conversation with author, December 1986.

51. Dailly, discussion, January 24, 2018.

52. Liese, discussion, February 8, 2018.

53. Kelly et al., "Impact Review of the Onchocerciasis Program: Ouagadougou, August 1985," US Agency for International Development, evaluation report no. 63, Washington, DC (1986), 7.

54. Kelly et al., "Impact Review," 34.

55. Onchocerciasis Fund Agreement, February 4, 1986, United Kingdom of Great Britain HMSO and the Secretary of State for Foreign and Commonwealth Affairs 1990, Gr. Brit. T.S. no. 62, 4–5.

56. Ebrahim M. Samba, *The Onchocerciasis Control Programme in West Africa: An Example of Effective Public Health Management* (Geneva: World Health Organization, 1994), 57.

57. Jan H. F. Remme (former Biostatistician for the OCP), discussion with the author, March 18, 2015.

58. Jan H. F. Remme, "Research for Control: The Onchocerciasis Experience," *Tropical Medicine and International Health* 9, no. 2 (2004): 244.

59. Remme, "Research for Control," 244.

60. Remme, discussion, March 18, 2015.

61. Onchocerciasis Fund Agreement 1986, supra note 40, 4–5.

62. Pound Sterling Live, "US Dollar to French Franc Spot Exchange Rates for 1975–2001 from the Bank of England," 2013–2018, http://www.poundsterlinglive.com/bank-of-england -spot/historical-spot-exchange-rates/usd/USD-to-FRF-1985; Pound Sterling Live, "US Dollar to Japanese Yen Spot Exchange Rates for 1975–2018 from the Bank of England," 2013–2018, http://www.poundsterlinglive.com/bank-of-england-spot/historical-spot-exchange-rates/usd /USD-to-JPY.

63. World Health Organization (WHO) Joint Programme Committee of the Onchocerciasis Control Programme, *Onchocerciasis Control Programme in West Africa*, 9th Sess., Annex 1, Agenda Item 14, at 28 (1988).

64. J. Mouchet and P. Guillet, *Insecticide Resistance in Blackfly of the Simulium Damnosum Complex in West Africa*, at 1–4, unpublished WHO doc. OCP/SWG/78.17 (July 3–7, 1978).

65. United States Environmental Protection Agency, "EPA R.E.D. Facts: Bacillus thuringiensis" (Government Archival Document, Washington DC, 1998), 5.

66. Davide Calamari et al., "Environmental Assessment of Larvicide Use in the Onchocerciasis Control Programme," *Parasitology Today* 14, no.12 (1998): 485, in *Thirty Years of Onchocerciasis Control in West Africa*, ed. Laurent Yaméogo et al. (Paris: IRD Éditions, 2003).

67. J. M. Hougard et al., "Criteria for the Selection of Larvicides by the Onchocerciasis Control Programme in West Africa," *Annals of Tropical Medicine and Parasitology* 87, no. 5 (1993): 437.

68. WHO Joint Programme Committee, annex 1, agenda item 15, 30.

69. Boakye A. Boatin, "Preface" in *Thirty Years of Onchocerciasis Control in West Africa*, ed. ed. Laurent Yaméogo, Christian Lévêque, and Jean-Marc Hougard (Paris: IRD Éditions, 2003), 11.

70. Calamari et al., "Environmental Assessment," 485.

71. Laurent Yaméogo et al., *Thirty Years of Onchocerciasis*, 43.

72. Calamari et al., "Environmental Assessment," 485.

73. Calamari et al., "Environmental Assessment," 486.

74. Calamari et al., "Environmental Assessment," 487.

75. Calamari et al., "Environmental Assessment," 487.

76. Bernhard Liese (former World Bank Principal Tropical Disease Specialist), discussion with the author, September 10, 2017.

77. Stacy Husion, "Intimate Encounters and the Politics of German Occupation in Belgium, 1940–44/45" (doctorate thesis, University of Toronto, 2015), 55–60.

78. Onchocerciasis Fund Agreement, February 25, 1992, United Kingdom of Great Britain HMSO and the Secretary of State for Foreign and Commonwealth Affairs 1997, Gr. Brit. T.S. no. 35, 5.

79. WHO Joint Programme Committee, annex 1, agenda item 14, 28.

80. WHO Joint Programme Committee, annex 1, agenda item 14, 28.

81. WHO Joint Programme Committee, annex 1, agenda item 14, 28.

82. WHO Joint Programme Committee, annex 1, agenda item 15, 30.

CHAPTER 4: **The Game Changer—Ivermectin**

1. William C. Campbell, "History of Avermectin and Ivermectin, with Notes on the History of other Macrocyclic Lactone Antiparasitic Agents," *Current Pharmaceutical Biotechnology* 13, no. 6 (2012): 854.

2. William C. Campbell, "Lessons from the History of Ivermectin and Other Antiparasitic Agents," *Annual Review of Animal Biosciences* 4 (2016): 197.

3. Campbell, "Lessons from the History," 196.

4. William C. Campbell (former Merck Senior Scientist in Parasitology), discussion with the author, July 22, 2015.

5. Darragh Murphy, "Meet Ireland's New Nobel Laureate, William C Campbell," *The Irish Times*, October 9, 2015.

6. Campbell, discussion, July 22, 2015.

7. Campbell, discussion, July 22, 2015.

8. Mark Siddall, "A Noble and Laudable Nobel Laureate: William C. Campbell," *The Huffington Post*, October 13, 2015.

9. Campbell, discussion, July 22, 2015.

10. Campbell (former Merck Senior Scientist in Parasitology), discussion, September 2, 2015.

11. John Lofflin, "The Miracle Molecule," *Veterinary Medicine* (2005): 47.

12. Campbell, "Lessons from the History," 203.

13. Roy Vagelos (former President of Merck Research Laboratories), discussion with the author, February 10, 2015.

14. Lofflin, "The Miracle Molecule," 44.

15. Campbell, "History of Avermectin," 856; Gerald Esch, *Parasites and Infectious Disease: Key Discoveries in Parasitology* (Cambridge: Cambridge University Press, 2007), 181.

16. Vagelos, discussion, January 18, 2015.

17. Andy Crump and Satoshi Ōmura, "Ivermectin, 'Wonder Drug' from Japan: The Human Use Perspective," *Proceedings of the Japan Academy, Series B Physical and Biological Sciences* 87, no. 2 (2011): 13.

18. Campbell, discussion, July 22, 2015.

19. Campbell, "History of Avermectin," 858.

20. Campbell, "History of Avermectin," 858.

21. Campbell, "History of Avermectin," 858.

22. World Health Organization (WHO), *Independent Commission on the Long-Term Prospects of the Onchocerciasis Control Programme*, at R27, (August 1981).

23. Campbell, "History of Avermectin," 859.

24. Bjorn Thylefors (former director of WHO's Office for the Prevention of Blindness and former ophthalmologist in the OCP EPI Unit, 1974), discussion with the author, March 25, 2015.

25. Thylefors, discussion, March 25, 2015.

26. Ken Brown (fomer executive director of anti-infectives and vaccines in Merck Research Laboratories), discussion with the author, February 3, 2015.

27. Brown, discussion, February 3, 2015.

28. Campbell, "History of Avermectin," 859.

29. Brown, discussion, February 3, 2015.

30. Vagelos, discussion, January 21, 2015.

31. Jerry Birnbaum, personal note sent to William C. Campbell, January 1980.

32. Brown, discussion, February 3, 2015.

33. Campbell, "History of Avermectin," 860.

34. Bruce M. Greene, Kenneth R. Brown, and Hugh R. Taylor, "Use of Ivermectin in Humans," in *Ivermectin and Abamectin*, ed. William C. Campbell (New York: Springer-Verlag, 1989), 311.

35. Campbell, "History of Avermectin," 860.

36. André Rougemont, "Ivermectin for Onchocerciasis," *The Lancet*, November 20, 1982.

37. Rougemont, "Ivermectin for Onchocerciasis," 1982.

38. Rougemont, "Ivermectin for Onchocerciasis," 1982.

39. Rougemont, "Ivermectin for Onchocerciasis," 1982.

40. Rougemont, "Ivermectin for Onchocerciasis," 1982.

41. Rougemont, "Ivermectin for Onchocerciasis," 1982.

42. Rougemont, "Ivermectin for Onchocerciasis," 1982.

43. Al Saah (former Merck scientist on Mectizan expert Committee), discussion with the author, January 29, 2015.

44. Vagelos, discussion, February 10, 2015.

45. Greene, Brown, and Taylor, "Use of Ivermectin," 312.

46. Yankum Dadzie (former OCP director), discussion with the author, July 16, 2016.

47. Greene, Brown, and Taylor, "Use of Ivermectin," 312–313.

48. Dadzie, discussion, July 16, 2016.

49. Greene, Brown, and Taylor, "Use of Ivermectin," 314.

50. Michel Pacqué (director of Sightsavers for Africa), discussion with the author, April 30, 2015.

51. Pacqué, discussion, April 30, 2015.

52. Pacqué, discussion, April 30, 2015.

53. Allen Foster (former chairman of the NGDO Coordination Group), discussion with the author, March 31, 2015.

CHAPTER 5: **Getting Mectizan to Africa, Concluding the OCP**

1. Charles Fettig (former director of Marketing for Cardiovascular Medications for Merck), discussion with the author, January 29, 2015.

2. Fettig, discussion, January 29, 2015.

3. Fettig, discussion, January 29, 2015.

4. Fettig, discussion, January 29, 2015.

5. Roy Vagelos (former CEO and chairman of the board, Merck and Co.), discussion with the author, January 15, 2015

6. Vagelos, discussion, January 15, 2015.

7. Vagelos, discussion, January 15, 2015.

8. William Foege (global health expert and former director for the Centers for Disease Control and Prevention), discussion with the author, November 20, 2014.

9. Vagelos, discussion, February 10, 2015.

10. "Merck Offers Free Distribution of New River Blindness Drug," *New York Times*, October 22, 1987.

11. Merck video of the press conference, MER-VID-VC 29–10 (4).

12. Bjorn Thylefors (former sirector of WHO's Office for the Prevention of Blindness and former ophthalmologist in the OCP EPI Unit, 1974), discussion with the author, March 25, 2015

13. Theodore M. Brown, Elizabeth Fee, and Victoria Stepanova, "Halfdan Mahler: Architect and Defender of the WHO 'Health for All by 2000' Declaration of 1978," *American Journal of Public Health* 106, no. 1 (2016): 1.

14. Fettig, discussion, January 29, 2015.

15. Vagelos, discussion, February 10, 2015.

16. Vagelos, discussion, January 15, 2015

17. Vagelos, discussion, January 15, 2015

18. Vagelos, discussion, January 15, 2015

19. Vagelos, discussion, January 15, 2015

20. Vagelos, discussion, January 15, 2015

21. Vagelos, discussion, February 10, 2015

22. Vagelos, discussion, February 10, 2015

23. Vagelos, discussion, January 15, 2015.

24. Vagelos, discussion, January 15, 2015.

25. Vagelos, discussion, January 15, 2015.

26. Vagelos, discussion, February 10, 2015.

27. Foege, discussion, November 20, 2014.

28. Foege, discussion, November 20, 2014.

29. Foege, discussion, November 20, 2014.

30. Foege, discussion, November 20, 2014.

31. William Foege, "10 Years of Mectizan," *Annals of Tropical Medicine and Parasitology* 92, no.1 (1998): s8.

32. Foege, discussion, November 20, 2014.

33. Foege, discussion, November 20, 2014.

34. De Sole et al., "Adverse Reactions After Large-Scale Treatment of Onchocerciasis with Ivermectin: Combined Results from Eight Community Trials," *Bulletin of the World Health Organization* 67, no. 6 (1989): 707.

35. J. Hans Remme (former manager, TDR Task Force for Onchocerciasis Operational Research), discussion with the author, October 1, 2018.

36. De Sole et al., "Adverse Reactions," 709.

37. De Sole et al., "Adverse Reactions," 711.

38. De Sole et al., "Adverse Reactions," 711.

39. Michael R. Reich, ed., *International Strategies for Tropical Disease Treatments: Experiences with Praziquantel* (Geneva: Action Programme on Essential Drugs, Division of Control of Tropical Diseases, 1998).

40. Azodoga Sékétéli (former APOC director), discussion with the author, October 3, 2015.

41. Onchocerciasis Control Program Phase IV, USAID doc., draft project paper 698-0485, 80

42. Allen Foster (former chairman of the Coordination Group), discussion with the author, March 31, 2015.

43. John Moores (philanthropist and software guru), discussion with the author, July 11, 2017.

44. Claudia Feldman, "A Forgotten Disease," *Houston Chronicle*, October 8, 2005, 5.

45. Allen Foster (former chair of Coordination Group), discussion with the author, March 31, 2015.

46. Foster, discussion, March 31, 2015.

47. Bob Pond, *Mass Distribution of Ivermectin: A Handbook for Community Treatment of Onchocerciasis* (Washington, DC: Africare, 1991), 38.

48. Michel Pacqué (director of Sightsavers for Africa), discussion with the author, April 30, 2015.

49. Pacqué, discussion, April 30, 2015.

50. Sékétéli, discussion, October 3, 2015.

51. Yankum Dadzie (former OCP director), discussion with the author, October 5, 2015.

52. Boakye Boatin, email to author, January 1, 2017.

53. Ebrahim Samba, "Compte Rendu de la Visite de Travail et de Sensibilisation du Dr. Ebrahim Samba, Directeur du Programme O.C.P., Dans le Cadre des Activities de Devolution de L'Aire Initiale du Programme au Mali" (internal document, July 16, 1992).

54. Sékétéli, discussion, October 3, 2015

55. Pacqué, discussion, April 30, 2015.

56. Pacqué, discussion, April 30, 2015.

57. Stefanie E. O. Meredith, Catherine Cross, and Uche V. Amazigo, "Empowering Communities in Combating River Blindness and the Role of NGOs: Case Studies from Cameroon, Mali, Nigeria, and Uganda," *Health Research Policy Systems* 10, no. 16 (2012): 6.

58. Meredith, Cross, and Amazigo, "Empowering Communities," 6.

59. Pacqué, discussion, April 30, 2015.

60. Pacqué, discussion, April 30, 2015.

61. Catherine Cross, email to author, February 4, 2017.

62. Pacqué, discussion, April 30, 2015.

63. Dadzie, discussion, October 5, 2016.

64. Ralph Henderson (WHO assistant director-general), discussion with the author, June 29, 2017.

65. "Community Directed Treatment with Ivermectin: Report of a Multi-Country Study," supra note 14, 79.

66. "Community Directed Treatment with Ivermectin," supra note 14, at 79.

67. Jan H. F. Remme, "Research for Control: The Onchocerciasis Experience," *Tropical Medicine and International Health* 9, no. 2 (2004): 253.

68. "Community Directed Treatment with Ivermectin," supra note 14, at 79.

69. "Community Directed Treatment with Ivermectin," supra note 14, at 80.

70. Remme, discussion, October 1, 2018.

71. Foege, discussion, November 20, 2014.

72. J. Remme, R. H. A. Baker, G. DeSole, K. Y. Dadzie, J. F. Walsh, M. A. Adams, E. S. Alley, and H. S. K. Avissey, "A Community Trial of Ivermectin in the Onchocerciasis Focus of asubende, Ghana.I. Effect on the Microfilarial Reservoir and the Transmission of *Onchocerca volvulus,*" *Tropical Medicine and Parasitology* 40 (1989): 367.

73. Remme, discussion, October 1, 2018.

74. Remme, discussion, October 1, 2018.

75. "Community-Directed Treatment of Lymphatic Filariasis in Africa: Report of a Multi-Centre Study in Ghana and Kenya," TDR/IDE/RP/CDTI/00.2 (2000), 1–2.

76. Meredith, Cross, and Amazigo, "Empowering Communities," 3.

77. Meredith, Cross, and Amazigo, "Empowering Communities," 3.

78. Onchocerciasis Fund Agreement, February 25, 1992, United Kingdom of Great Britain HMSO and the Secretary of State for Foreign and Commonwealth Affairs 1997, Gr. Brit. T. S. no. 35, 3.

79. Onchocerciasis Control Program, "25 Years of OCP" (Government Document, Ouagadougou, Burkina Faso, 1999), 20.

80. Koroma et al., "Impact of Three Rounds of Mass Drug Administration on Lymphatic Filariasis in Areas Previously Treated for Onchocerciasis in Sierra Leone," *PLoS Neglected Tropical Diseases* 7, no. 6 (2013): 6.

81. Koroma et al., "Impact of Three Rounds," 1.

82. Koroma et al., "Impact of Three Rounds," 7.

83. Onchocerciasis Fund Agreement, supra note 64, 1992, 4–5.

84. World Health Organization (WHO) Joint Programme Committee of the Onchocerciasis Control Programme, *Onchocerciasis Control Programme in West Africa*, sixteenth sess., annex 5, agenda item 4, 34 (1995).

85. WHO Joint Programme Committee, supra note 73, agenda item 11, 17.

86. Dadzie, discussion, October 6, 2015.

87. Boakye Boatin, e-mail to author, June 26, 2019.

88. Gro Harlem Brundtland, "Onchocerciasis Control Programme: Closure Ceremony" (speech, Ouagadougou, Burkina Faso, December 5, 2002).

89. Brundtland, "Closure Ceremony," December 5, 2002.

90. Brundtland, "Closure Ceremony," December 5, 2002.

91. Brundtland, "Closure Ceremony," December 5, 2002.

92. Brundtland, "Closure Ceremony," December 5, 2002.

93. Brundtland, "Closure Ceremony," December 5, 2002.

CHAPTER 6: **A Closer Look at Socioeconomic Development**

1. "Onchocerciasis Control in the Volta River Basin Area: Report of the Preparatory Assistance Mission to the Governments of: Dahomey, Ghana, Ivory Coast, Mali, Niger, Togo, Upper Volta," UNDP/FAO/IBRD/WHO internal doc. 73.1, 1973.

2. Jim Kelly et al., "Impact Review of the Onchocerciasis Program: Ouagadougou, August 1985," US Agency for International Development Evaluation Report no. 63 (Washington DC, 1986),

3. Della E. McMillan et al., "Settlement and Development in the River Blindness Control Zone," in *Series on River Blindness Control in West Africa*, World Bank Technical Paper no. 192, December 1992, xiv–xv.

4. John Elder and Laura Cooley, "Sustainable Settlement and Development of the Onchocerciasis Control Program Area, Proceedings of a Ministerial Meeting," World Bank Technical Paper no. 310 (1995), 128.

5. Elder and Cooley, *Sustainable Settlement*, 133.

6. Katherine Marshall, *Back-to-Office Report: Ministerial Meeting on Sustainable Settlement and Development of the Onchocerciasis (Riverblindness) Controlled Areas*, World Bank Archives, Paris (1994), para. 2.

7. Della E. McMillan, *Sahel Visions: Planned Settlement and River Blindness Control in Burkina Faso* (Tucson: University of Arizona Press, 1995).

8. J. Remme et al., "The Predicted and Observed Decline in Onchocerciasis Infection during 14 Years of Successful Control of *Simulium* spp. in West Africa," *Bulletin of the World Health Organization* 3, no. 68 (1990): 331–39.

9. McMillan, *Sahel Visions*, 15.

10. McMillan, *Sahel Visions*, 163.

11. McMillan, *Sahel Visions*, 166.

12. Elder and Cooley, *Sustainable Settlement*, 46.

13. Elder and Cooley, *Sustainable Settlement*, 44.

14. Elder and Cooley, *Sustainable Settlement*, 44.

15. Elder and Cooley, *Sustainable Settlement*, 44.

16. Elder and Cooley, *Sustainable Settlement*, 46.

17. McMillan, *Sahel Visions*, 16.

18. McMillan, Della E., Jean-Baptiste Nana, and Kimseyinga Savadogo. "Settlement and Development in the River Blindness Control Zone Case Study Burkina Faso." In *Series on River Blindness Control in West Africa*, World Bank Technical Paper no. 200, June 1993.

19. McMillan et al., "Settlement and Development," 1993, 8.

20. Committee for International Cooperation in National Research in Demography and Food and Agriculture Organization of the United Nations (CICRED/FAO), *Population Dynamics in Rural Areas Freed from Onchocerciasis in Western Africa* (1999), 19.

21. CICRED/FAO, *Population Dynamics in Rural Areas*, 53.

22. CICRED/FAO, *Population Dynamics in Rural Areas*, 53.

23. J. H. F. Remme, and J. B. Zongo, "Demographic Aspects of the Epidemiology and Control of Onchocerciasis in West Africa," in *Demography and Vector-Borne Diseases*, ed. Michael W. Service (Boca Raton, FL: CRC Press, 1989), 32.

24. CICRED/FAO, *Population Dynamics in Rural Areas*, 58.

25. Remme and Zongo, "Demographic Aspects," 32.

26. Remme and Zongo, "Demographic Aspects," 32.

27. McMillan et al., "Settlement and Development," 1993.

28. United States Department of Agriculture, "Index Mundi, Burkina Faso Cotton Production and Exports by Year, 1965–2018," https://www.indexmundi.com/agriculture/?country=bf&commodity=cotton&graph=production.

29. McMillan et al., "Settlement and Development," 1992, 26.

30. Jeffrey Vitale, *Economic Importance of Cotton in Burkina Faso*, Food and Agriculture Organization of the United Nations (Rome: 2018), 29.

31. Vitale, *Economic Importance*, 2–3.

32. Vitale, *Economic Importance*, 2.

33. CICRED/FAO, *Population Dynamics in Rural Areas*, 96.

34. CICRED/FAO, *Population Dynamics in Rural Areas*, 96.

35. CICRED/FAO, *Population Dynamics in Rural Areas*, 103.

36. Harounan Kazianga et al., "Disease Control, Demographic Change and Institutional Development in Africa," *ELSVIER, Journal of Development Economics* (2014): 5.

37. Kazianga, "Disease Control," 13.

38. Kazianga, "Disease Control," 13.

39. CICRED/FAO, *Population Dynamics in Rural Areas*, 55–57.

40. CICRED/FAO, *Population Dynamics in Rural Areas*, 57.

41. CICRED/FAO, *Population Dynamics in Rural Areas*, 37.

42. CICRED/FAO, *Population Dynamics in Rural Areas*, 40.

43. CICRED/FAO, *Population Dynamics in Rural Areas*, 36.

44. "Innovation for Sustainable Agricultural Growth in Togo," *Forum for Agricultural Research in Africa (FARA) and Center for Development Research*, University of Bonn (ZEF), October 2017, 27.

45. CICRED/FAO, *Population Dynamics in Rural Areas*, 51.

46. McMillan, "Settlement and Development," 26.

47. CICRED/FAO, *Population Dynamics in Rural Areas*, 67.

48. Census data from Institut National de la Statistique, Guinea, for 1983 and 1996.

49. CICRED/FAO, *Population Dynamics in Rural Areas*, 67.

50. Remme, "Demographic Aspects," 23.

51. Nicholas Prescott and André Prost, "Cost-Effectiveness of Blindness Prevention by the Onchocerciasis Control Program in Upper Volta," PHN Technical Note, The World Bank, Washington DC, November 1983.

52. B. Benton and E. D. Skinner, "Cost-Benefits of Onchocerciasis Control," *Acta Leiden* 59, no. 1–2 (1990).

53. Benton and Skinner, "Cost-Benefits of Onchocerciasis Control."

54. Aehyung Kim and Bruce Benton, "Cost-Benefit Analysis of the Onchocerciasis Control Program (OCP)," World Bank Technical Paper no. 282, 1995, 4.

55. Kim and Benton, "Cost-Benefit Analysis."

56. Kim and Benton, "Cost-Benefit Analysis," 7.

57. Kim and Benton, "Cost-Benefit Analysis," 7.

58. Kim and Benton, "Cost-Benefit Analysis," 8.
59. Benton and Skinner, "Cost-Benefits of Onchocerciasis Control," table 2.
60. Kim and Benton, "Cost-Benefit Analysis," 10.
61. Kim and Benton, "Cost-Benefit Analysis," 12.
62. Kim and Benton, "Cost-Benefit Analysis," 12.
63. Kim and Benton, "Cost-Benefit Analysis," 15.
64. Kim and Benton, "Cost-Benefit Analysis," 15.

CHAPTER 7: **Widening the Effort to All of Africa**

1. World Health Organization Expert Committee on Onchocerciasis, "Technical Report Series 852" (Geneva: 1995), 28.
2. Adrian Hopkins (medical director of the NGDO, Christoffel-Blindenmission in the Democratic Republic of the Congo), discussion with author, April 7, 2015.
3. World Health Organization (WHO), "Report of the Meeting on Strategies for Ivermectin Distribution through Primary Health Care Systems" (Geneva: April 1991), 17.
4. H. R. Taylor, B. O. Duke, and B. Munoz, "The Selection of Communities for Treatment of Onchocerciasis with Ivermectin," *Tropical Medicine and Parasitology* 43 (1992): 267.
5. P. Ngoumou and J. F. Walsh, "A Manual for Rapid Epidemiological Mapping of Onchocerciasis" (Geneva: World Health Organization, 1993), 2.
6. J. H. F. Remme, "Research for Control: The Onchocerciasis Experience," *Tropical Medicine and International Health* 9, no. 2 (2004): 249.
7. African Programme for Onchocerciasis Control (APOC), *Charting the Lion's Stare: The Story of River Blindness Mapping in Africa* (Burkina Faso: World Health Organization, 2009) , 25.
8. APOC, *Charting the Lion's Stare*, 25.
9. APOC, *Charting the Lion's Stare*, 25.
10. Mounkaila Noma et al., "The Geographic Distribution of Onchocerciasis in the 20 Participating Countries of the African Programme for Onchocerciasis Control: (1) Priority Areas for Ivermectin Treatment," *Parasites & Vectors* 7, no. 325 (2014): 2.
11. APOC, *Charting the Lion's Stare*, 11.
12. Noma et al., "Geographic Distribution of Onchocerciasis," 7.
13. Noma et al., "Geographic Distribution of Onchocerciasis," 5.
14. Noma et al., "Geographic Distribution of Onchocerciasis," 11.
15. Noma et al., "Geographic Distribution of Onchocerciasis," 11.
16. Noma et al., "Geographic Distribution of Onchocerciasis," 11.
17. Noma et al., "Geographic Distribution of Onchocerciasis," 11.
18. Noma et al., "Geographic Distribution of Onchocerciasis," 11.
19. Mounkaila Noma, email to author, August 10, 2018.
20. L. E. Coffeng et al., "African Programme for Onchocerciasis Control 1995–2015: Model-Estimated Health Impact and Cost," *PLoS Negl Trop Dis* 7, no. 1 (2013): 3.
21. M. E. Murdoch et al., "Onchocerciasis: The Clinical and Epidemiological Burden of Skin Disease in Africa," *Annals of Tropical Medicine & Parasitology* 96, no. 3 (2002): 283.
22. Murdoch et al., "Burden of Skin Disease," 283.

23. Murdoch et al., "Burden of Skin Disease," 283.

24. Remme, "Research for Control," 247.

25. Murdoch et al., "Burden of Skin Disease," 283.

26. World Bank Group (WBG), "Defeating Riverblindness: Success in Scaling Up and Lessons Learned," in *Global Learning Process on Scaling Up Poverty Reduction Conference*, Shanghai, May 22, 2004, 8 (Washington, DC: World Bank, 2004)

27. World Health Organization/African Programme for Onchocerciasis Control (WHO/APOC), *1995–2010: 15 Years of Working with Communities to Eliminate River Blindness* (internal document, 2011), 8; Amazigo et al., "Ivermectin Improves the Skin Condition and Self-Esteem of Females with Onchocerciasis," *Animals of Tropical Medicine & Parasitology* 98, no. 5 (2004): 533–37.

28. African Programme for Onchocerciasis Control (APOC). "Memorandum for the African Programme for Onchocerciasis Control (APOC): Phase I (1996–2001), Part II." April 17, 1996.

29. James D. Wolfensohn, *Voice for the World's Poor: Selected Speeches and Writings of World Bank President James D. Wolfensohn, 1995–2005* (Washington, DC: World Bank Publications, 2005), 35.

30. Wolfensohn, *Voice for the World's Poor*, 37–39.

31. Wolfensohn, *Voice for the World's Poor*, 32.

32. Wolfensohn, *Voice for the World's Poor*, 30.

33. APOC Launch Conference, World Bank Archives, tape 2, December 5, 1995.

34. APOC Launch, tape 2, 1995.

35. APOC Launch, tape 2, 1995.

36. APOC Launch, tape 2, 1995.

37. APOC Launch, tape 2, 1995.

38. APOC Launch, tape 2, 1995.

39. APOC Launch, tape 2, 1995.

40. APOC Launch, tape 2, 1995.

41. APOC Launch, tape 2, 1995.

42. APOC Launch, tape 2, 1995.

43. APOC Launch, tape 2, 1995.

44. M. Sauerbrey, "The Onchocerciasis Elimination Program for the Americas (OEPA)," *Ann Trop Med Parasitol* 102, suppl. 1 (2008): 25–29.

45. J. Blanks et al., "The Onchocerciasis Elimination Program for the Americas: A History of the Partnership," *Pan Am J Public Health* 3, no. 6 (1998): 371.

46. Y. Dadzie et al., "Is Onchocerciasis Elimination in Africa Feasible by 2025," *Infectious Diseases of Poverty* (July 2018): 8; F. O. Richards et al., "The Positive Influence the Onchocerciasis Elimination Program for the Americas Has Had on Africa Programs." *Infect Dis Poverty* 8, no. 52 (2019); E. Cupp et al., "Elimination of Onchocerciasis in Africa by 2025: The Need for a Broad Perspective, *Infect Dis Poverty* 8, no. 50 (2019).

47. Committee for Sponsoring Agencies (CSA), "African Programme for Onchocerciasis Control: Programme Document," JAF/CSA internal document (December 1996): 34

48. CSA, "African Programme for Onchocerciasis Control," 10.

49. African Programme for Onchocerciasis Control—Tenth Session of the Joint Action Forum (APOC), *Final Communique December 7–9, 2004*, Kinshasa, Democratic Republic of Congo, 5.

50. World Health Organization African Programme for Onchocerciasis Control Joint Action Forum (WHO/APOC), "Year 2005 Progress Report: 1st September 2004–31 August 2005," JAF internal doc. 11.5 (September 2005): 7

51. WHO/APOC, "Year 2005 Progress Report," 11.

52. WHO/APOC, "Year 2005 Progress Report," 7.

53. World Bank Group (WBG), "Defeating Riverblindness," 20.

54. Sékétéli, discussion, October 3, 2015.

55. Sékétéli, discussion, October 3, 2015.

56. Sékétéli, discussion, October 3, 2015.

57. Sékétéli, discussion, October 3, 2015.

58. Sékétéli, discussion, October 3, 2015.

59. WHO/APOC, "Year 2005 Progress Report," 7.

60. WHO/APOC, "Year 2005 Progress Report," 7.

61. WHO/APOC, "Year 2005 Progress Report," 7.

62. WHO/APOC, "Year 2005 Progress Report," 7.

63. Michel Boussinesq (ORSTOM researcher) email to author, November 11, 2018.

64. "WHO Drug Information," *World Health Organization* 5, no. 3 (1991).

65. US Food and Drug Administration, "What Is a Serious Adverse Event?" https://www.fda.gov/safety/reporting-serious-problems-fda/what-serious-adverse-event.

66. Global Health-Division of Parasitic Diseases, "Parasites—Loiasis—Disease," Centers for Disease Control and Prevention, January 20, 2015. https://www.cdc.gov/parasites/loiasis/disease.html.

67. Boussinesq, email, November 11, 2018.

68. Mectizan Donation Program, "Central Nervous System (CNS) Complications of Loiasis and Adverse CNS Events Following Treatment: Report of an Invited Consultation, 2–3 October 1995," (Atlanta: MDP, 1996), 14, table 2.

69. M. Ducorps et al., "Secondary Effects of the Treatment Of Hypermicrofilaremic Loiasis Using Ivermectin," *Bulletin de la Société de Pathologie Exotique* 88 (1995): 105–12.

70. Ducorps et al., "Secondary Effects," 105. Author's translation.

71. Michael Heisler (Mectizan Donation Program director), discussion with author, January 2, 2019.

72. Mectizan Donation Program, "CNS Complications of Loiasis," 2.

73. Mectizan Donation Program, "CNS Complications of Loiasis," 3.

74. Mectizan Donation Program, "CNS Complications of Loiasis," 4.

75. Mectizan Donation Program, "CNS Complications of Loiasis," 6.

76. Mectizan Donation Program, "CNS Complications of Loiasis," 7.

77. Mectizan Donation Program, "CNS Complications of Loiasis," 8.

78. Mectizan Donation Program, "CNS Complications of Loiasis," 8.

79. Boussinesq, email, November 11, 2018.

80. Jacques Gardon et al., "Serious Reactions after Mass Treatment of Onchocerciasis with Ivermectin in an Area Endemic for *Loa loa* Infection," *The Lancet* 350, no. 9070 (1997): 18.

81. Gardon et al., "Serious Reactions after Mass Treatment," 21.

82. Gardon et al., "Serious Reactions after Mass Treatment," 21.

83. Gardon et al., "Serious Reactions after Mass Treatment," 22.

84. Boussinesq, email, November 11, 2018.

85. D. Addiss, minutes of the MDP-sponsored meeting on "Central Nervous Disorders following treatment with Mectizan® in areas co-endemic for onchocerciasis and loiasis," France: University of Tours, October 7–8, 1999.

86. Brian O. L. Duke, "Overview: Report of a Scientific Working Group on Serious Adverse Events Following Mectizan® Treatment of Onchocerciasis in *Loa loa* Endemic Areas." *Filarial Journal* 2, suppl. 1 (October 2003).

87. African Programme for Onchocerciasis Control—Fifth Session of the Joint Action Forum (APOC/JAF 5), *Report December 8–10, 1999* (The Hague), 6.

88. Mectizan Expert Committee (MEC), "Recommendations for the Treatment of Onchocerciasis with Mectizan in Areas Co-Endemic for Onchocerciasis and Loiasis," (Atlanta: MEC, 2000): 1.

89. MEC, "Recommendations for the Treatment," 1–2.

90. MEC, "Recommendations for the Treatment," 2–3.

91. MEC, "Recommendations for the Treatment," 3.

92. Mectizan Program notes, no. 26, Spring 2001, 2.

93. Nana A. Y. Twum-Danso, "*Loa-loa* Encephalopathy Temporally Related to Ivermectin Administration Reported from Onchocerciasis Mass Treatment Programs from 1989 to 2001: Implications for the Future," *Filaria Journal* 2 (2003): 1.

94. Global Health-Division of Parasitic Diseases, "Parasites—Loiasis—Disease."

95. WHO/APOC, "Year 2005 Progress Report," supra note 70, 15.

96. Duke, "Report of a Scientific Working Group."

97. Nancy J. Haselow et al., "Programmatic and Communication Issues in Relation to Serious Adverse Events Following Ivermectin Treatment in areas Co-Endemic for Onchocerciasis and Loiasis," *Filarial Journal* 2, suppl. 1 (2003): 2.

98. Haselow et al., "Programmatic and Communication Issues," 2.

99. Boussinesq, email, December 12, 2018.

100. Michel Boussinesq et al., "Relationships between the Prevalence and Intensity of *Loa Loa* Infection in the Central Province of Cameroon," *Annals of Tropical Medicine & Parasitology* 95, no. 5 (2001): 495.

101. Innocent Takougang et al., "Rapid Assessment Method for Prevalence and Intensity of *Loa-loa* Infection," *Bulletin of the World Health Organization* 80, no. 11 (2002).

102. H. G. Zouré, S. Wanji, M. Noma, U. V. Amazigo, P. J. Diggle, A. H. Tekle, and J. H. Remme, "The Geographic Distribution of *Loa loa* in Africa: Results of Large-Scale Implementation of the Rapid Assessment Procedure for Loiasis (RAPLOA)," *PLOS Neglected Tropical Diseases* 5, no. 6 (2011): 3.

103. Zouré et al., "The Geographic Distribution of *Loa loa*," 3.

104. The Mectizan Expert Committee and The Technical Consultative Committee [MEC/TCC], "Recommendations for the Treatment of Onchocerciasis with Mectizan in Areas Co-Endemic for Onchocerciasis and Loiasis" (2004).

105. Zouré et al., "The Geographic Distribution of *Loa loa*," 1.

106. Zouré et al., "The Geographic Distribution of *Loa loa*," 7.

107. Zouré et al., "The Geographic Distribution of *Loa loa*," 7.

108. Afework Hailemariam Tekle et al., "Integrated Rapid Mapping of Onchocerciasis and Loiasis in the Democratic Republic of Congo: Impact on Control Strategies," *Acta Tropica* 120, suppl. 1 (2011): S88.

109. Tekle, "Integrated Rapid Mapping," S89.

110. Boussinesq, email, October 17, 2019

111. Duke, "Report of a Scientific Working Group."

112. Duke, "Report of a Scientific Working Group," 10.

113. Brett Israel, "A Cellphone-Based Microscope for Treating River Blindness," *Berkeley News*, November 9, 2017.

114. Joseph Kamgno et al., "A Test-and-Not-Treat Strategy for Onchocerciasis in *Loa loa*–Endemic Areas," *New England Journal of Medicine* 10 (2017): 1.

115. Boussinesq et al., "Relationships between the Prevalence and Intensity of *Loa loa*," 498.

116. Kamgno et al., "A Test-and-Not-Treat Strategy," 1.

117. Maria Rebollo Polo (Team Leader for the NTD Elimination Effort), discussion with author, December 19, 2018.

118. Kamgno et al., "A Test-and-Not-Treat Strategy," 1.

119. World Health Organization, "Weekly Epidemiological Record, no. 91/43" (2016): 507.

120. David Addiss (director of the Focus Area for Compassion and Ethics), discussion with author, December 4, 2018.

121. Bill Foege (global health expert and former director for the Centers for Disease Control and Prevention), discussion with author, November 20, 2014.

122. Addiss, discussion, December 14, 2018.

123. Merck, "Corporate Responsibility Report 2017/2018," (2018).

124. E. A. Ottesen, B. O. Duke, M. Karam, and K. Behbehani, "Strategies and Tools for the Control/Elimination of Lymphatic Filariasis," *Bulletin of the World Health Organization* 75, no. 6 (1997): 491–503.

125. Malcolm Dean, *Lymphatic Filariasis: The Quest to Eliminate a 4000-Year-Old Disease* (London: Hollis, 2001), 15–16.

126. World Health Organization (WHO), *Bulletin of the World Health Organization* 85, no. 6 (June 2007).

127. WHO, *Bulletin 85*, 421.

128. United States Agency International Development, "Lymphatic Filariasis," last modified 2018. https://www.neglecteddiseases.gov/usaid-target-diseases/lymphatic-filariasis.

129. "CDC—Lymphatic Filariasis—General Information—Frequently Asked Questions." Centers for Disease Control and Prevention (2018), 2, https://www.cdc.gov/parasites/lymphaticfilariasis/gen_info/faqs.html.

130. "CDC Frequently Asked Questions," 3; Shona Wynd, Wayne D. Melrose, David N. Durrheim, Jaime Carron, and Margaret Gyapong, "Understanding the Community Impact of Lymphatic Filariasis: A Review of the Sociocultural Literature," *Bulletin of the World Health Organization* 85, no. 6 (2007): 422–423.

131. E. A. Ottesen et al., "The Role of Albendazole in Programmes to Eliminate Lymphatic Filariasis," *Parasitology Today* 15, no. 9 (1999): 382–386.

132. Bjorn Thylefors (MDP director in 2001), discussion with author, March 25, 2015.

133. "Lymphatic Filariasis, Treatment and Prevention," World Health Organization, https://www.who.int/lymphatic_filariasis/epidemiology/treatment_prevention/en/.

134. Thylefors, discussion, March 25, 2015.

135. Eric Ottesen (senior advisor, Neglected Tropical Diseases Support Center, Task Force for Global Health), email to author, March 10, 2019.

136. Thylefors, discussion, March 25, 2015.

137. Andy Wright (former vice president, Global Health Programmes, GlaxoSmith-Kline), discussion with author, April 7, 2015.

138. Wright, discussion, April 7, 2015.

139. Wright, discussion, April 7, 2015.

140. Wright, discussion, April 7, 2015.

141. Hans Remme (former manager, TDR Task Force for Onchocerciasis Operational Research), discussion with author, October 1, 2018.

142. World Health Organization (WHO), "Attack Poverty the Global Alliance to Eliminate Lymphatic Filariasis Proceedings of the First Meeting," Department of Communicable Diseases Control, Prevention and Eradication (2000), 4.

143. APOC/JAF 5, *Report*, 26.

144. APOC/JAF 5, *Report*, 32.

145. Dean, *Lymphatic Filariasis*, 18.

146. APOC/JAF 5, *Report*, 32.

147. APOC/JAF 5, *Report*, 1.

148. APOC/JAF 5, *Report*, 1.

149. APOC/JAF 5, *Report*, 32.

150. APOC/JAF 5, *Report*, 28–29.

151. APOC/JAF 5, *Report*, 33.

152. APOC/JAF 5, *Report*, 33.

153. "Report of the APOC Committee of Sponsoring [Agencies, 87th [ad hoc] session," Ouagadougou (March 6–7, 2000), annex 1.

154. African Programme for Onchocerciasis Control—Sixth Session of the Joint Action Forum (APOC/JAF 6), *Progress Report December 11–13, 2001*, Yaoundé, Cameroon.

155. David Heymann (WHO executive director for communicable diseases) email to author, March 17, 2000.

156. WHO, "Attack Poverty," 16.

157. World Health Organization, "Weekly Epidemiological Record, no. 90/38," September 2015, 493. http://www.who.int/wer.

158. APOC/JAF 6, *Progress Report*, 29.

159. APOC/JAF 6, *Progress Report*, 29.

160. Yankum Dadzie (NGDO Coordinator and Director of OCP), discussion with author, October 6, 2015.

161. World Health Organization Global Programme to Eliminate Lymphatic Filariasis (WHO/GPELF), "Progress Report 2000–2009 and Strategic Plan 2010–2020" (2010), 50.

162. World Health Organization, "WHO Annual Report on Lymphatic Filariasis" (2003), 17.

163. WHO/GPELF, "Progress Report," 11.

164. WHO/GPELF, "Progress Report," 49.

165. World Health Organization Regional Committee for Africa, "Progress Report on the Implementation of the Resolution on Neglected Tropical Diseases" (May 2017), 1.

166. John Gyapong and Boakye Boatin, *Neglected Tropical Diseases—Sub-Saharan Africa* (New York: Springer, 2016), 2.

167. David Molyneux, email to author, September 13, 2019.

CHAPTER 8: **Deepening and Widening the Objective**

1. Ok Pannenborg (former World Bank Chief Health Advisor and Chief Health Scientist), discussion with author, March 6, 2019.

2. Bernhard Liese (former World Bank Principal Tropical Disease Specialist), discussion with author, March 3, 2019.

3. Liese, discussion, March 3, 2019; Laurent Yameogo (former Coordinator, APOC), discussion with author, March 11, 2019.

4. Liese, discussion, March 4, 2019.

5. Ousmane Bangoura, email to author, June 13, 2005.

6. African Programme for Onchocerciasis Control—Eleventh Session of the Joint Action Forum (APOC/JAC 11), *Final Communique December 6–9, 2005*, Paris, France.

7. APOC/JAF 11, *Final Communiqué*, 2.

8. World Health Organization African Programme for Onchocerciasis Control (WHO/APOC), "Final Evaluation Report," JAF doc. 21.6 (October 2015), 58.

9. Donald Bundy (former APOC Coordinator, World Bank), discussion with author, June 3, 2015.

10. International Bank for Reconstruction and Development, "Agreement Providing for the Amendment and Restatement of the Memorandum for the African Programme for Onchocerciasis Control for Phase II and for the Phrasing-Out Period," December 5, 2007, 6.

11. International Bank for Reconstruction and Development, "Memorandum for the African Programme for Onchocerciasis for Phase II," 12.

12. WHO/APOC, "Final Evaluation Report," 43

13. Kenneth Gustavsen (former Manager, Global Health Partnerships, Merck & Co., Inc.), discussion with author, March 21, 2019.

14. African Programme for Onchocerciasis Control—Thirteenth Session of the Joint Action Forum (APOC/JAF 13), *Final Communique December 4–7, 2007*, Brussels, Belgium, 8.

15. Uche Amazigo (former director, APOC), discussion with author, November 4, 2015.

16. Amazigo, discussion, January 20, 2016.

17. World Bank, APOC II Trust Fund Programme, "Forecasted Statement of Cash Receipts, Disbursements, and Fund Balance," (January 1, 2002–December 31, 2015).

18. African Programme for Onchocerciasis Control—Fourteenth Session of the Joint Action Forum (APOC/JAF 14), *Final Communique December 8–11, 2008*, Kampala, Uganda.

19. World Health Organization (WHO), "Weekly Epidemiological Record, no. 49/50," December 2012, 497. http://www.who.int/wer.

20. WHO, "Weekly Epidemiological Record, no. 49/50," 497.

21. World Health Organization African Programme for Onchocerciasis Control, "Vector Elimination, Itwara, Uganda," https://www.who.int/apoc/vector/itwara/en/.

22. R. Garms et al., "The Elimination of the Vector *Simulium neavei* from the Itwara Onchocerciasis Focus in Uganda by Ground Larviciding," *Acta Trop.* 111, no. 3 (September 2009): 203–10.

23. Garms et al., "Elimination of the Vector *Simulium neavei*," 203.

24. Garms et al., "Elimination of the Vector *Simulium neavei*," 203.

25. Garms et al., "Elimination of the Vector *Simulium neavei*," 203.

26. T. L. Lakwo et al., "Transmission of *Loa loa* and Prospects for the Elimination of its Vector, the Blackfly *Simulium neavei* in the Mpamba-Nkusi Focus in Western Uganda," *Med Vet Entomol.* 20, no. 1 (March 2006): 93–101.

27. T. L. Lakwo et al., "Successful Interruption of the Transmission of Onchocerciasis volvulus in Mpamba-Nkusi Focus, Kibaale District, Mid-Western Uganda," *East African Medical Journal* 92 (August 2015): 401–7.

28. Lakwo et al., "Successful Interruption," 401.

29. World Health Organization African Programme for Onchocerciasis Control (WHO/APOC), "Vector Elimination Tukuyu, United Republic of Tanzania," https://www.who.int/apoc/vector/tukuyu/en/.

30. S. Traore et al., "The Elimination of the Onchocerciasis Vector from the Island of Bioko as a Result of Larviciding by the WHO African Programme for Onchocerciasis Control," *Acta Trop.* 111, no. 3 (September 2009): 211–208.

31. Z. Herrador et al., "Interruption of Onchocerciasis Transmission in Bioko Island: Accelerating the Movement from Control to Elimination in Equatorial Guinea," *PLoS Neglected Tropical Diseases* 12, no. 5 (May 2018): 1.

32. World Health Organization African Programme for Onchocerciasis Control (WHO/APOC), "Report of the External Evaluation," October 2005.5.

33. Laurent Yaméogo (former Coordinator, APOC), discussion with author, March 15, 2019.

34. Yaméogo, discussion, March 15, 2019.

35. World Health Organization African Programme for Onchocerciasis Control—Committee of Sponsoring Agencies (WHO/APOC), "A Strategic Overview of the Future of Onchocerciasis Control in Africa," September 2006, iv.

36. World Health Organization African Programme for Onchocerciasis Control (WHO/APOC), "Yaoundé Declaration on Onchocerciasis Control in Africa," September 2006, 2.

37. APOC/JAF 13, *Final Communiqué*, 9.

38. APOC/JAF 11, *Final Communiqué*, 9.

39. WHO/APOC, "Strategic Overview," 18.

40. WHO/APOC, "Strategic Overview," 20.

41. African Programme for Onchocerciasis Control—Twelfth Session of the Joint Action Forum (APOC/JAF 12), *Final Communique December 5–8, 2006*, Dar-es-Salaam, Tanzania.

42. International Bank for Reconstruction and Development, "Memorandum for the African Programme for Onchocerciasis for Phase II."

43. WHO/APOC, "Strategic Overview," 18–21.

44. African Programme for Onchocerciasis Control—Seventeenth Session of the Joint Action Forum (APOC/JAF 17), *Final Communique December 12–14, 2011*, Kuwait City, Kuwait, 9.

45. World Health Organization Special Programme for Research and Training in Tropical Diseases (WHO/TDR), "Community Directed Interventions for Major Health Problems in Africa," 2008.

46. WHO/TDR, "Community Directed Interventions," 19.

47. WHO/TDR, "Community Directed Interventions," 5.

48. WHO/TDR, "Community Directed Interventions," 5.

49. WHO/TDR, "Community Directed Interventions," 56.

50. WHO/TDR, "Community Directed Interventions," 56.

51. WHO/TDR, "Community Directed Interventions," 6.

52. WHO/TDR, "Community Directed Interventions," 6.

53. WHO/TDR, "Community Directed Interventions," 7.

54. World Health Organization (WHO), "Report of the External Mid-Term Evaluation of the African Programme for Onchocerciasis Control," JAF doc. 16.8, October 2010, 11.

55. WHO, "Mid-Term Evaluation," 8.

56. WHO, Mid-Term Evaluation," 8.

57. L. Diawara et al., "Feasibility of Onchocerciasis Elimination with Ivermectin Treatment in Endemic Foci in Africa: First Evidence from Studies in Mali and Senegal," *PLoS Negl Trop Dis* 3, no. 7 (July 2009): e497.

58. M. O. Traoré et al., "Proof-of-Principle of Onchocerciasis Elimination with Ivermectin Treatment in Endemic Foci in Africa: Final Results of a Study in Mali and Senegal," *PLoS Negl Trop Dis* 6, no. 9: e1825 (September 2012): 1.

59. Traoré et al., "Proof-of-Principle," 1.

60. Traoré et al., "Proof-of-Principle," 2.

61. Traoré et al.,, "Proof-of-Principle," 11.

62. Yankum Dadzie et al., "Is Onchocerciasis Elimination in Africa Feasible by 2025?" *Infectious Diseases of Poverty* 7, no. 63 (July 2018): 8.

63. Dadzie et al., "Onchocerciasis Elimination," 9.

64. APOC/JAF 13, *Final Communiqué*, 8.

65. International Bank for Reconstruction and Development, "Memorandum for the African Programme for Onchocerciasis for Phase II," 10.

66. APOC/JAF 14, *Final Communiqué*, 2.

67. Traoré et al., "Proof-of-Principle," 13.

68. Traoré et al., "Proof-of-Principle," 13.

69. World Health Organization (WHO), "Informal Consultation on Elimination of Onchocerciasis Transmission with Current Tools in Africa" (February 2009): 7.

70. WHO, "Informal Consultation," 4.

71. African Programme for Onchocerciasis Control—Fifteenth Session of the Joint Action Forum (APOC/JAF 15), *Final Communique December 8–10, 2009*, Tunis, Tunisia, 4.

72. World Health Organization African Programme for Onchocerciasis Control (WHO/APOC), "Conceptual and Operational Framework of Onchocerciasis Elimination with Ivermectin Treatment," (September 2010): 12–14.

73. Dadzie, "Onchocerciasis Elimination," 8.

74. Dadzie, "Onchocerciasis Elimination," 8.

75. APOC/JAF 14, *Final Communiqué*, 4.

76. APOC/JAF 17, *Final Communiqué*, 4.

77. APOC/JAF 17, *Final Communiqué*, 4.

78. African Programme for Onchocerciasis Control—Eighteenth Session of the Joint Action Forum (APOC/JAF 18), *Final Communique December 11–13, 2012*, Bujumbura, Burundi, 4.

79. APOC/JAF 18, *Final Communiqué*, 6.

80. APOC/JAF 18, *Final Communiqué*, 6.

81. World Health Organization (WHO), "Accelerating Work to Overcome the Global Impact of Neglected Tropical Diseases: A Roadmap for Implementation" (2012): 3.

82. Uniting to Combat Neglected Tropical Diseases, "London Declaration on Neglected Tropical Diseases" (January 2012).

83. The Henry J. Kaiser Family Foundation, "The U.S. Government and Global Neglected Tropical Disease Efforts" (January 2019): 6.

84. United States Agency International Development, "USAID Neglected Tropical Disease Program 2016 Evaluation" (March 2018): xi, 97.

85. African Programme for Onchocerciasis Control—Sixteenth Session of the Joint Action Forum (APOC/JAF 16), *Final Communique December 7–9, 2010*, Abuja, Nigeria.

86. APOC/JAF 17, *Final Communiqué*, 1.

87. APOC/JAF 17, *Final Communiqué*, 2.

88. WHO, "Mid-Term Evaluation," 12.

89. APOC/JAF 17, *Final Communiqué*, 7.

90. APOC/JAF 17, *Final Communiqué*, 7.

91. APOC/JAF 17, *Final Communiqué*, 7.

92. African Programme for Onchocerciasis Control (APOC), "Concept Note Transforming APOC into a new regional entity for Oncho & LF elimination and support to other PC/NTD," JAF 19.7, (November 2013): 17.

93. World Health Organization African Programme for Onchocerciasis Control (WHO/APOC), "Programme for the Elimination of Neglected Diseases in Africa (PENDA)," JAF 19.8. (November 2013): 64.

94. WHO/APOC, "PENDA," 22.

95. WHO/APOC, "PENDA," 23.

96. WHO/APOC, "PENDA," 21–22.

97. WHO/APOC, "PENDA," 13–14.

98. WHO/APOC, "PENDA," 44.

99. Emily Wainwright (USAID) and Darin Evans (USAID), discussion with author, October 19, 2015.

100. African Programme for Onchocerciasis Control—Nineteenth Session of the Joint Action Forum (APOC/JAF 19), *Final Communique for December 11–13, 2013*, Brazzaville, Congo, 4

101. APOC/JAF 19, *Final Communique*, 5.

102. APOC/JAF 19, *Final* Communique, 6.

103. A. Beattie, and R. Johnson, African Programme for Onchocerciasis Control, "APOC Management Review Final Report," (July 2014): 9.

104. U.K. Department for International Development and U.S. Agency for International Development (DFID/USAID), "Joint Statement on Support for Onchocerciasis Elimination in Africa," (October 2014): 1.

105. DFID/USAID, "Joint Statement," 1.

106. DFID/USAID, "Joint Statement," 1.

107. DFID/USAID, "Joint Statement," 1.

108. Wainwright, discussion, October 19, 2015.

109. Evans, discussion, October 9, 2015.

110. Evans, discussion, October 19, 2015.

111. J. Hans Remme (former Manager, TDR Task Force for Onchocerciasis Operational Research), discussion with author, April 10, 2019.

112. Patrick Lammie (Task Force for Global Health), discussion with author, June 30, 2017.

113. FY14 Development Grant Facility (DGF), "A Consolidated Report on the World Bank's Grant Making Facilities for FY14," Annex 8.

114. Ok Pannenborg (former World Bank Chief Health Advisor & Chief Health Scientist), discussion with author, July 29, 2019.

115. Adrian Hopkins (Director of the Mectizan Donation Program), discussion with author, April 7, 2015.

116. Christian Bailly (former Oncho representative in the French Ministry of Cooperation), discussion with author, March 25, 2015.

117. Wainwright, discussion, October 19, 2015.

118. Wainwright, discussion, October 19, 2015.

119. Wainwright, discussion, October 19, 2015.

120. WHO/APOC, "Final Evaluation Report," 55.

121. World Health Organization (WHO), "The Expanded Special Project for Elimination of Neglected Tropical Diseases (ESPEN) 2017 Annual Report," (2017): 26.

122. WHO, "ESPEN 2017 Annual Report," 30.

123. WHO, "ESPEN 2017 Annual Report," 7.

124. World Health Organization (WHO), "WHO AFRO Launches New Project to Help African Countries Control and Eliminate Neglected Tropical Diseases," press release, Geneva (May 2016).

125. World Health Organization (WHO), "Weekly Epidemiological Record, no. 47," November 2018, 633, http://www.who.int/wer.

126. WHO, "Weekly Epidemiological Record, no. 47," 638.

127. WHO, "Weekly Epidemiological Record, no. 47," 638.

128. African Programme for Onchocerciasis Control—Twenty-First Session of the Joint Action Forum (APOC/JAF 21), *Progress Report December 15–16, 2015*, Kampala, Uganda.

129. A. Tekle et al., "Progress towards Onchocerciasis Elimination in the Participating Countries of the African Programme for Onchocerciasis Control: Epidemiological Evaluation Results," *Infectious Diseases of Poverty* 5, no. 66 (2016): 18.

130. Tekle et al., "Onchocerciasis Elimination," 18.

131. Tekle et al., "Onchocerciasis Elimination," 18.

132. Tekle et al., "Onchocerciasis Elimination," 18.

133. Tekle et al., "Onchocerciasis Elimination," 18.

134. Tekle et al., "Onchocerciasis Elimination," 22.

135. APOC/JAF 21, "Final Communiqué".

136. Tekle et al., "Onchocerciasis Elimination," 18.

137. Tekle et al., "Onchocerciasis Elimination," 18.

138. World Health Organization, "Weekly Epidemiological Record, no. 45," November 2017, 683. http://www.who.int/wer.

CHAPTER 9: **Learning from the Past, Looking to the Future**

1. Hans Remme (former manager, TDR Task Force for Onchocerciasis Operational Research), email to author, July 18, 2019.

2. Hans Remme, discussion with author, April 21, 2019.

3. African Programme for Onchocerciasis Control—Seventeenth Session of the Joint Action Forum (APOC/JAF 17), "Report of the CSA Advisory Group on Onchocerciasis Elimination," *Final Communique December 12–14, 2011*, Kuwait City, Kuwait.

4. APOC/JAF 17, "Report of the CSA," 4.

5. APOC/JAF 17, "Report of the CSA," 5.

6. Remme, discussion, April 10, 2019.

7. Remme, discussion, April 10, 2019.

8. Y. Dadzie et al., "Is Onchocerciasis Elimination in Africa Feasible By 2025," *Infectious Diseases of Poverty* 7, no. 63 (July 2018): 2.

9. Maria P. Rebollo et al., "Onchocerciasis: Shifting the Target from Control to Elimination Requires a New First Step—Elimination Mapping" (Oxford University Press: 2017).

10. World Health Organization, "Weekly Epidemiological Record, no. 47," November 2018, 635, http://www.who.int/wer.

11. W. David Hong, "A New Cure for River Blindness and Elephantiasis," *BioMedCentral* (January 2019): 1.

12. John Moores (philanthropist and software executive), discussion with author, July 16, 2018.

13. Moores, discussion, July 16, 2018.

14. Author's presentation to the World Bank Executive Directors, April 11, 2002; African Programme for Onchocerciasis Control—Nineteenth Session of the Joint Action Forum (APOC/JAF 19) *Final Communique for December 11–13, 2013*, Brazzaville, Congo, 9; $268 million is based on the last known World Bank report of total APOC receipts and pledges from donors. The World Bank official responsible for APOC at its closure, Andy Tembon, was unable to provide the total amount of transfers from the Oncho Trust Fund to APOC, which was requested by the author in emails, Benton to Tembon, dated March 9, 2019, March 27, 2019, June 13, 2019, June 17, 2019, and June 18, 2019.

15. Brenda Colatrella (Associate Vice President for Corporate Responsibility, Merck), email to author, April 21, 2019.

16. L. E. Coffeng, W. A. Stolk, H. G. M. Zouré, J. L. Veerman, K. B. Agblewonu, et al., "African Programme for Onchocerciasis Control 1995–2015: Model-Estimated Health Impact and Cost," *PLoS Negl Trop Dis* 7, no. 1 (2013).

17. World Health Organization, "Weekly Epidemiological Record, no. 45," November 2017, 681–700. http://www.who.int/wer.

18. World Health Organization African Programme for Onchocerciasis Control (WHO/APOC), "Year 2005 Progress Report: 1st September 2004–31 August 2005," (2005), 11.

19. B. Benton, "Economic Impact of Onchocerciasis Control through the African Programme for Onchocerciasis Control: An Overview," *Annals of Tropical Medicine & Parasitology* 92, suppl. 1 (1998): S38.

20. Benton, "Economic Impact of Onchocerciasis Control," S38.

21. Coffeng et al., "African Programme for Onchocerciasis Control 1995–2015," 8.

22. Emily Wainwright (USAID), discussion with author, October 19, 2015.

23. USAID, "Working to Protect Against Neglected Tropical Diseases Fact Sheet" (2017).

24. Mark Rosenberg et al., *Real Collaboration: What It Takes for Global Health to Succeed* (Berkeley: University of California Press, 2010).

25. Rosenberg, *Real Collaboration*, 6.

26. Rosenberg, *Real Collaboration*, 125.

27. Remme, discussion, April 21, 2019.

28. Remme, discussion, April 21, 2019.

29. World Health Organization African Programme for Onchocerciasis Control, "Final Evaluation Report," JAF doc. 21.6, October 2015.

30. WHO/APOC, "Final Evaluation Report," 46.

31. WHO/APOC, "Final Evaluation Report," 31–32.

32. WHO/APOC, "Final Evaluation Report," annex 1, 67, 89.

33. Ferroni, Marco, *Regional Public Goods in Official Developments Assistance*, Inter-American Development Bank (November 2001): 10.

34. Ferroni, *Regional Public Goods*, 10.

35. African Programme for Onchocerciasis Control—Twenty-First Session of the Joint Action Forum, *Progress Report December 15–16, 2015*, Kampala, Uganda, slide 18; World Health Organization, "Weekly Epidemiological Record, no. 49," December 4, 2015, 664. https://www.who.int/wer/2015/wer9049.pdf?ua=1.

36. Wainwright, discussion, October 19, 2015.

37. United States Agency International Development, "USAID Neglected Tropical Disease Program 2016 Evaluation" (March 2018): 23.

38. USAID, "2016 Evaluation," 36.

39. FY14 Development Grant Facility (DGF), "A Consolidated Report on the World Bank's Grant Making Facilities for FY14," annex 8.

40. Birger Fredriksen (former World Bank Director for Human Development for Africa), discussion with author, June 5, 2019.

41. Fredriksen, discussion, June 5, 2019.

42. Moores, discussion, July 16, 2018.

43. Moores, discussion, July 11, 2017.

44. *Compassion in Global Health*, produced by A Richard Stanley Production (The Task Force for Global Health, 2011), DVD, 30 min.

45. Azodoga Sékétéli (former APOC Director), discussion with author, October 3, 2015.

46. World Health Organization/African Programme for Onchocerciasis Control (WHO/APOC), *1995–2010: 15 Years of Working with Communities to Eliminate River Blindness* (internal document, 2011), 9.

47. APOC Launch Conference Wrap-Up Session, "JAF APOC—Tape 2—Jimmy Carter—Uche Amazigo—United States—James Wolfensohn" IN129501BET 12/5/1995, Folder ID: 30161621, World Bank Group Archives, Washington, DC, United States.

48. Craig McNamara, discussion with author, October 31, 2019.

49. Kenneth Frazier (Merck CEO), discussion with author, January 14, 2015.

50. Frazier, discussion, January 14, 2015.

51. Merck Press Release, "Merck Remains Steadfast in its Commitment to Supporting International Response Efforts to the Ebola Outbreak in the Democratic Republic of the Congo (DRC)" (April 2019).

52. Frazier, discussion, January 14, 2015.

53. Frazier, discussion, January 14, 2015.

54. Frazier, discussion, January 14, 2015.

55. Special Presidential Award citation to Bruce Benton on November 1, 2000.

Bibliography

African Programme for Onchocerciasis Control. *Charting the Lion's Stare: The Story of River Blindness Mapping in Africa*. Burkina Faso: World Health Organization, 2009. https://apps.who.int/iris/bitstream/handle/10665/275759/WHO-APOC-MG-09-2 -eng.pdf.

African Programme for Onchocerciasis Control. "Concept Note: Transforming APOC into a new regional entity for Oncho & LF elimination and support to other PC/ NTD." JAF 19.7, November 2013.

African Programme for Onchocerciasis Control. "Memorandum for the African Programme for Onchocerciasis Control (APOC): Phase I (1996–2001), Part II." April 17, 1996.

African Programme for Onchocerciasis Control—Eighteenth Session of the Joint Action Forum. *Final Communique December 11–13, 2012*. Bujumbura, Burundi.

African Programme for Onchocerciasis Control—Eleventh Session of the Joint Action Forum. *Final Communique December 6–9, 2005*. Paris, France.

African Programme for Onchocerciasis Control—Fifteenth Session of the Joint Action Forum. *Final Communique December 8–10, 2009*. Tunis, Tunisia.

African Programme for Onchocerciasis Control—Fifth Session of the Joint Action Forum. *Report December 8–10, 1999*. The Hague, The Netherlands.

African Programme for Onchocerciasis Control—Fourteenth Session of the Joint Action Forum. *Final Communique December 8–11, 2008*. Kampala, Uganda.

African Programme for Onchocerciasis Control—Nineteenth Session of the Joint Action Forum. *Final Communique for December 11–13, 2013*. Brazzaville, Congo.

African Programme for Onchocerciasis Control—Seventeenth Session of the Joint Action Forum. *Final Communique December 12–14, 2011*. Kuwait City, Kuwait.

African Programme for Onchocerciasis Control—Seventeenth Session of the Joint Action Forum. "Report of the CSA Advisory Group on Onchocerciasis Elimination." *Final Communique December 12–14, 2011*. Kuwait City, Kuwait.

African Programme for Onchocerciasis Control—Sixteenth Session of the Joint Action Forum. *Final Communique December 7–9, 2010*. Abuja, Nigeria.

African Programme for Onchocerciasis Control—Sixth Session of the Joint Action Forum. *Progress Report December 11–13, 2001*. Yaoundé, Cameroon.

African Programme for Onchocerciasis Control—Tenth Session of the Joint Action Forum. *Final Communique December 7–9, 2004*. Kinshasa, Democratic Republic of Congo.

African Programme for Onchocerciasis Control—Thirteenth Session of the Joint Action Forum. *Final Communique December 4–7, 2007.* Brussels, Belgium.

African Programme for Onchocerciasis Control—Twelfth Session of the Joint Action Forum. *Final Communique December 5–8, 2006.* Dar-es-Salaam, Tanzania.

African Programme for Onchocerciasis Control—Twenty-First Session of the Joint Action Forum. *Progress Report December 15–16, 2015.* Kampala, Uganda.

Agreement Governing the Operations of the Onchocerciasis Control Programme in the Volta Basin Area. November 1, 1973. 1126 U.N.T.S. 17537.

Amazigo, U.V., E. Nnoruka, C. Maduka, J. Bump, B. Benton & A. Sékétéli. "Ivermectin Improves the Skin Condition and Self-Esteem of Females with Onchocerciasis: A Report of Two Cases." *Annals of Tropical Medicine & Parasitology* 98, no. 5 (2004): 533–537.

Amazigo, Uche, Mounkaila Noma, Jesse Bump, Bruce Benton, Bernhard Liese, Laurent Yaméogo, Honorat Zouré, and Azodoga Sékétéli. "Onchocerciasis." In *Disease and Mortality in Sub-Saharan Africa*, edited by Dean T. Jamison, Richard G. Feachem, Malegapuru W. Makgoba, Eduard R. Bos, Florence K. Baingana, Karen J. Hofman, and Khama O. Rogo, 215–222. Washington, DC: The International Bank for Reconstruction and Development / The World Bank, 2006.

Bahman, A.M. "Investment Costs of Developing Irrigated Land." *International Journal of Development Research* 5, no. 11 (2015): 6082–6087.

Basáñez, M-G., S.D.S. Pion, T.S. Churcher, L.P. Breitling, M.P. Little, and M. Boussinesq. "River Blindness: A Success Story under Threat?" *PLoS Med* 3, no. 9 (2006): e371. https://doi.org/10.1371/journal.pmed.0030371.

Bastawrous, Andrew, Philip I. Burgess, Abdull M. Mahdi, Fatima Kyari, Matthew J. Burton, and Hannah Kuper. "Posterior Segment Eye Disease in Sub-Saharan Africa: Review of Recent Population-Based Studies." *Tropical Medicine and International Health* 19, no. 5 (2014): 600–609.

Beattie, Allison, and Richard Johnson. "APOC Management Review Final Report." African Programme for Onchocerciasis Control, July 2014, JAF20/INF/Doc.1.

Benton, B., J. Bump, A. Sékétéli, and B. Liese. "Partnership and Promise: Evolution of the African River-Blindness Campaigns." *Annals of Tropical Medicine & Parasitology* 96, suppl. 1 (2002).

Benton, B., and E.D. Skinner. "Cost-Benefits of Onchocerciasis Control." *Acta Leiden* 59, no. 1–2 (1990): 405–411.

Benton, Bruce. "Defeating Riverblindness (*onchocerciasis*) in Africa." Presentation at the World Bank Directors Meeting, Washington, DC, December 2001.

Benton, Bruce. "Defeating Riverblindness (onchocerciasis) in Africa." Presentation, The World Bank, Washington, DC, June 2002.

Benton, B. "Economic Impact of Onchocerciasis Control through the African Programme for Onchocerciasis Control: An Overview." *Annals of Tropical Medicine & Parasitology* 92, suppl. 1 (1998): S33–S39.

Benton, Bruce. "The Onchocerciasis (Riverblindness) Program's Visionary Partnerships." *Africa Region Findings & Good Practice Infobriefs*, no. 174. Washington, DC: World Bank, 2001.

Benton, Bruce. "The World Bank Group Archives: Oral History Program." Interview by Robert P. Grathwol. The World Bank, Washington, DC, May 9 and 16, June 13 and 27, 2006: 1–123.

Blanks, J., F. Richards, F. Beltrán, R. Collins, E. Alvarez, G. Zea Flores, B. Bauler, et al. "The Onchocerciasis Elimination Program for the Americas: A History of the Partnership." *Pan Am J Public Health* 3, no. 6 (1998): 367–74.

Blinkhorn, Thomas, and Jamie Martin, producers. *A Plague Upon the Land*. Burkina Faso: World Bank / International Finance Corporation, 1984, VHS.

Blinkhorn, Thomas A. "The Making of a World Bank Movie: Troubles Plague 'A Plague Upon the Land' Amateur Filmmakers but Everything Turns Out All Right in the End." Bank notes, October 6, 1973.

Blinkhorn, Thomas A. "The World Bank Group Archives: Oral History Program." Interview by Robert P. Grathwol, The World Bank, Washington, DC, June 16–18, 2008: 1–83.

Boakye, A. Boatin. Preface to *Thirty Years of Onchocerciasis Control in West Africa*, ed. Laurent Yaméogo, Christian Lévêque, and Jean-Marc Hougard. Paris: IRD Éditions, 2003.

Boussinesq M., J. Gardon, J. Kamgno, S.D.S. Pion, N. Gardon-Wendel and J.P. Chippaux. "Relationships between the Prevalence and Intensity of *Loa Loa* Infection in the Central Province of Cameroon." *Annals of Tropical Medicine & Parasitology* 95, no. 5 (2001): 495–507.

Brown, Theodore M., Elizabeth Fee, and Victoria Stepanova. "Halfdan Mahler: Architect and Defender of the WHO 'Health for All by 2000' Declaration of 1978." *American Journal of Public Health* 106, no. 1 (2016): 38–39.

Brundtland, Gro Harlem. "Onchocerciasis Control Programme: Closure Ceremony." Speech given in Ouagadougou, Burkina Faso, December 2002.

Bump, Jesse Boardman. "The Lion's Gaze: African River Blindness from Tropical Curiosity to International Development." PhD dissertation, Johns Hopkins University, 2004.

Bump, Jesse. "The Crosskey-Davies Experiment and Onchocerciasis in West Africa." *PLoS Neglected Tropical Diseases*, 8, no. 10 (2014): 1–4. https://www.ncbi.nlm.nih.gov/pmc/articles/PMC4191949/.

Bynum, Helen. *Success in Africa: The Onchocerciasis Control Programme in West Africa, 1974–2002*. Geneva: World Health Organization, 2002.

Calamari, Davide, Laurent Yaméogo, Christian Lévêque, and Jean-Marc Hougard. "Environmental Assessment of Larvicide Use in the Onchocerciasis Control Programme." *Parasitology Today* 14, no. 12 (1998): 485–489. In *Thirty Years of Onchocerciasis Control in West Africa*, ed. Laurent Yaméogo, Christian Lévêque, and Jean-Marc Hougard, 67–71. Paris: IRD Éditions, 2003.

Campbell, William C. "History of Avermectin and Ivermectin, with Notes on the History of other Macrocyclic Lactone Antiparasitic Agents." *Current Pharmaceutical Biotechnology* 13, no. 6 (2012).

Campbell, William C. "Lessons from the History of Ivermectin and Other Antiparasitic Agents." *Annual review of Animal Biosciences* 4 (2016).

"CDC—Lymphatic Filariasis—General Information—Frequently Asked Questions." Centers for Disease Control and Prevention. Last modified March 2018. https://www.cdc.gov/parasites/lymphaticfilariasis/gen_info/faqs.html.

Chaufournier, Roger. "The World Bank/IFC Archives Oral History Program." Interview by Robert W. Oliver. The World Bank, Washington, DC, July 22, 1986: 1–74.

Coffeng, L.E., W.A. Stolk, H.G.M. Zouré, J.L. Veerman, K.B. Agblewonu, et al. "African Programme for Onchocerciasis Control 1995–2015: Model-Estimated Health Impact and Cost." *PLoS Negl Trop Dis* 7, no. 1 (2013).

Coles, John. *Blindness and the Visionary: The Life and Work of John Wilson.* London: Giles de la Mare, 2006.

Committee for International Cooperation in National Research in Demography (CICRED) and Food and Agriculture Organization of the United Nations (FAO). *Population Dynamics in Rural Areas Freed from Onchocerciasis in Western Africa.* 1999.

Committee for Sponsoring Agencies. "African Programme for Onchocerciasis Control: Programme Document." JAF/CSA internal doc., December 1996.

"Community Directed Treatment with Ivermectin: Report of a Multi-Country Study." WHO doc. TDR/AFR/RP/96.1, 1996.

"Community-Directed Treatment of Lymphatic Filariasis in Africa: Report of a Multi-Centre Study in Ghana and Kenya." TDR/IDE/RP/CDTI/00.2, 2000.

Compassion in Global Health. Produced by A Richard Stanley Production, The Task Force for Global Health, 2011. DVD, 30 min.

Crump, A., Carlos M. Morel, and Satoshi Ōmura. "The Onchocerciasis Chronicle: From the Beginning to the End?" *Trends in Parasitology* 28, no. 7 (2012): 280–288.

Crump, Andy, and Satoshi Ōmura. "Ivermectin, 'Wonder Drug' from Japan: The Human Use Perspective." *Proceedings of the Japan Academy, Series B Physical and Biological* 87, no. 2 (2011).

Cupp, E., M. Sauerbrey, V. Cama et al. "Elimination of Onchocerciasis in Africa by 2025: The Need for a Broad Perspective. *Infect Dis Poverty* 8, no. 50 (2019).

Dadzie, Yankum, Uche V. Amazigo, Boakye A. Boatin, and Azodoga Sékétéli. "Is Onchocerciasis Elimination in Africa Feasible By 2025: A Perspective Based on Lessons Learnt from the African Control Programmes," *Infectious Diseases of Poverty* 7, no. 63 (July 2018).

De Sole, G., J. Remme, K. Awadzi, S. Accorsi, E.S. Alley, O. Ba, K.Y. Dadzie, J. Giese, M. Karam, and F.M. Keita. "Adverse Reactions After Large-Scale Treatment of Onchocerciasis with Ivermectin: Combined Results from Eight Community Trials." *Bulletin of the World Health Organization* 67, no. 6 (1989): 707–719.

Dean, Malcolm. *Lymphatic Filariasis: The Quest to Eliminate a 4000-Year-Old Disease.* London: Hollis Publishing Company, 2001.

Diawara, L., M.O. Traoré, A. Badji, Y. Bissan, K. Doumbia, S.F. Goita, L. Konaté et al. "Feasibility of Onchocerciasis Elimination with Ivermectin Treatment in Endemic Foci in Africa: First Evidence from Studies in Mali and Senegal." *PLoS Neglected Tropical Diseases* 3, no. 7 (July 2009): e497.

Ducorps, M., N. Gardon-Wendel, S. Ranque, W. Ndong, M. Boussinesq, J. Gardon, D. Schneider, and J.P. Chippaux. "Secondary Effects of the Treatment of Hypermicrofilaremic Loiasis Using Ivermectin." *Bulletin de la Société de Pathologie Exotique* 88 (1995): 105–112.

Duke, Brian O.L. "Overview: Report of a Scientific Working Group on Serious Adverse Events Following Mectizan® Treatment of Onchocerciasis in *Loa loa* Endemic Areas." *Filarial Journal* 2, suppl. 1 (October 2003).

Easom, Donald. "River Blindness Foundation Newsletter." 1992.

Economic Community of West African States. "Agricultural Potential in West Africa." February 2008.

Elder, John, and Laura Cooley. "Sustainable Settlement and Development of the Onchocerciasis Control Program Area, Proceedings of a Ministerial Meeting." World Bank Technical Paper no. 310, 1995.

Esch, Gerald. *Parasites and Infectious Disease: Key Discoveries in Parasitology.* United Kingdom: Cambridge University Press, 2007.

Feldman, Claudia. "A Forgotten Disease," *Houston Chronicle*, October 2005.

Ferroni, Marco. *Regional Public Goods in Official Development Assistance.* Inter-American Development Bank, November 2001.

Foege, William. "10 Years of Mectizan." *Annals of Tropical Medicine and Parasitology* 92, no. 1 (1998): s7–s10.

FY14 Development Grant Facility. "A Consolidated Report on the World Bank's Grant Making Facilities for FY14." Supplementary Information as Part of the DGF Section of the Report.

Gardon, Jacques, Nathalie Gardon-Wendel, Demanga-Ngangue, Joseph Kamgno, Jean-Philippe Chippaux, and Michel Boussinesq. "Serious Reactions After Mass Treatment of Onchocerciasis with Ivermectin in an Area Endemic for *Loa loa* Infection." *The Lancet* 350, no. 9070 (July 1997): 18–22.

Garms, R., J.F. Walsh, and J.B. Davies. "Studies of the Reinvasion of the OCP in the Volta River Basin by *Simulium damnosum* s.l. with Emphasis on the South-Western Areas" *Tropenmed Parasitol* 30 (1979): 345–362.

Garms, R., T.L. Lakwo, R. Ndyomugyenyi, W. Kipp, T. Rubaale, E. Tukesiga, J. Katamanywa, R.J. Post, and U.V. Amazigo. "The Elimination of the Vector *Simulium neavei* from the Itwara Onchocerciasis Focus in Uganda by Ground Larviciding." *Acta Tropica* 111, no. 3 (September 2009): 203–210.

Global Health-Division of Parasitic Diseases, "Parasites—Loiasis—Disease," Center for Disease Control and Prevention, January 20, 2015. https://www.cdc.gov/parasites/loiasis/disease.html.

Goddard, Jerome. "Black Flies and Onchocerciasis," *Infectious Medicine* 18, no. 6 (2001).

Greene, Bruce M., Kenneth R. Brown, and Hugh R. Taylor. "Use of Ivermectin in Humans." In *Ivermectin and Abamectin*, ed. William C. Campbell, 311–323. New York: Springer-Verlag, 1989.

Gyapong, John, and Boakye Boatin, eds. *Neglected Tropical Diseases—Sub-Saharan Africa.* New York: Springer, 2016.

Haselow, Nancy J., Julie Akame, Cyrille Evini, and Serge Akongo. "Programmatic and Communication Issues in Relation to Serious Adverse Events Following Ivermectin Treatment in Areas Co-Endemic for Onchocerciasis and Loiasis." *Filarial Journal* 2, suppl. 1 (October 2003).

Herrador, Zaida, Belén Garcia, Policarpo Ncogo, Maria Jesus Perteguer, Jose Miguel Rubio, Eva Rivas, Marta Cimas et al. "Interruption of Onchocerciasis Transmission in Bioko Island: Accelerating the Movement from Control to Elimination in Equatorial Guinea." *PLoS Neglected Tropical Diseases* 12, no. 5 (May 2018).

Hong, W. David. "A New Cure for River Blindness and Elephantiasis." *BioMedCentral* (January 29, 2019).

Hopkins, Adrian, and Boakye A. Boatin. "Onchocerciasis." In *Water and Sanitation-Related Diseases and the Environment: Challenges, Interventions, and Preventative Measures*, edited by Janine M.H. Selendy, 133–149. New Jersey: John Wiley & Sons, Inc., 2011.

Hougard, J.M., P. Poudiougo, P. Guillet, C. Back, L.K.B. Akpoboua, and D. Quillévéré. "Criteria for the Selection of Larvicides by the Onchocerciasis Control Programme in West Africa." *Annals of Tropical Medicine and Parasitology* 87, no. 5 (1993): 435–442.

Husion, Stacy. "Intimate Encounters and the Politics of German Occupation in Belgium, 1940-44/45." Doctorate thesis, University of Toronto, 2015.

"Innovation for Sustainable Agricultural Growth in Togo." *Forum for Agricultural Research in Africa (FARA) and Center for Development Research*. University of Bonn (ZEF), October 2017.

International Bank for Reconstruction and Development. "Agreement Providing for the Amendment and Restatement of the Memorandum for the African Programme for Onchocerciasis Control for Phase II and for the Phrasing-Out Period" (December 2007).

Israel, Brett. "A Cellphone-Based Microscope for Treating River Blindness." *Berkley News*, November 9, 2017.

Joint Coordinating Committee of the Onchocerciasis Control Program. "Onchocerciasis Control Program: Economic Review Mission," fifth sess., pt. 2. In *Evaluation Report: Economic Aspects*, October 25, 1978.

Joseph Kamgno et al. "A Test-and-Not-Treat Strategy for Onchocerciasis in *Loa loa*–Endemic Areas." *The New England Journal of Medicine* 10 (2017): 1.

Kazianga, Harounan, William A. Masters, and Margaret S. McMillan. "Disease Control, Demographic Change and institutional Development in Africa." *ELSVIER, Journal of Development Economics*, April 2014.

Kelly, Jim, Clive Shiff, Howard Goodman, Larry Dash, Antoinette Brown, and Ali Khalif Galaydh. "Impact Review of the Onchocerciasis Program: Ouagadougou, August 1985." U.S. Agency for International Development Evaluation Report no. 63, Washington, DC, 1986.

Kim, Aehyung, and Bruce Benton. "Cost-Benefit Analysis of the Onchocerciasis Control Program (OCP)," World Bank Technical Paper no. 282, May 1995.

Knox, David. "Opening Statement: Meeting of Contributors to the Onchocerciasis Fund." Speech given in Paris, October 11–12, 1982, World Bank Archives, Washington, DC, 1300674.

Koroma, Joseph B., Santigie Sesay, Mustapha Sonnie, Mary H. Hodges, Foday Sahr, Yaobi Zhang, and Moses J. Bockarie. "Impact of Three Rounds of Mass Drug Administration on Lymphatic Filariasis in Areas Previously Treated for Onchocerciasis in Sierra Leone." *PLoS Neglected Tropical Diseases* 7, no. 6 (2013): 1–13.

Lakwo, T.L., R. Garms, T. Rubaale, M. Katabarwa, F. Walsh, P. Habomugisha, D. Oguttu et al. "The Disappearance of Onchocerciasis from the Itwara Focus, Western Uganda After Elimination of the Vector *Simulium neavei* and 19 Years of Annual Ivermectin Treatments." *Acta Tropica* 126, no. 3 June 2013: 218–221.

Lakwo, T.L., et al. "Transmission of *Loa loa* and Prospects for the Elimination of its Vector, the Blackfly *Simulium neavei* in the Mpamba-Nkusi Focus in Western Uganda." *Med Vet Entomol.* 20, no. 1 (March 2006): 93–101.

Lakwo, T.L., R. Garms, E. Tukahebwa, A.W. Onapa, E. Tukesiga, J. Ngorok, J. Katamanywa et al. "Successful Interruption of the Transmission of Onchocerciasis volvulus in Mpamba-Nkusi Focus, Kibaale District, Mid-Western Uganda." *East African Medical Journal* 92, no. 8 (August 2015): 401–407.

Le Berre, René. "Contribution a L'Étude Biologique et Écologique de *Simulium damnosum*." Dissertation, Docteur ès Science Naturelles: Maître de Recherches à L'ORSTOM, 1966.

Lofflin, John. "The Miracle Molecule." *Veterinary Medicine* (2005).

Marshall, Katherine. *Back-to-Office Report: Ministerial Meeting on Sustainable Settlement and Development of the Onchocerciasis (Riverblindness) Controlled Areas.* Paris: World Bank Office, April 12–14, 1994.

McMillan, Della E. *Sahel Visions: Planned Settlement and River Blindness Control in Burkina Faso.* Tucson: University of Arizona Press, 1995.

McMillan, Della E., Jean-Baptiste Nana, and Kimseyinga Savadogo. "Settlement and Development in the River Blindness Control Zone Case Study Burkina Faso." In *Series on River Blindness Control in West Africa*, World Bank Technical Paper no. 200, June 1993.

McMillan, Della E., Thomas Painter, and Thayer Scudder. "Settlement and Development in the River Blindness Control Zone." In *Series on River Blindness Control in West Africa*, World Bank Technical Paper no. 192, December 1992.

McNamara, Robert S. "To the Board of Governors, Washington, D.C. September 30, 1968." In *The McNamara Years at the World Bank: Major Policy Addresses of Robert S. McNamara, 1968–1981.* Washington, DC: World Bank, 1981.

McNamara, Robert. "The World Bank's Venture into the Onchocerciasis Program." In *Roger Chaufournier and the Onchocerciasis Program: A Tribute to One of Its Founding Fathers.* Working paper, 1994.

Mectizan Donation Program. "Central Nervous System (CNS) Complications of Loiasis and Adverse CNS Events Following Treatment: Report of an Invited Consultation, 2–3 October 1995." Atlanta: MDP, 1996.

Mectizan Expert Committee. "Recommendations for the Treatment of Onchocerciasis with Mectizan in Areas Co-Endemic for Onchocerciasis and Loiasis." Atlanta: MEC, May 2000.

Merck, George. "Medicine is for the Patient, Not for the Profits." Speech given at the Medical College of Virginia, Richmond, VA, December 1950.

"Merck Offers Free Distribution of New River Blindness Drug," New York Times, October 22, 1987.

Merck & Co. "Merck Remains Steadfast in its Commitment to Supporting International Response Efforts to the Ebola Outbreak in the Democratic Republic of the Congo [DRC]." Press release, April 9, 2019.

Meredith, Stefanie E.O., Catherine Cross, and Uche V. Amazigo. "Empowering Communities in Combating River Blindness and the Role of NGOs: Case Studies from Cameroon, Mali, Nigeria, and Uganda." *Health Research Policy Systems* 10, no. 16 (2012): 1–20.

Mouchet, J., and Guillet, P. *Insecticide Resistance in Blackfly of the Simulium damnosum Complex in West Africa.* Unpublished WHO doc. OCP/SWG/78.17, July 3–7, 1978.

Murdoch, M.E., M.C. Asuzu, M. Hagan, W.H. Makunde, P. Ngoumou, K.F. Ogbuagu, D. Okello, G. Ozoh, and J. Remme. "Onchocerciasis: The Clinical and Epidemiological Burden of Skin Disease in Africa." *Annals of Tropical Medicine & Parasitology* 96, no. 3 (2002): 283–296.

Murphy, Darragh. "Meet Ireland's New Nobel Laureate, William C Campbell," *The Irish Times*, October 9, 2015.

Nana A.Y. Twum-Danso. "*Loa-loa* Encephalopathy Temporally Related to Ivermectin Administration Reported from Onchocerciasis Mass Treatment Programs from 1989 to 2001: Implications for the Future." *Filaria Journal* 2 (2003).

Ngoumou, P., and J.F. Walsh. "A Manual for Rapid Epidemiological Mapping of Onchocerciasis." Switzerland: World Health Organization, 1993.

Noma, Mounkaila, Honorat G.M. Zouré, Afework H. Tekle, Peter Al Enyong, Bertram E.B. Nwoke, and Jan H.F. Remme. "The Geographic Distribution of Onchocerciasis in the 20 Participating Countries of the African Programme for Onchocerciasis Control: (1) Priority Areas for Ivermectin Treatment." *Parasites & Vectors* 7, no. 325 (2014): 1–15.

OECD Sahel and West Africa Club. "The Socio-Economic and Regional Context of West African Migrations." Paris, November 2006.

Onchocerciasis Control Program. "25 Years of OCP." Government document, Ouagadougou, Burkina Faso, 1999.

"Onchocerciasis Control Program Phase IV," USAID doc., draft project paper, 698–0485.

"Onchocerciasis Control in the Volta River Basin Area: Report of the Preparatory Assistance Mission to the Governments of: Dahomey, Ghana, Ivory Coast, Mali, Niger, Togo, Upper Volta." UNDP/FAO/IBRD/WHO internal doc. 73.1, 1973.

Onchocerciasis Fund Agreement, February 4, 1986. United Kingdom of Great Britain HMSO and the Secretary of State for Foreign and Commonwealth Affairs 1990, Gr. Brit. T. S. no. 62.

Onchocerciasis Fund Agreement. February 25, 1992. United Kingdom of Great Britain HMSO and the Secretary of State for Foreign and Commonwealth Affairs 1997, Gr. Brit. T. S. no. 35.

Ottesen, E.A., B.O. Duke, M. Karam, K. and Behbehani. "Strategies and Tools for the Control/Elimination of Lymphatic Filariasis." *Bull World Health Organ* 75, no. 6 (1997): 491–503.

Ottesen, E.A., M.M. Ismail, and J. Horton. "The Role of Albendazole in Programmes to Eliminate Lymphatic Filariasis." *Parasitology Today* 15, no. 9 (September 1999): 382–386.

Pond, Bob. *Mass Distribution of Ivermectin: A Handbook for Community Treatment of Onchocerciasis.* Washington, DC: Africare, 1991.

Pound Sterling Live. "US Dollar to French Franc Spot Exchange Rates for 1975–2001 from the Bank of England." https://www.poundsterlinglive.com/bank-of-england -spot/historical-spot-exchange-rates/usd/USD-to-FRF-1985.

Pound Sterling Live. "US Dollar to Japanese Yen Spot Exchange Rates for 1975–2018 from the Bank of England." https://www.poundsterlinglive.com/bank-of-england -spot/historical-spot-exchange-rates/usd/USD-to-JPY.

Prescott, Nicholas, and André Prost. "Cost-Effectiveness of Blindness Prevention by the Onchocerciasis Control Program in Upper Volta." PHN Technical Note, The World Bank, Washington DC, November 1983.

Rebollo, Maria P., Honorat Zouré, Kisito Ougoussan, Yao Sodahlon, Eric A. Ottesen, and Paul T. Cantey. "Onchocerciasis: Shifting the Target from Control to Elimination Requires a New First Step—Elimination Mapping." Oxford University Press on behalf of Royal Society of Tropical Medicine and Hygiene, 2017.

Reich, Michael R., ed. *International Strategies for Tropical Disease Treatments: Experiences with Praziquantel.* Cambridge: Harvard University, WHO/DAP/CTD/98.5, 1998.

Remme, J., G. De Sole, and G.J. van Oortmarssen. "The Predicted and Observed Decline in Onchocerciasis Infection during 14 Years of Successful Control of *Simulium* spp. in West Africa." *Bulletin of the World Health Organization* 68, no. 3 (1990): 331–339.

Remme, J., R.H.A. Baker, G. DeSole, K.Y. Dadzie, J.F. Walsh, M.A. Adams, E.S. Alley, and H.S.K. Avissey. "A Community Trial of Ivermectin in the Onchocerciasis Focus of Asubende, Ghana. I. Effect on the Microfilarial Reservoir and the Transmission of *Onchocerca volvulus*." *Tropical Medicine and Parasitology* 40 (1989): 367–374.

Remme, J.H.F. "The Burden of Onchocerciasis in 1990." *World Health Organization* (2004): 1–26.

Remme, J.H.F., and J.B. Zongo. "Demographic Aspects of the Epidemiology and Control of Onchocerciasis in West Africa." In *Demography and Vector-Borne Diseases*, 17–36. Boca Raton, FL: CRC Press, 1989.

Remme, J.H.F. "Research for Control: The Onchocerciasis Experience." *Tropical Medicine and International Health* 9, no. 2 (2004): 243–254.

Richards, F.O., B.E.B Nwoke, I. Zarroug et al. "The Positive Influence the Onchocerciasis Elimination Program for the Americas Has Had on Africa Programs." *Infect Dis Poverty* 8, no. 52 (2019).

Rosenberg, Mark, Elisabeth Hayes, Margaret McIntyre, and Nancy Wall Neill. *Real Collaboration: What It Takes for Global Health to Succeed.* Berkeley: University of California Press, February 2010.

Rougemont, André. "Ivermectin for Onchocerciasis." *The Lancet*, November 20, 1982.

Samba, Ebrahim. "Compte Rendu de la Visite de Travail et de Sensibilisation du Dr. Ebrahim Samba, Directeur du Programme O.C.P., dans le Cadre des Activities de Devolution de L'Aire Initiale du Programme au Mali." Unpublished manuscript, July 16, 1992.

Samba, Ebrahim M. *The Onchocerciasis Control Programme in West Africa: An Example of Effective Public Health Management.* Geneva: World Health Organization, 1994.

Sauerbrey, M. "The Onchocerciasis Elimination Program for the Americas (OEPA)." *Ann Trop Med Parasitol* 102, suppl. 1 (September 2008): 25–29. doi:10.1179/136485908X337454.

Siddall, Mark. "A Noble and Laudable Nobel Laureate: William C. Campbell," *The Huffington Post*, October 13, 2015.

Takougang, Innocent, Martin Meremikwu, Samuel Wandji, Emmanual V. Yenshu, Ben Aripko, Samson B. Lamlenn, Braide L. Eka, Peter Enyong, Jean Melo, Oladele Kale, and Jan H. Remme. "Rapid Assessment Method for Prevalence and Intensity of *Loa loa* Infection." *Bulletin of the World Health Organization* 80, no. 11 (2002).

Taylor, H.R., B.O. Duke, and B. Munoz. "The Selection of Communities for Treatment of Onchocerciasis with Ivermectin." *Tropical Medicine and Parasitology* 43 (1992): 267–270.

Tekle, Afework Hailemariam, Honorat Zouré, Samuel Wanji, Stephen Leak, Mounkaila Noma, Jan H.F. Remme, and Uche Amazigo. "Integrated Rapid Mapping of Onchocerciasis and Loiasis in the Democratic Republic of Congo: Impact on Control Strategies." *Acta Tropica* 120, suppl. 1 (September 2011): S81-S90.

Tekle, Afework H., Honorath G. M. Zouré, Mounkaila Noma, Michel Boussinesq, Luc E. Coffeng, Wilma A. Stolk, and Jan H. F. Remme. "Progress towards Onchocerciasis Elimination in the Participating Countries of the African Programme for Onchocerciasis Control: Epidemiological Evaluation Results." *Infectious Diseases of Poverty* 5, no. 66 (2016).

Traoré, S., Mamadou O., Moussa D. Sarr, Alioune Badji, Yiriba Bissan, Lamine Diawara, Konimba Doumbia, Soula F. Goita et al. "Proof-of-Principle of Onchocerciasis Elimination with Ivermectin Treatment in Endemic Foci in Africa: Final Results of a Study in Mali and Senegal." *PLoS Neglected Tropical Diseases* 6, no. 9 (2012): 1–14.

Traoré S., M.D. Wilson, A. Sima, T. Barro, A. Diallo, A. Aké, S. Coulibaly et al. "The Elimination of the Onchocerciasis Vector from the Island of Bioko as a Result of Larviciding by the WHO African Programme for Onchocerciasis Control." *Acta Tropica* 111, no. 3 (September 2009): 211–218.

U.K. Department for International Development and U.S. Agency for International Development [DFID/USAID]. "Joint Statement on Support for Onchocerciasis Elimination in Africa." October 2014.

U.S. Food and Drug Administration. "What Is a Serious Adverse Event?" https://www.fda.gov/safety/reporting-serious-problems-fda/what-serious-adverse-event.

United States Agency International Development. "Lymphatic Filariasis." Last modified 2018. https://www.neglecteddiseases.gov/usaid-target-diseases/lymphatic-filariasis.

United States Agency International Development. "USAID Neglected Tropical Disease Program 2016 Evaluation." March 2018.

United States Department of Agriculture, "Index Mundi, Burkina Faso Cotton Production and Exports by Year, 1965–2018," https://www.indexmundi.com/agriculture/?country=bf&commodity=cotton&graph=production.

United States Environmental Protection Agency. "EPA R.E.D. Facts: *Bacillus thuringiensis.*" Government archival document, Washington, DC, 1998.

Useem, Michael. *The Leadership Moment.* New York: Times Books, 1998.

Vagelos, P. Roy, and Louis Galambos. *Medicine, Science, and Merck.* New York: Cambridge University Press, 2004.

Vitale, Jeffrey. *Economic Importance of Cotton in Burkina Faso.* Food and Agriculture Organization of the United Nations, Rome, 2018.

Webb, Gerald, John Wilson, Basile Adjou-Moumouni, Lawrence Dash, Paul Lechuga, Steven Smits, and George Tsalikis. "External Review of the Onchocerciasis Control Program." Unpublished external review, October 1990.

"WHO Drug Information." *World Health Organization* 5 no. 3 (1991).

Wigg, David. "And Then Forgot to Tell Us Why . . . A Look at the Campaign Against River Blindness in West Africa." A World Bank development essay, Washington, DC: The World Bank Group, 1993,

Wilson, John. "Blind Eyes and Seeing Hands." *West African Review* 1392, no. 3 (1950). In "The Lion's Gaze: African River Blindness from Tropical Curiosity to International Development," by Jesse Bump. Dissertation, John Hopkins University, 2004: 202.

Wilson, John Foster. *Travelling Blind*. London: Hutchinson, 1963.

Wolfensohn, James D. "Address to the Board of Governors." In *The Annual Meeting of the World Bank and the International Monetary Fund*, Washington DC, October 10, 1995.

Wolfensohn, James D. *Voice for the World's Poor: Selected Speeches and Writings of World Bank President James D. Wolfensohn, 1995–2005*. Washington, DC: World Bank Publications, 2005, 35.

World Bank. Press release. Paris, October 16, 1985.

World Bank. "Meeting of the Executive Directors of the Bank and IDA held on Tuesday, May 1, 1973: Onchocerciasis in Western Africa." Board transcript, Washington, DC: World Bank Group, May 1, 1973. http://documents.worldbank.org/curated/en/51362149 6833276816/Transcript-of-meeting-of-the-Executive-Directors-of-the-Bank-and-IDA -held-on-Tuesday-May-1-1973-Onchocerciasis-in-Western-Africa.

World Bank Group. "Defeating Riverblindness: Success in Scaling Up and Lessons Learned," in Global Learning Process on Scaling Up Poverty Reduction Conference, Shanghai, May 22, 2004, 8. Washington, DC: World Bank.

World Health Organization. "Accelerating Work to Overcome the Global Impact of Neglected Tropical Diseases: A Roadmap for Implementation." Geneva, 2012.

World Health Organization. "Attack Poverty: The Global Alliance to Eliminate Lymphatic Filariasis. Proceedings of the First Meeting," Department of Communicable Diseases Control, Prevention and Eradication, May 2000.

World Health Organization. *Bulletin of the World Health Organization* 85, no. 6 (June 2007).

World Health Organization. "Independent Commission on the Long-Term Prospects of the Onchocerciasis Control Programme." August 1981.

World Health Organization, "Informal Consultation on Elimination of Onchocerciasis Transmission with Current Tools in Africa." February 2009.

World Health Organization. "Lymphatic Filariasis, Treatment and Prevention." https:// www.who.int/lymphatic_filariasis/epidemiology/treatment_prevention/en/.

World Health Organization. "Onchocerciasis Control Programme in the Volta River Basin Area, pt. 1." Evaluation report, OCP doc. 78.2, 1979.

World Health Organization. "Report of the External Mid-Term Evaluation of the African Programme for Onchocerciasis Control." JAF doc. 16.8, October 2010.

World Health Organization. "Report of the Meeting on Strategies for Ivermectin Distribution through Primary Health Care Systems." Geneva, April 1991.

World Health Organization. "TDR's Contribution to the Development of Ivermectin for Onchocerciasis: Third External Review." Prepared by Tomoko Fujisaki and Michael Reich in the Takemi Program in International Health, Harvard School of Public Health, reference doc. 3. n.p: World Health Organization, 1998.

World Health Organization. "WHO Annual Report on Lymphatic Filariasis." 2003.

World Health Organization. "The Expanded Special Project for Elimination of Neglected Tropical Diseases (ESPEN) 2017 Annual Report." 2017.

World Health Organization. "Weekly Epidemiological Record, no. 45." November 2017, 681–700. http://www.who.int/wer.

World Health Organization. "Weekly Epidemiological Record, no. 47." November 2018, 633–648. http://www.who.int/wer.

World Health Organization. "Weekly Epidemiological Record, no. 49/50." December 2012, 493–508. http://www.who.int/wer.

World Health Organization. "Weekly Epidemiological Record, no. 49." December 4, 2015, 661–680. https://www.who.int/wer/2015/wer9049.pdf?ua=1.

World Health Organization. "Weekly Epidemiological Record, no. 90/38." September 2015, 489–504. http://www.who.int/wer.

World Health Organization. "Weekly Epidemiological Record, no. 91/43." October 2016, 501–516. http://www.who.int/wer.

World Health Organization. "WHO AFRO Launches New Project to Help African Countries Control and Eliminate Neglected Tropical Diseases." Press release, Geneva, May 2016.

World Health Organization/African Programme for Onchocerciasis Control, *1995–2010: 15 Years of Working with Communities to Eliminate River Blindness*. Internal document, 2011, 9.

World Health Organization African Programme for Onchocerciasis Control. "Conceptual and Operational Framework of Onchocerciasis Elimination with Ivermectin Treatment." September 2010.

World Health Organization African Programme for Onchocerciasis Control. "Final Evaluation Report." JAF doc. 21.6, October 2015.

World Health Organization African Programme for Onchocerciasis Control. "Programme for the Elimination of Neglected Diseases in Africa (PENDA)." JAF doc. 19.8, November 2013.

World Health Organization African Programme for Onchocerciasis Control. "Progress Report." PowerPoint presentation, JAF doc. 21, Kampala, Uganda, December 15–16, 2015.

World Health Organization African Programme for Onchocerciasis Control. "Report of the External Evaluation." October 2005.

World Health Organization African Programme for Onchocerciasis Control. "Vector Elimination, Itwara, Uganda." https://www.who.int/apoc/vector/itwara/en/.

World Health Organization African Programme for Onchocerciasis Control. "Vector Elimination, Tukuyu, United Republic of Tanzania." https://www.who.int/apoc/vector/tukuyu/en/.

World Health Organization African Programme for Onchocerciasis Control. "Yaoundé Declaration on Onchocerciasis Control in Africa." September 2006.

World Health Organization African Programme for Onchocerciasis Control. "Year 2005 Progress Report: 1st September 2004–31 August 2005." JAF internal doc. 11.5. September 2005.

World Health Organization African Programme for Onchocerciasis Control—Committee of Sponsoring Agencies. "A Strategic Overview of the Future of Onchocerciasis Control in Africa." September 2006.

World Health Organization Expert Committee on Onchocerciasis. "Technical Report Series 852." Geneva, 1995.

World Health Organization Global Programme to Eliminate Lymphatic Filariasis. "Progress Report 2000–2009 and Strategic Plan 2010–2020." 2010, 1–78.

World Health Organization Joint Programme Committee of the Onchocerciasis Control Programme. *Onchocerciasis Control Programme in West Africa, Ninth Session.* November 29–December 2, 1988. Dakar, Senegal.

World Health Organization Joint Programme Committee of the Onchocerciasis Control Programme. *Onchocerciasis Control Programme in West Africa, Sixteenth Session.* December 6–8, 1995. Washington, DC.

World Health Organization Regional Committee for Africa. "Progress Report on the Implementation of the Resolution on Neglected Tropical Diseases." May 2017, 1–12.

World Health Organization Special Programme for Research and Training in Tropical Diseases. "Community Directed Interventions for Major Health Problems in Africa." 2008.

Wynd, Shona, Wayne D. Melrose, David N. Durrheim, Jaime Carron, and Margaret Gyapong. "Understanding the Community Impact of Lymphatic Filariasis: A Review of the Sociocultural Literature." *Bulletin of the World Health Organization* 85, no. 6 (June 2007): 421–500.

Yaméogo, Laurent, Christian Lévêque, and Jean-Marc Hougard. *Thirty Years of Onchocerciasis Control in West Africa.* Paris: IRD Éditions, 2003.

Zouré, H. G., S. Wanji, M. Noma, U.V. Amazigo, P.J. Diggle, A.H. Tekle, and J.H. Remme. "The Geographic Distribution of *Loa loa* in Africa: Results of Large-Scale Implementation of the Rapid Assessment Procedure for Loiasis (RAPLOA)." *PLOS Neglected Tropical Diseases* 5, no. 6 (June 2011).

Index